Dedications

This book is dedicated to all cancer victims and their families who experience needless suffering and loss of loved ones because they have been denied knowledge and use of effective cancer cures.

This book is also dedicated to Dr. Hulda Regehr Clark, PH.D. N.D. for telling the world how to cure and prevent cancer and other diseases that plague humankind.

Oct 2, 2001

Sumily.

Buster,

Here's to a new era in cancer care.

Ron Sdonshi

Publisher's Information

CANCER: Cause, Cure and Cover-up

© Ronald Gdanski, Grimsby, Canada, 2000

Nadex Publishing, Division of Nadex Industries Ltd.

P.O. Box 307, Grimsby, Ontario, Canada, L3M 4G5

ISBN 0-9685665-0-2

Printed and bound in Canada

10 9 8 7 6 5 4 3

Ordering information: Visa and Master Card by phone

Phone or fax 800-656-7606   (905)-945-2180

For complete details, please check our web page at

www.newvisionsinc.org *(may be under construction)*

How infections cause cancer

Cancer occurs most often in membrane walls of storage vessels and ducts such as the lungs, colon, breast, prostate, lymphatic system and so on. The problem starts with a break in a membrane due to nutritional deficiencies, chemical toxins, viral growths, physical injury, or parasites.

Repair of injury is a natural process controlled by the autonomic nervous system. Electrical energy called the *'current of injury'* is increased to make DNA replicate.

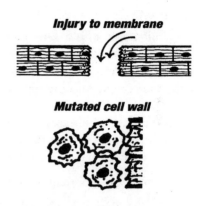

Injury to membrane

Mutated cell wall

Normally, adjacent cells of the injured membrane multiply to repair the injury and stop multiplying when the injury is repaired.

Out-of-control replication occurs when the new cells fail to connect with old cells. The medical problem of a skin graft that does not take is similar to cancer. In both cases, new cells that do not knit with old cells fail to repair the membrane injury.

Rejected cells form tumors

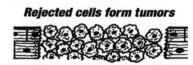

If cells that multiply are infected, the microbes inside these cells also multiply within the cytoplasm of the cell. During the formation of new cell-wall membranes, (mitosis), microbial cell-wall proteins mutate the new cell-wall membranes. These daughter cells with mutated cell walls, part human, part microbial, are rejected by the original membrane cells and the injury is not repaired.

Additional adjacent cells are called upon to multiply. These in turn are mutated, rejected, and so on. For each old normal cell that multiplies, we end up with two cancer cells and one less normal cell. That's how microbial infection switches human cells to non-productive cancer cells, consumes normal membrane cells, and forms a tumor.

Cancer is the continuous multiplication, mutation, and rejection of membrane cells that fail to repair an injury. The problem is not genetic. The problem occurs during the normal several-hour process of mitosis.

Leukemia, liver and bone cancer are also caused by new cells with mutated cell wall traits, caused by infection of cells during mitosis.

Cautionary Statement and Disclaimer

The author is a reporter, not a doctor. The conclusions drawn from the research and personal observations are largely theoretical. What you do with this information is up to you and is not his responsibility.

This book is sold for educational purposes and to promote freedom of choice in health care. Any of the information imparted herein is not medical advice, diagnosis, or prescription. Data have been provided only to support recognition of the need for immediate reform of the health care system. If you have a health problem, you are warned to seek healing solutions and guidance from qualified health-care professionals. Alternative therapies can be effective but self-treatment can be hazardous. Cures for cancer are discussed in general terms, and these may or may not apply to your situation.

This book represents information obtained from authentic and highly regarded sources. Every reasonable effort has been made to use only reliable data and information, but the author and the publisher cannot assume responsibility for the validity of all materials or for the consequences of their use.

The opinions expressed in this book are those of the author alone and do not necessarily reflect the position of any other person, group, or business with which the author may be associated. Neither the publisher nor printer is responsible for damages or other liabilities.

This book is not intended to be disruptive of available health services. Rather, it is intended to conserve medical funds and save lives by recognizing the true microbial cause of cancer and other diseases. It is time to apply medical research about the parasitic cause of disease to prevent and cure disease. It is time to stop misinformation and medical abuse of the health care system.

If you do not wish to be bound by the above conditions, you may return your purchase to the publisher for refund.

About the author

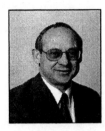

Have you ever felt compelled to share your experiences with another person because you thought you could help someone achieve something, or avoid making a serious mistake? You knew it would bother you if you didn't try even though it wasn't your place to get involved.

What if you firmly believed you knew how to help someone prevent and possibly cure cancer? Wouldn't you feel compelled to tell him or her? I find myself in this situation as I write this text. So many people are being denied access to valuable information about cancer and alternative therapies that a book of this nature must be written.

Most people simply do not believe in alternative therapies and refuse to even consider them because of medical propaganda. Through my research on the cause of cancer, I have personally interviewed a good number of people who have been cured of cancer by using alternative therapies. I now believe I know how cancer starts and how to achieve remission. If the information in this book will encourage you to consider cancer as an infectious disease treatable with natural health products and lifestyle changes, my main goal will have been achieved.

People who have already been cured of cancer because someone advised them to try these methods know how wonderful it was that someone had spoken up when it counted. I realize I do not have all the answers concerning cancer, but there is enough here to make this book well worth reading.

I also realize there is a significant credibility gap, as I am not a medical doctor or cancer specialist. Why should you believe me? All I ask is that you consider the references. Rely on the sources of the information quoted and your own logic to uncover the truth. Review the logic in current unproductive theories and compare that to the logic in suppressed cancer cures. Weigh the evidence and come to your own conclusion.

My educational background includes two stimulating years with Father Athol *(Pere)* Murray at Notre Dame College in Wilcox, Saskatchewan in the late 1950's. This inspiring educator motivated thousands of students to believe in traditional human values and stand up for what they believe in. I received a B.A. from the University of Ottawa (majoring in Philosophy), studied English and free-lance writing at Carleton University in Ottawa, and Education at Queens University, in Kingston. While in Ottawa, I worked at the National Research Council in Applied Biology where I cultured and processed yeast for scientific analysis. I also taught both public and high school for several years. For the past 33 years, I have been in private business producing and marketing inventions in the field of office products and herbal products in the field of alternative health. While writing this text, I enjoyed my 60th birthday, in excellent health, with friends and family.

Business success has provided me with discretionary income and abundant free time. With a large personal library and the Internet, I am a full-time dabbler in the arts and sciences. I have been a member of the Rotary Club of Grimsby, Ontario, for twenty years. I was recently awarded the Paul Harris Award that is given annually to a member exhibiting outstanding "Service above Self." It is with this background and public spirit that I researched and organized this information.

After watching an older brother die of cancer, I became interested in knowing the cause of cancer in order to avoid it. I began by researching the herbal tea formula developed by Rene Caisse called essiac and later started marketing it under the business name of *New Action Products (NAP)*. After reading Dr. Hulda Clark's book *The Cure for All Cancers* in 1993, I focused my cancer research on the study of parasites as the cause of cancer and herbal remedies as the treatment. By combining the herbal formulas of Dr. Clark and Rene Caisse, with the guidance of a professional herbalist, I produced a number of unique herbal formulas for the Canadian marketplace. Through sale of these food-supplements, I have received first-hand information from cancer patients who have used them with considerable success.

Some of the *NAP* products are now listed in the "Sources" section of Dr. Clark's books. To so qualify for listing, these products must pass stringent tests for purity and quality.

We recently exported a shipping-container load of these products with over three million capsules of parasite-cleansing herbs to a Chinese pharmaceutical company. Before obtaining a license to import these products, the importer had to prove to Chinese authorities that these products would kill cancer cells in vitro. Obviously they do. The products were tested with cancer patients at a 500-bed cancer-research hospital for a two-year period before qualifying for import. Permission to import herbs into China is not easily achieved, especially by a very small business. Obviously, these products have significant value in stopping cancer or import permits would not have been issued and our products would not have been selected over competitive products. Please realize these herbs are only part of a cancer treatment used to kill fungi and parasites.

The brochure below shows how our Canadian-made products, based on the research of Canadian born Dr. Hulda Regehr Clark, Ph.D., N.D., and Canadian nurse Rene Caisse, are promoted and distributed by mainstream medicine in mainland China for the treatment of cancer.

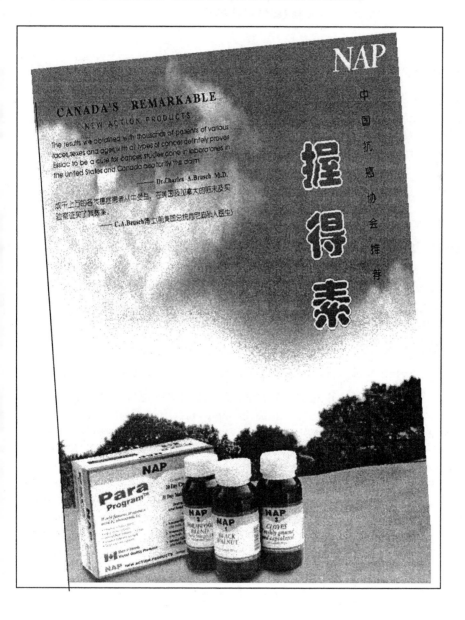

Book purpose, structure and conclusion

This book has three major themes that are intricately involved. The first explains how microbes cause cancer, the second explains how and why effective cancer cures are possible and the third describes how effective cancer cures are being ignored and suppressed. The last chapter looks optimistically into the future, due to the possibility of creating a new vision for our political-economic-medical system.

Information is organized into three roughly equal sections.

1. The *CAUSE* of cancer. (Chapters 1-9)

2. *PREVENTION* of and *CURE* for cancer. (Chapters 10-19)

3. *SUPPRESSION* and *COVER-UP* *of cures that work.* (Chapters 20-30)

The conclusion is deeply disturbing. Before we can hope to have early cancer detection programs and effective cancer cures in public use, we must *FIRST* stop suppression of existing methods for early diagnoses, available cancer cures, and information about them. We are being robbed of our health and economic wealth by abuses of the health care system by medical authorities.

Suppression of effective health care and exploitation of tax revenue is entrenched in conventional health care and politics. The medical monopoly of health care paid for with public funds through taxes ensures that large-scale tax abuse will occur. These abuses must be stopped. The system is now destroying our economy, social safety net, and health care services. Raising taxes is not the answer. Raising taxes destroys human incentive and creates an underground economy resulting in less tax revenue. Abusive waste of tax revenue must be stopped by correcting the fundamental cause of the problem—by eliminating the medical monopoly on health care.

The Table of Contents with major sub-headings listed below will provide you with an overview of this book. Many different sources were required to uncover and describe the *Cause, Cure, and Cover-up* of cancer and to establish that the evidence of suppressed cancer cures is also evident in the treatment of other major diseases.

Table of Contents

Introduction

In this introduction, I will describe how I came upon information regarding the cause of cancer and the effectiveness of alternative cancer treatments. I am the first to admit it seems incredible for me to claim I know the cause of cancer when thousands of researchers have failed to find it. The simple truth is that I did not *discover* it; I *uncovered* and *disclosed* it. All of the information is available in medical texts, books, or the Internet. Through extensive research, I have been able to connect it all together. The big question now is what to do with this knowledge.

In 1992, I experienced my first emotional face-to-face meeting with cancer as I observed my brother living with and dying from prostate cancer. His suffering and death served as a powerful wake-up call for me. I went looking for answers in order to avoid a similar fate. And, given that mainstream medicine has such a high rate of failure, I turned my focus to alternative cancer treatments. Close to eight years of reading, observation and reflection are tied up in this report.

Cancer caused by microbes and parasites

Although there are many conflicting theories regarding the cause of cancer, this report is limited to these two opposing theories: (a) defective genes cause cancer, as *promoted* by mainstream medicine; and (b) cancer microbes cause cancer, as *suppressed* by mainstream medicine.

By attending health fairs across North America and visiting cancer clinics in Mexico, I very quickly learned there are many cancer treatments suppressed in both Canada and the USA. This information came as a shock to me and it is still difficult to accept. None of my personal doctors could possibly be involved in such a horrible act. Still, why do we not have any significant advancement in cancer cures? Why are we losing the war on cancer? Why are some cancer cures suppressed?

The ongoing persecution of the prominent Toronto physician, Dr. Joseph Krop, is a good example of present-day persecution used by the Canadian enforcers of conventional medical practice against any medical doctor who steps out of line and uses alternative therapies. Obviously, all doctors are not involved in the suppression of effective cures.

Public indoctrination in the value of chemotherapy for treating bone cancer is so profound that the Province of Saskatchewan issued a court order to force 13-year-old Tyrell Dueck to accept amputation of his leg against his will and that of his loving parents. What ever happened to freedom of choice? Why was Tyrell not permitted to leave Canada for treatments he wanted in Mexico until he was considered incurable? If you are a child with cancer, does that mean you are no longer free to travel outside of Canada? That's scary.

We have seen remarkable recoveries from people all across Canada, including people with bone cancer, who have followed Dr. Hulda Clark's program to eliminate or cleanse the body of parasites. The combination of products used to eliminate parasites from the body is referred to as a parasite cleanse. Herbal remedies and electromagnetic devices, used as directed, are both effective and safe for eliminating parasites.

The Internet helps makes this report possible

With modern technology a dedicated researcher can find and review a considerable volume of research material in a short time. Searching the Internet or a multimedia encyclopedia with key words such as 'growth hormones,' 'cell-wall membrane', 'bacteria' and 'enzymes' gives one instant access to information that formerly would have taken months to find and review. One does not search for new information on cancer in medical books because their focus is limited to drugs, genetics, and suppression of alternatives. Useful information will be found only in biology, microbiology, and the physical sciences.

Access to research data in this report would not be possible without the freedom of the Internet. Since all of the sciences are covered on the Internet, censorship by any one group is impossible. Microbiology provides more answers for cancer information than does medicine. In my opinion, cancer is a microbial disease and the study of microbial physiology and metabolism is the key to understanding and controlling cancer.

Tracing the process in which the cell-wall components of fungi and bacteria are woven into the cell-wall membrane of human cells will identify the complete cancer process.

Modern medicine should be called *Applied Pharmaceuticals* due to the limited focus of applying drugs and surgery for treatment. As such, it fails to evaluate the significance of nutrition for vital energy, cellular environment, oxidation, pollutants, or parasites. The possibility that cancer can be prevented and cured by removing the cause is seldom considered.

In this text, you will learn that all cancer cells have impaired respiration, leading to fermentation of blood sugars. This research was published by Dr. Otto Warburg of Germany more than 70 years ago. Impaired respiration that stops the oxidative process leads to continuous mutated and division of cells.

When you recognize that Dr. Otto Warburg identified one of the causes of cancer about seventy years ago, you will understand why we have a more serious problem than just finding a cure for cancer. We must find a way to have mainstream medicine accept and use it.

Metabolism is the process in which cells produce energy from food nutrients. There are two kinds of metabolism in human cells: with oxygen and without oxygen. What makes fully developed healthy human cells switch from one form of metabolism to another? The answer to this question will give us the functional cause of cancer.

I believe that this report will provide you with a clear understanding of how cancer occurs through the action of normal cells responding to a polluted cellular environment and the influence of microbial enzymes. Enzymes are tools that cause events to occur within living things. Microbial enzymes cause cellular mutations leading to cancer. Infected cells do not have to be inflamed in order to become cancer cells as a non-inflammatory infection can cause mutation of cell-wall membranes.

The theory that microbial enzymes cause cancer by mutating the cell wall and cell function, explains these mysteries about cancer:

- why the natural process for repair of damaged skin, or the natural growth process itself, starts replication that ends up as cancer.

- why the essential difference between normal cells and cancer cells is how well or poorly they knit together to form new membranes

- why defective genes do not cause cancer

- why cancer *appears* to be hereditary in some cases

- why viruses cannot cause cancer directly or mutate genes

- why we do not have cancer of the heart or arteries

- why up to 96% of cancers occur in cells adjacent to storage vessels and ducts such as lung, colon, breast and prostate

- why cancer tumors develop in infants and children

- how spontaneous remissions can occur with a change in lifestyle

- why tumor membrane tissue resembles the material that forms the outer membrane of mushrooms (a fungus).

The other theories about the cause of cancer do not explain these mysteries about cancer, nor can they explain rapid growth. The defective-gene theory is obviously wrong, as you shall see. If it were not for medical propaganda supporting the defective-gene theory, there would be no reason to even theorize that defective genes cause rapid and uncontrolled growth. This false theory is the cornerstone of the cancer industry for economic reasons.

Rate of growth is dependent upon the capacity of cells to metabolize nutrients for production of energy. To say defective genes cause cancer is to say defective genes cause rapid or out of control metabolism. Normal metabolism is dependent on the availability of oxygen, on minerals for production of enzymes, on food nutrients, and on removal of carbon dioxide. None of these are supplied or controlled by genes. They are controlled by what we do and by the decisions we make in choosing our life-style. To a large extent, the products required for rapid growth and good health on one hand, or cancer growth on the other, are controlled by our personal choices.

Rapid growth is also a result of cells losing human traits and becoming more microbial in nature.

Written for the public

The language level and content of this book is written for the general reader, however health professionals who want to know the true cause of cancer should read this book. Since I do not have a medical career, I can speak openly about the cause of cancer. I do not hold a license to be revoked nor do I have hospital privileges to lose. I have funded my own research and am free to express all facts as I see them within the Canadian Charter of Rights and Freedom of Speech. In order to defend this cause-of-cancer theory against would-be detractors, I have tried to be both clear and scientific.

I have researched the cancer problem with a completely open mind. People who have made up their minds about an issue often fail to follow up on hunches or clues. They become a product of their training and only see what they already believe or what they have been taught. Since I have not attended medical classes, I believe what I see, rather than see what I believe or have been taught to believe. I do not discredit observations or hunches simply because they disagree with my training.

I routinely question every source of information and look for some logic in it. "Why should I believe you?" is my favorite question. By looking for hidden motives and evidence of indoctrination, I have uncovered numerous references of false information written to deceive the public. I now believe that *misinformation* is regularly and purposely published by mainstream medicine. Numerous examples are quoted throughout the text. The defective-gene theory is only one of many.

I have stayed focused on the problem so I have read, or otherwise observed a significant amount of information in a rather brief period. After my brother's death from cancer, when I still believed that inherited defective genes caused cancer, I thought it would be my death sentence too. Living with the fear of hereditary cancer due to defective genes is very stressful. There's nothing you can do to change heredity. I understand why women diagnosed with 'so-called' defective breast genes are having their healthy breasts removed in order to prevent cancer.

The sad truth is that effective cancer cures are available outside of mainstream medicine. Breast cancer —a common storage-vessel cancer —is easy to understand, treat, and prevent. That is why women should take a keen interest in reading this book.

The mental and emotional relief that comes from knowing the true cause of cancer is hard to describe. I sincerely hope this information will bring you peace of mind and help you through any suspicion or personal diagnosis of cancer. I also hope that you will take an active part in establishing your right to early diagnosis, and effective treatments to prevent and cure this frightful disease for you and your loved ones.

Since I did research in the fields of medicine, biology, biochemistry, microbiology, human genetics and physics, and since I do not hold university level training in any of these fields, I support all major statements with direct reference to texts. I have elected to identify the source of each quotation with the quotation, rather than as footnotes, so that you can evaluate the reference as you read it. Page references are also given in case you want to look up these references for clarification and for more information.

In order to understand the basic cause of cancer we must first familiarize ourselves with terms relating to metabolism, enzymes, and genes. These words will appear throughout the text and must be understood to obtain full meaning of what follows.

Definition of important concepts

Metabolism is a collective term for the entire range of enzyme-driven processes that take place in the body. Metabolism is divided into *catabolism* and *anabolism.*

In *catabolism,* a complex substance is *broken down* into simpler ones, usually with a *release of energy.* Enzymes are required to break down the molecules and eliminate the wastes. All chemical actions inside living things are controlled or *catalyzed* by enzymes.

In the *anabolic process* complex substances such as amino acids, digestive enzymes, immune system defenses, and cell-wall membranes are *assembled* from simpler components, with the *consumption of energy.* Both enzymes and energy are required in this process. Adequate cellular energy is the key to a strong immune system and control of microbial infectious agents or 'pathogens'. Adequate oxygen is required to produce energy by aerobic metabolism.

Three concepts that serve as keys to understanding metabolism are based on the use of oxygen and glycogen. Glycogen is a sugar stored in tissue to be converted to energy as required.

Glycolysis, meaning the metabolism or breakdown of glycogen molecules to release energy for cells.

aerobic glycolysis meaning with free oxygen; and

anaerobic glycolysis, meaning without free oxygen.

Capacity to metabolize glycogen with or without oxygen determines the difference between aerobic and anaerobic life forms. The capacity for the human cell to *switch* from one to the other is the reason we have cancer and out-of-control replication. It is a genetic capacity but not a genetic defect or fault. Defective genes are not involved.

When the switch in metabolism occurs before cells divide and multiply, fungi and bacteria are allowed to contaminate the assembly process of new cells. The immune system cannot eliminate parasites in the cells from the process of cell reproduction. Each normal human cell that divides produces two new cancer cells simply because microbial cell-wall components mutate the cell during the assembly process. Microbial enzymes and growth hormones modify the assembly process.

Where do enzymes come from? How are they made? What do genes have to do with enzymes? Let's start with the definition of a gene.

The present scientific definition of a gene is *"a sequence of nucleotides in DNA that codes for a functional product."* Genes are strings of DNA molecules within the nucleus of our cells.

In biochemistry, the duplication of genes is called *replication;* the synthesis of a copy of DNA into messenger RNA (mRNA) is called *transcription.* The subsequent synthesis of a protein molecule from the mRNA is called *translation.* Duplication of new daughter cells is called *mitosis, or division* or *multiplication* because a cell must first divide in order to form two new cells. Please make a mental note of *mitosis, replication, transcription,* and *translation.* See glossary for more information.

Enzymes are copies of our DNA structure. Production of enzymes is like having a stamp with your name and address and an inkpad. You can make copies of your name and address without limitation as long as you keep ink in the inkpad. It is the same with enzymes. Genes will *transcribe* mRNA and *translate* enzymes without limitation as long as we supply essential needs through nutrition.

Unfortunately, parasites and microbes will translate enzymes as long as we nourish them with carbon found in sugar. The majority of human disease comes from feeding fungi too much carbon and allowing fungal enzymes to 'stamp out' our enzymes or substitute their proteins for ours. Most primitive life forms have cell walls that contain a sugar/protein combination called *chitin,* whereas most human cells walls contain phosphates and *lipids* (dissolve like fats). The replacement of lipids in the cell wall by chitin leads to cancer, autoimmune and degenerative diseases.

Human cells evolved from earlier life forms that had cell walls made of chitin. It follows that human cells have dormant genes for forming chitin. In addition, some human cells have active genes for forming chitin because parts of our body, such as the colon, fingernails and cuticles, are formed from chitin. If any cells inside our body have active genes for forming chitin parasites in these cells could produce chitin growth hormones that would result in increased production of chitin with new cells having bizarre traits. It may well be that cancer initiates only in cells with active chitin forming genes. With each new generation of cells, cancer cells could express more chitin forming genes resulting in progressive changes that explain cancer progression. The common ancestry between human cells and parasitic cells explains why infection of cells during replication causes cell wall mutation. The genes are not defective. The genes are responding normally to enzymes and hormones, but to the microbial growth hormone message that is identical to the human cell message.

Enzymes are produced according to the genetic makeup of the cell as well as the environment of the cell. Genes are like a factory making thousands of different products. The assembly line starts when orders come in for new enzymes based on the needs of the cell. The enzyme capacity you inherit limits the variety of enzymes your cells can produce. Regulator genes sense the cellular environment, activate or turn on the genes required and produce functional products to serve the cell, based on the environment of the cell.

Just as an assembly line needs raw materials and tools to hold pieces in place or move them about, the assembly of enzymes requires raw materials from food and tools to hold atoms in place and move them about. These holding tools in metabolism are called *substrates.*

Substrates are essential for metabolism because they provide the capacity for enzymes to break down large molecules of food nutrients. Substrates are important to understanding cancer because they control or limit the metabolic process and therefore control rate of growth. A blotter used for soaking up excess ink or other liquids is an example of a substrate. In the metabolic process, substrates absorb excess atoms and release them for another process.

In order to reduce or break down large molecules of carbohydrates, fat or protein, the molecule must be reduced to manageable pieces. In most cases, hydrogen bonds are broken to allow removal of smaller sections of the molecule. Some enzymes are *substrates* that grip active hydrogen molecules until they can be used elsewhere or combined with other molecules to be safely removed. For example, two atoms of hydrogen combined with one atom of oxygen produce water (H_2O) that is used by the cell or excreted as waste. The process works fine until essential minerals are missing and the process breaks down with microbial infection.

Gene expression and gene repression explained

The process of turning gene dominance "on" and "off" is referred to as *"gene expression"* and *"gene repression."* The only active genes capable of transcribing enzymes or functional proteins are *expressed* genes. In a zipper that is partially unzipped, the open sides are like expressed genes. Either side may transcribe mRNA. Repressed genes are like the closed portion of the zipper. Repressed genes are also referred to as dormant genes, although they may be active as regulatory genes. The total gene package is referred to as the *genome*. Amazingly, only about 2% to 3% of the total gene package encodes genetic information used for producing functional products.

About forty-five per cent of the human genome that encodes genetic information contains genes identical to those found in microbes like fungi and bacteria that rely on fermentation of glucose for energy. It is therefore possible for human cells to revert to an earlier form of metabolism without oxygen simply by expressing dormant genes. Through progressive doubling, these cancer cells can also express dormant genes to produce more chitin cell-wall membrane material and develop more aggressive cancer traits. If any cancer genes exist, they will probably be nothing more than the expression of dormant genes for production of chitin or genes that somehow mutate the cell-wall membrane. Cancer is a mutated cell-wall membrane disease due to microbial genes in parasites, or the expression of dormant genes.

Now, let's review how microbes cause cancer by modifying the environment of the cell, causing a change in metabolism, and mutating the cell-wall membrane and cell function during normal replication.

Section ONE: The CAUSE of Cancer

1. How virus, bacteria, fungi and parasites cause cancer

This chapter describes how infections cause cancer. The cancer process is described in terms of cell wall components, microbial enzymes, metabolism, and repair of injury. Subsequent chapters will add more detail and deal with false information that shapes public opinion and perceptions about cancer. This one very long chapter will help you to understand the cause of and cure for cancer.

We must understand the conflict between human enzymes and parasitic enzymes in order to understand the cancer process. Cancer depends upon the enzymes that are in control of metabolism and replication. Normal cells produce enzymes to oxidize nutrients. Cancer cells produce enzymes to ferment nutrients. Normal cells produce energy for the body. Cancer cells guard energy for cellular replication and growth. That's the simple energy basis for rapid growth of cancer cells.

We must also understand why DNA replicates out-of-control. All adult cancers that form tumors begin with damaged tissue. The normal repair mechanism that causes skin cells to multiply to repair injury is the reason why DNA begins to replicate. To repair an injury, the body produces a measurable ionic field called the *current of injury*. This is the force and source of energy that causes DNA to replicate, cells to divide, and new growth to repair the damage. The mechanics of the process will be described in detail later.

In normal circumstances, when the injury is repaired the current of injury shuts down, and replication stops. Cancer occurs when these newly assembled cell-wall membranes are mutated by the microbial enzymes during cell division. These cells with traits of single-celled microbes do not knit with existing membrane. They fail to repair the injury and the current of injury fails to shut down. The result is continuous out-of-control replication and mutation of cells. Defective genes have nothing to do with the process of cancer.

Cancer is known to occur in bone fractures that do not heal, because the current of injury does not shut down. Bones contain rapidly multiplying blood cells in bone marrow. Broken bones are capable of healing because bone is a living substance, even though bones are firm and solid. The effectiveness of electromagnetic fields to increase the rate of bone repair has been demonstrated and accepted by mainstream medicine. A specialized electromagnetic device produces a weak direct current that mimics the normal current of injury and increases rate of growth. An energy field, not enzymes, is the cause of increased rate of replication. It follows that that genes, defective or not, are not related to the process of initiating cancer in bone cells. Microbes cause cancer in bones and cells by mutating the cell wall during mitosis.

Cancer in infants and children does not require injury because the life stage of children is such that cells are replicating rapidly for growth. Similarly, body parts that mature later in life, such as reproductive organs, can become cancerous without injury. Infection of these rapidly growing cells by fungi and bacteria results in cancer that forms tumors, or if white blood cells (leukocytes) are mutated, leukemia results. Since mutated white blood cells do not function to eliminate invaders, the body continues to produce more of them, resulting in high blood counts and loss of immune system function. Contamination of replicating cells with microbial enzymes, lipids and proteins can account for all human cancers and eliminate the mysteries relating to cancer.

Back in your high school days or in recent health-related material you probably learned about digestive enzymes such as *proteases*, that digest protein, *amalases*, that digest starch, and *lipases*, that digests fat. You probably learned how the immune system produces defensive cells, and defensive cells produce defensive enzymes to destroy invaders. We also have **metabolic enzymes** that run our bodies; repair damaged cells, and guides the cell-replication process. The enzymes that guide replication are shared by all living things and these can be transferred across species without loss of function. That is why microbes can cause cancer in humans by mutating cell-wall membranes.

The key to understanding cancer is that DNA cannot replicate unless a very specific enzyme called *DNA polymerase* is available. The enzyme could be compared to a special tool that speeds assembly of DNA. The enzyme used by scientists to cause human DNA to replicate in test tubes is harvested from bacteria. It follows without question that bacteria in our cells can also produce this enzyme and cause cell mutation during normal replication or tissue repair. Cancer is a microbial disease caused by microbial enzymes modifying or taking control of normal processes during assembly of cell components.

Parasites become involved in adult cancers because parasites force their way through epithelial cells, cause injury and turn on the current of injury that causes these cells to divide. Fungi and bacteria, associated with larger parasites, contaminate the injured tissue and cause cancer. Parasites cause cancer by turning on the current of injury in membrane cells that protect our organs, or in cells that form our storage vessels and ducts.

In bone cancer, bones do not grow out of control. Bones are consumed by fungi and bacteria. Microbes do not have bones, and cannot produce bone-growth factors. Even bone cancer is caused by enzymes from parasitic microbes in our body and can be cured the same way as any other cancer. There is actually only one type of cancer, and that is mutated cell function and cell-wall membrane cancer. Different parasites may cause cancer and their various contributions to the cell wall membrane results in the variety of appearance in cancer cells. Appearances are due to the variety of changes in the cell-wall membrane and are not a result of genetic changes.

All that information we've been told about defective genes, oncogenes, suppressor genes, viral mutated genes and genetic defects during replication is false information. Defective genes cause defective human parts, not cancer. Errors in replication that cause cancer do not occur without the direct mutation of normal replicating cells by microbial growth factors from parasites. Parasites cause cancer by infecting cells and injuring tissues in the body that leads to the defective repair process.

What are parasites?

Parasites include all life forms living inside the tissues or on the skin's surface of another creature called the 'host', without the host receiving any benefit in return for providing food and shelter. Human parasites range in size from twenty-foot tape worms to thousands of varieties of microscopic life-forms. Fungi and bacteria living in our tissues and organs are called parasites because they live off our body without benefiting us in return.

'Microbe' is a general term referring to living forms that can be viewed only through a microscope. In the cancer process, we will be dealing with fungi and bacteria that are microscopic parasites. Viruses will be studied in detail to prove that they do not cause cancer nor do they modify genes to cause cancer. Viruses cause benign growths that lead to cancer. In this text, 'microbes' will be used to refer to either fungi or bacteria equally. The word 'fungi' is the plural form and refers to the group that includes yeasts and molds. Fungus, the singular form, refers to a specific type of fungi. Larger parasites in our body are hosts to fungi and bacteria so that the spread and proliferation of large parasites includes a corresponding spread and proliferation of fungi and bacteria. These microbes thrive inside parasitic hosts because they are beyond the reach of the human immune system. Large parasites are like army tanks and personnel carriers protecting and distributing microbial parasites in the wake of their injury to tissue and organ cells.

I am now certain that most cancer growths start from injury to a mass of skin or epithelial tissue that results in internal bleeding or an injury that will not heal, such as a fractured bone. That is why the majority of cancers occur in storage vessels and ducts. Cancer does not start from a single cancer cell because the unique reduced respiration of cancer cells can only occur within a large group of cells. It takes a large mass of cells to mutate simultaneously to defeat the immune system defenses. A colony of fermenting cells must be formed before a tumor can develop. A quantity of trapped blood in a storage vessel or duct feeds fungi and bacteria, and provides the initial toxins that alter the environment and metabolism of adjacent cells allowing cancer to start.

Fungi and bacteria thrive in the blood clots and succeed in modifying the environment of adjacent cells so that fungi and bacteria can survive in these cells as well. The body's attempt to repair the damaged tissue initiates new growth and starts the replication process of these infected cells. Fungi produce toxins that reduce oxygen levels in cells and destroy human enzymes required for metabolism. Fungi cannot gain control of the replicating cells without the safe haven and energy supply of trapped blood sugars. This is why benign growths and infections lead to cancer.

Cancer can also start from sports or any physical injury where epithelial tissue is damaged and blood becomes trapped in connective tissue or bone fragments. Also, blood can become trapped due to hardening of the arteries with a break in the plaque, or weakening of the arteries due to nutritional deficiencies. Varicose veins are a good example of internal bleeding with blood trapped within the body.

In the past, the concept that microbes cause cancer was rejected by cancer researchers because cancer microbes taken from cancer cells could not initiate cancer in healthy animals. Researchers did not realize that the current of injury was not turned on and the oxygen levels were too high for anaerobic microbes to thrive. Consequently, it was assumed that bacteria observed in cancer cells were secondary or coincidental. Another cause was deemed necessary to cause replication, so virus and defective genes became the prime targets of research. This subject will be developed further in the next chapter.

The fact that bacteria have been observed and photographed in cancer cells is more than coincidence. Since enzymes from bacteria are essential for replication of DNA in the DNA polymerase chain reaction, bacterial enzymes are obviously capable of controlling cell wall assembly after normal DNA is replicated. That's why researchers cannot find any defective genes in cancer cells. Cancer occurs during assembly of cell-wall membranes and the defect is not in the genes. The defect is in the cytoplasm and the cell-wall membrane.

In order to clearly understand the cause of cancer we must take time to learn about fungi, bacteria, enzymes, and metabolism. We must also learn to use specific terms for concise and accurate communication of ideas. Just as you cannot discuss computer functions without using terms such as bits and bytes, you cannot discuss the cause of cancer without using related scientific terms. The enclosed glossary will help you master these terms.

A book called *The Science Class You Wish You Had* by Arnold and David Brody, Ph.D., gives us a frame of reference to help visualize the size of an atom and how easy it is to become confused with understanding atoms and molecules (Page 78):

> ...The diameter of the nucleus (in an atom) is about one hundred thousands of the diameter of the whole atom. The volume of the nucleus is one trillionth of the whole atom. To put this in another perspective, if the earth were enlarged to the incredible size of 93 million miles in diameter (the distance from here to the sun), the nucleus of even the largest atom, increased proportionately, would still be microscopic. The basic characteristics of the atom seem so bizarre and foreign to everyday experience that it is difficult to conceptualize.

The minute size of viruses and DNA nucleotides are also hard to imagine. Dr. Guyton informs us that a cell has a *diameter* of about 1000 times that of the smallest virus and a *volume* about one billion times that of the smallest virus.

Cells host to virus, fungi, or bacteria can continue to maintain normal metabolic functions and replication, incurring only a small amount of cell wall mutation and loss of function with each new generation. This is why we have degenerative diseases and so-called autoimmune diseases.

It helps to understand why the defective gene theory is wrong when we realize that the entire DNA body of nucleotides making up all of the chromosomes in our body is less than a teaspoon in amount. Cancer is a problem of the cell wall and membrane dysfunction, not defective genes.

The concept that we probably have new cancer cells every day is based on the false theory of defective replication of genes. Cancer doesn't start at the single cell level. It starts with a large group of mature cells parasitized by fungi and bacteria or other parasites. We don't experience new cancer cells every day. When the internal environment allows cancer to start, it will not stop until the all microbes in adjacent cells are killed and the current of injury shuts down due to satisfactory repair of membrane injury.

Here are several important characteristics about fungi and bacteria relating to cancer. This information supports the concept that cell-wall membranes on new daughter cells will be mutated by microbial cell-wall material known as chitin.

Fungi cells are closely related to animal cells

There are about *500,000* fungal species on Earth. *Biologically, they are closely related to both the plant and animal kingdoms.* Due to the structure of their cell walls, as well as their type of nutrients, they are positioned between plants and bacteria and form the *fungal kingdom.* Fungi are not plants because they lack the vascular tissues (phloem and xylem) that form the true roots, stems, and leaves of higher plants. Fungi also lack chlorophyll for photosynthesis and must therefore live as parasites. Their function on earth is to break down dead and dying matter for renewal. **Fungi also attack living tissue and survive by producing toxins and enzymes to defeat the host's immune system.**

The monthly scientific magazine "EXPLORE", published in Germany and USA, contains articles by alternative health care professionals and publishes research in support of microbes as the cause of cancer. An article in Volume 5, Numbers 5 & 6, 1994, by Dr. K. Mueller-Christiansen, provides valuable insights into the difference between yeast and fungi. (Page 20-21). *(From this point forward, please recognize bold type within a quotation as my method for emphasis. Italics will be used for explanatory material and comments.)*

Morphologically considered, one differentiates two large groups, namely the thread or filamentous *fungi* and the *yeast.* Mushrooms are filamentous fungi. The actual fungus consists of a subterranean network that is irregularly branched out and formed by interweaving cell threads, the so-called mycelia. Among the filamentous fungi are also the dermatomyces, which attack the skin, as well as the mould fungi known from the household.

Yeasts are unicellular fungi

Yeasts, whether round or oval shaped, are unicellular fungi with a distinct cell wall, which form a psydomycel in contrast to the thread fungi *(psydomycel look like a chain of sausages or narrow balloons twisted into shapes).* **Yeasts multiply vegetatively by**

sprouting and/or splitting. Yeast ferments sugar into alcohol under anaerobic *(without oxygen)* conditions. Another yeast called *Penicillum* produces the antibiotic penicillin used to fight bacterial infections.

Fungi nutrition is carbon in dead and living organisms

Clinically important is that yeasts do not always behave like yeasts, and thread fungi do not always behave like thread fungi. For instance, *Candida Albicans,* a genuine yeast, can also invade the mucous membrane of a human body as a thread fungus while pathogenic fungi of the species *Histoplasm* can spread within tissue like yeasts. **The source of nutrition for all fungi is the organically bound carbon of dead and living organisms.**

Candida Albicans is a yeast form common to all living creatures. No one is immune to yeast and fungi in the body. The Columbia Encyclopedia gives additional important data regarding the physical description of fungi as follows:

Their bodies (fungi) consist of slender, cottony filaments called *hyphae;* a mass of hyphae is called a *mycelium.* **The mycelium carries on all the processes necessary for the life of the organism, including, in most species, that of sexual reproduction.**

A third significant detail regarding function of fungi and bacteria in cancer comes from the Internet. While searching under Biochemistry, Genetics, and Molecular Biology, I found several references to cloning of DNA. **The enzyme required to cut genes into manageable units comes from bacteria, which normally use this enzyme to cut and destroy the genes of invading viruses.**

A fourth significant detail, and probably the most important of all that ties fungi to the cancer process comes from *The Canadian Medical Association, Home Medical Encyclopedia,* under Fungi:

Some fungi are able to invade and form colonies within the lungs, in the skin, beneath the skin, or sometimes in various tissues throughout the body, leading to conditions ranging from mild skin irritations to severe, even fatal illness.

Fungi that can invade membrane (skin) cells to form colonies will damage the membrane wall, initiate a current of injury, multiply along with the normal cells to repair the injury, and mutate these cells during the assembly process. Is cancer the "fatal illness"?

In addition, the most commonly used source of chromosome material comes from yeast. It is referred to as *Yeast Artificial Chromosome* because it has all of the four DNA bases needed to make up complete human chromosomes. Bacterial enzymes are used to cut fungal mycelia into useful molecules *(called nucleotides)* to promote replication. Genetic researchers use the same enzymes to promote DNA cloning. Cancer microbes are therefore capable of the same process in human cells as that of DNA cloning in test tubes. It follows that the obvious close tie between fermentation and rapid cancer growth is the rapid development of DNA nucleotides in fungal mycelia. *(Nucleotides are molecules used by the cell to construct DNA much like bricks are used by a homebuilder to build a wall.)*

Cancer and fungi have been associated through visual documentation as well as statistical information gathered by the World Health Organization (WHO). The direct one-to-one relationship of fungi and cancer are recorded in books called Fungalbionics, by a group of doctors working for the WHO. They also find that all effective treatments for cancer are antifungal.

Visual documentation, based on the use of high quality microscopes, shows that all cancer cells are parasitized. According To Dr. Costantini, the scientific study of fungi is *fungalbionics*. The Greek word *mykes* means fungus, from which comes the word *mycotoxins*, or the study of the toxins produced by fungi. Mycotoxins are biologically active substances, like enzymes, that enable fungi to survive in a hostile world. A fungus in central Michigan is considered to be the largest living thing in the world.

In my research, I have found that the connection between cancer, fungi and parasites is through the cell-wall membrane. All living things produce membranes to protect organs, or in the case of microbes, to form body parts. In primitive life forms, the cell-wall material is called chitin, and you can observe the physical characteristics of chitin in the exoskeleton of flies, spiders, or the skin of a mushroom. The crunchy sound heard from stepping on cockroaches or other insects is the sound of chitin breaking. Chitin gives cancer tumor membranes the characteristics and appearance of primitive life forms.

Researchers have recently identified genes that produce chitin in yeast such as *Candida albicans*, and *Saccharomyces cerevisiae*. All primitive living things have these genes, because chitin is common to all primitive life. (See Internet Adams, Causier et al. 1993, or just search under "chitin and fungus") The above yeast cells are commonly associated with cancer. Why are researchers looking for these genes? Could they be planning to produce a drug that would stop chitin production in order to cure cancer? If so, do they already know the true cause of cancer?

It follows that when human chromosomes and DNA are induced to replicate by the current of injury or natural growth, the DNA of parasites in the cells will also replicate simultaneously. The greater the number of microbes within the cell, the greater the amount of microbial cell-wall chitin components will be produced and the faster cancer will spread.

During the assembly process of the two daughter cells, these chitin-forming molecules produced by normal parasitic DNA, will be incorporated into the cell-wall membrane of both new cells. The mutated cells form a new membrane combination, part phospho-lipid, part chitin. The chitin portions, formed from glucose, break the plasma field of the cell. A break in the plasma field results in rejection by the body, leads to attack by the auto immune system, and allows for further infection. The many different cancers, based on appearance and form, are a result of the combination of a specific type of fungi and a specific type of original cell. Although there are many types of cancer, based on properties of the combination, there is still only one type of cancer based on cause. **All human cancers are caused by the incorporation of chitin into the cell-wall membrane of human cells during mitoses.**

Note these six features of fungi and bacteria:

1. Fungi rely on carbon in dead and **living** things for nutrition.

2. Mycelia can *invade* the mucus membrane of a human cell. The consequent injury to tissue will initiate the human repair process and develop a current of injury to cause DNA replication.

3. Fungal mycelia bring into the cell all the processes necessary for microbial life–*including reproduction.*

4. Fungi also attack living tissue and survive by producing toxins and enzymes to *defeat the host's immune system.*

5. Bacteria resident in human cells as parasites can produce enzymes to *cut nucleic acids from fungal mycelia.*

6. Fungi have genes that produce cell-wall membrane material called chitin that mutates the cell-wall membrane of normal cells during assembly.

In conclusion, fungal mycelia invade human cells to cause cancer. Invasion of epithelial *(skin)* cells by fungal mycelium explains why up to 96% of cancers occur in epithelial cells adjacent to lymphatic fluids. Fungi gain strength in trapped body fluids and modify the environment of adjacent cells, allowing microbes to thrive.

Damage to skin tissue by flukes and other parasites causes internal bleeding with loss of oxygen in the resulting blood clot. Fermentation of glucose in blood or lymphatic fluid enables fungi to thrive and empowers mycelia to invade adjacent tissue. Bacteria resident in cells as parasites produce the enzymes that controls how cells differentiate and mycelia provide combinations of molecules for rapid growth as well.

The reference to fungal nutrition relying on organically bound carbon should also be noted, as yeast and fungi rely on carbohydrates and sugars for nutrition. Consider for a moment how we make bread, beer, and wine. Sugar and yeast are required. Sugar is always added so that yeast will multiply. When we consume excess sugar, we feed yeast and fungi in our body. When I worked at growing and processing yeast in the laboratory, we used trays filled with liquid glucose. Nothing but glucose was required to grow hundreds of floating pads of mycelia, about ¼ inch thick, to be used for DNA analysis. Growth stopped when the glucose supply was depleted.

One of the most recent cures for cancer is to inject insulin into cancer patients so that all of the glucose is consumed by the body. As a result, fungi and cancer cells starve to death. Another cure for cancer is metabolic therapy that eliminates sugar from the diet and eliminates cancer cell growth over a longer period.

Sugar comes in three main forms called sucrose, maltose, and fructose. These are converted by the body to glycogen and stored for energy. Refined sugars consumed as food are absorbed quickly by the body. Consuming large amounts of these sugars results in an imbalance of too little oxygen and the inability of the body to metabolize these sugars. These sugars contaminate blood and lymph fluids. Fungi and yeast thrive on these excess sugars leading to an imbalance and shortage of essential minerals needed for other enzymes. Consequently, disease can occur in any part of the body, and the personality of the person can be modified due to lack of functional enzymes controlling mood and emotions. Children who consume too much sugar are often hyperactive, overweight, and unruly. They also tend to experience disease conditions more frequently than others.

Have you ever noticed that flu outbreaks occur just after periods of heavy sugar consumption such as Christmas and Easter? The sugar fermentation process creates a downward health spiral leading to loss of enzyme function, loss of metabolic function, loss of immune system function, increase in yeast and parasitic life-forms, more loss of enzymes and so on. If fermentation continues, supported by wrong food choices, disease progresses from normal health to a functional disease such as personality disorders and chronic fatigue, to organ diseases such as diabetes and benign cysts, warts and tumors, to a tissue disease such as cancer. Cancer doesn't start in healthy well-oxidized cells due to replication errors nor is it due to genetic defects. Nutrition and parasites, as well as fungi and bacteria have a major part to play in the cancer process.

Bacteria are closely related to animal cells

Bacteria have cell-wall membranes closely similar to human cell walls and share the same enzymes that cause cell-wall membranes to form. This enzyme is called epidermal growth factor (EGF) because it controls epidermal cell growth. The enzyme is also referred to as *growth hormone* because it is produced in humans only in the pituitary gland. A hormone is a fluid that exits the source without access to a duct. An enzyme exits the source where it is produced through a duct, such as bile exits through the bile duct. Other than that, there appears to be no difference between an enzyme and a hormone as both are produced by duplication of patterns in DNA. Bacteria produce growth factors within the cell wall in enzymes, whereas humans produce growth factors in the pituitary gland. Creatures with billions of cells making up one body control growth factors by producing them in a special gland so that growth will conform to the life-force or shape of the species. Replication of DNA is controlled by an ionic field of energy produced by the body so that body parts do not grow out of proportion.

The following reference on composition of bacterial cells come from *McGraw-Hill Multimedia of Science and Technology*. Page references are not available because this reference is from a computer disk.

The overall chemical composition of the bacterial cell is very similar to that of all other types of cells of animal, plant, and microbial origin, which are capable of growth and replication. **Bacteria thus possess the protein ribonucleic acid (RNA) and deoxyribonucleic acid (DNA), which are the major classes of chemical constituents for replication.**

Obviously, bacterial parasites in our body are capable of producing the vital DNA polymerase enzyme required to speed DNA replication and mutate cells during assembly of cell contents and the cell-wall membrane. Defective genes and viral oncogenes are not required to explain cancer.

Bacterial metabolism

The following reference is also taken from the McGraw-Hill Multimedia of Science and Technology. This reference establishes that bacterial cells are very masterful, and similar to animal cells in form and content. *(Italics were used in the original text for explanatory material.)*

Anabolism *(metabolism or breakdown of a nutrient)* is an immensely complex phenomenon. This is clear from the fact that many bacteria can live and multiply in a simple inorganic medium supplied with but a single organic substrate, such as acetate. These organisms can synthesize all of their cell constituents–carbohydrates, fats, proteins, enzymes, nucleic acids, and so on–from the single substrate. So bewildering are the number and diversity of the components of a bacterial cell that it seems hopeless to attempt an explanation of the manner in which the necessary syntheses are accomplished.

Of what is a bacterial cell composed? In addition to water, which accounts for about 70% of the cell's total weight, there are present over 3000 different molecules *(which account for some 15% of the total weight)* deoxyribonucleic acid [DNA] *(one of two kinds, about 1% of the total weight)*, ribonucleic acid [RNA] (some 1000 different molecular species, totaling 6% of the weight), carbohydrates *(perhaps 50 different kinds, 3% of cell weight)*, lipids *(about 50 different kinds, 2% of total cell weight)*, the building blocks of molecules of the intermediary metabolism *(500 kinds, 2% of total cell weight)*, and inorganic ions (about 12 kinds, 1% of cell weight).

Bacteria have the capacity to survive, thrive and multiply in a solution of acetic acid (vinegar) made by a fungus called the vinegar plant. Acetate is an acid containing acetic acid made up only of hydrogen, carbon, and oxygen atoms. It is theoretically impossible for bacteria to produce all of the cell components from these three molecules, but they do. Obviously, there is a lot we do not know about biochemistry.

Bacteria have also been found miles deep inside the earth's crust and scientists believe these bacteria live off minerals in rocks. Bacteria have also been found in pools of oil formed millions of years ago. It is now assumed that natural gas is a by-product of microbial metabolism of previous plant life.

This amazing capacity of bacteria to thrive on fungal-produced vinegar supports a theory that bacteria can thrive in human cells on products produced by fungi through fermentation of glucose. For example, lactic acid used as food by bacteria is produced by fermentation in human cells. There is good reason to believe bacteria use modified human cells to ferment glucose and produce products which bacteria use for growth and replication. Cancer is not an accident or genetic problem but a natural occurrence orchestrated by fungi and bacteria for their mutual benefit.

Microbial cells are far more resilient, mysterious and powerful than I had believed before I started this research into cancer. These cells are similar to human cells in DNA and cytoplasm, but the cell-wall membrane is different. This cell wall difference is the key to understanding how an infection leads to cancer.

A common denominator of all anaerobic parasites is that they produce defensive toxins and enzymes to reduce the oxygen level in the tissue or cells that they invade. Malonic acid has been identified as one of the major oxygen-reducing toxins that help anaerobic microbes to survive in an aerobic host. Plants also use malonic acid to control oxygen levels. Malonic acid can be found in root crops that store well, such as carrots, because the malonic acid reduces oxidation.

The key to understanding microbial infection and disease is to understand how oxygen levels are controlled at the cellular level, how oxygen-free microspheres and tumors are formed and how the oxidative metabolism process is shut down. A tumor creates an environment that serves as a microsphere for anaerobic life. *Microspheres* are like enclosed football stadiums capable of supporting a vast number of microbes and cancer cells within a reduced oxygen protected environment. The complexity of what microbial cells are capable of doing brings up a question. How do they do it? They must have some form of 'intelligence'. How do they 'think'?

Microbes demonstrate intelligence

Doctors claim that most modern antibiotics do not work because the microbes have 'outsmarted' the antibiotics. Does that mean microbes have intelligence, or is 'outsmarted' being used metaphorically? At first, I assumed it simply meant that natural selection processes allowed some microbes to survive, and these became resistant to the drugs, however natural selection cannot explain many aspects of microbial behavior. Why do they produce defensive enzymes to cut opposing viral enemies to pieces? How could they do what they do without some limited form of "intelligence"?

Do microbes think? Could a bacterial cell, without some form of intelligence, produce thousands of cellular components from a single substrate such as acetate just by chance or crystal-like growth? Could bacteria produce defensive enzymes without knowing why? Not likely! Some people consider microbes as being super intelligent. We cannot even understand how they do what they do, let alone duplicate it.

Where is the seat of microbial intelligence? Where is its memory and sensory apparatus? How does it store knowledge? What is the source of wave energy for thinking? Is it an ionic field like the current of injury? Could it all be in the tiny amount of DNA? Does it have access to some form of universal intelligence? Maybe, someday, we will unravel these mysteries. With our present limited knowledge about life and thought processes, we must consider all living things to have some intelligence. We must therefore deal with them as "intelligent" beings.

Bacteria can survive in a single substrate such as acetate, to produce all of their thousands of cellular parts. They have thrived for millions of years, miles below the surface of the earth in rocks and oil. Bacteria consume minerals. Bacteria deplete the body of minerals too. It is highly probable that bacteria cause cancer for a reason. Given the opportunity, they will produce growth factors that mutate a cell-wall membrane so that the cell functions to its advantage. For example, an increase in growth hormone receptors on the cell wall would increase rate of mitosis. *(Mitosis includes all steps in cell division and multiplication.)*

Just as we use captive microbes to ferment products that we use, such as bread, beer, wine, and vinegar, *perhaps* microbes use captive human cells to ferment products that they use. The unlimited growth of human cells serves a valuable purpose for the unlimited growth of microbes, and explains the fundamental reason why cancer exists. Cancer is not an accident or an adaptation of human cells to survive in a harsh environment. Cancer is caused by microbes and directed by them to serve their needs. Bacteria are farming our cells to feed themselves and feeding our DNA nucleotides during replication with molecules cut from fungal mycelia. That is why cancer growth is so rapid.

Professor Joe Tsien at Princeton University has genetically engineered 'smart mice' by inserting an extra gene into their DNA. According to a newspaper article (Hamilton Spectator, Sept. 2, 1999):

> In his research Tsien found the improved learning and memory came from increased production of a brain protein called NR2B and its effect on brain-cell switches called NMDA receptors....It is quite possible there are other key molecules also involved in learning and memory.

Tsien's research shows a direct relationship between nutrition and intelligence through protein production. Microbes make proteins. Do these contain memory? Perhaps microbes have more intelligence in some ways than humans because they have been around for a much longer time. They also have a better physical 'view' of the atomic structure and how enzymes work to perform metabolic functions. Obviously, they have no problem adapting to their environment and modifying their environment to suit their needs. That is why they have survived for billions of years and can evade the majority of antibiotics used in medicine.

There is plenty of evidence in microbiology to prove that microbes are able to produce proteins similar to those of human cells. In addition, microbes use the same 'postal code system' to deliver proteins to a specific location as is used by human cells. Bacteria and fungi are capable of controlling human cellular functions as well as mutating cell-wall membranes during cell division.

War of the enzymes: man verses microbe

The 1999 Nobel Prize in Physiology or Medicine was won by cell-biologist Guenther Blobel for his discovery of how proteins are positioned in cellular structures using an amino acid address system

In the review material on the Internet at http://www.nobel.se, we are given the following details. I have summarized the more significant points, in point form, to discuss how this research relates to an understanding of cancer.

1. An adult human being is made up of approximately 100,000 billion cells. Every cell contains about one billion protein molecules. Proteins are used for cell components and as enzymes to facilitate chemical activity.

2. Proteins are directed to the proper locations within cells by an amino acid address system (like a postal code) that is universal in "**yeast, plant, and animal cells.**"

3. The discovery helps explain how the immune system functions and the reason for the onset of several kinds of inherited diseases. In cystic fibrosis, for example, the signal is changed so that some proteins end up in the wrong place. In the immune system, proteins are formed by human cells to block "invader" cell function. Similarly, both bacteria and fungi produce defensive enzymes to protect their territory and counter human enzymes.

4. Blobel's research makes it possible to construct new drugs that are targeted to a particular cell section or component to correct the specific defect. Yeast cells can be modified by genetic engineering into protein factories to produce the desired proteins.

The universal protein address system is shared by "**yeast, plant, and animal cells.**" Microbial cells have sufficient "intelligence" to deliver proteins to the proper parts of their structure and could deliver these proteins to the human cell structure. About forty-five per cent of the human genome is identical to ancestral microbial genes so some of the dormant genes may be capable of forming primitive cell-wall protein called chitin. Microbes have the capacity to produce competitive proteins, deliver them to the proper position in the cell, and block delivery of normal human proteins as well.

The information available on Blobel's discovery does not address the problem of how, when, or why the address system fails. Rather, the information will be used by pharmaceutical companies as an opportunity to engineer new drugs to solve the problem of human degenerative diseases. Here we go again! More drugs.

Why not focus on correcting the address system? What causes it to fail? If yeast cells can be harvested to correct the problem, doesn't it make sense to assume that yeast and fungi in our body can cause the problem? The cure for disease should be not in administering anything to block the symptom or pathway, but in *removal of the cause* from the body. The simple solution is to eliminate the foreign proteins or enzymes by eliminating the fungi and bacteria that produce them. The first step is to do research to find out how the cause can be eliminated. What is the pathway that causes disease?

A path is a route one follows to go from point A to point B. For example, a ladder is a path that one uses to get from level A to level B. A pathway is a mental path that one follows to get from concept A to concept B. If some of the rungs are missing in your ladder, the path is broken, and non-functional. Similarly, if some of the key concepts are missing in your pathway, the theory or statement is non-functional.

When one makes statements such as stress causes cancer, there are a few rungs missing in the pathway. Stress, as a concept, exists only in the mind, much like the concepts of truth and beauty. Cancer, however, is a physical condition. There are too many steps missing between these two points. The same principle applies to saying defective genes or virus cause cancer as well as to saying the breakdown of the immune system causes cancer. The complete pathway should be identified, described clearly, and proven or supported by observations.

Similarly, a statement saying microbes or parasites cause cancer is a pathway with a few rungs missing. Which parasites, which microbes, and which enzymes do they use? How exactly, do they do it? This research fills in most, if not all, of the missing rungs. I don't think it really matters at this time if we know exactly which species of fungi and bacteria cause cancer. Perhaps they all do. Does it really matter, if all of them can be eliminated by the same method? If they can survive as parasites and have genes that produce primitive membrane material such as chitin, then they can mutate a cell wall during assembly. If they can gain a foothold in injured tissue or trapped blood, then they can probably cause cancer.

The metabolic pathway that leads to degenerative diseases such as cancer, inherited diseases and so-called autoimmune diseases is *the replacement of human proteins by fungal proteins in cellular tissue or the lack of human proteins due to nutritional deficiencies.* The cure is to replace the deficiencies, or remove microbes to stop production of foreign proteins. Drugs are not the only answer unless these drugs are antifungal or nutritional. Improved nutrition and parasite cleansing are ultimately the final answer. As far as we know, minerals cannot be made in the body. If we do not correct the essential mineral nutritional deficiencies, and eliminate the bacterial colonies that consume minerals causing additional deficiencies, disease follows.

Replication cycles of DNA in cells is initiated only by the life-force that dominates the cell. In human bodies, replication began with conception, and replication begins to repair damage to cells as soon as injury occurs. The cause of cancer starts with normal mitosis of cells, due to growth or repair, and flows from fungal proteins that mutate the repair process during assembly of the new cells.

If replication for repair or growth occurs *within normal oxygen levels* and cells are not infected, then replication follows a pathway leading to development of two new human cells.

However, if replication takes place in a *low-oxygen environment* with immune suppressed cells infected with fungi or bacteria, the repair process is mutated by fungal and bacterial proteins. These cells gain more characteristics of primitive life forms, the cells are rejected by the body, and repair, or growth, does not take place. The resulting cells become cancer tumors without function for the body and out-of-control growth continues.

If replication occurs *within low oxygen levels*, replication takes place to produce two cells that express genes to maintain the fermentation process. Without sufficient oxygen and energy in the form of ATP, human cells cannot assemble cell-wall components or direct growth. When microbes create a low-oxygen microsphere of a group of cells, they literally take over the cells by controlling energy production. Microbes manage the rapid replication and growth we call cancer. Microbes contaminate human cells with the enzyme DNA polymerase that supports cell division and replication. That's all there is to out-of-control replication. Defective genes or viruses are not involved.

Cancer begins with the invasion of immune suppressed cells by fungal mycelia. Cells that are immune suppressed cannot stop the fungal mycelia from invading the cell. Invasion is the forceful entry of the mycelia through the cell wall. You will recall that fungi thrive on carbon in dead and living cells, and that mycelia invade mucus membranes. Fermentation of trapped blood sugars, in ducts and storage vessels, or connective tissue, enables a mass of mycelia to invade a mass of cells, simultaneously, enabling a cancer tumor to start. Fermentation of blood sugars and proteins produces the toxins that suppress the immune system of adjacent cells allowing fungal mycelia to invade the cells.

Cancer may also start when a group of cells are invaded by fungal mycelia or parasites ingested in food. In 1913, stomach cancers were created in the laboratory by feeding cockroaches infected with parasitic worm larvae to laboratory rats. We will review this in detail later. In cases where apparently healthy people suddenly develop stomach or , it could be caused by parasites in food.

One of my friends died of cancer a few months after having acquired food poisoning from eating fresh imported berries. I wonder how many cases of cancer occur from food poisoning such as this. Presently, it appears that no one compiles and publishes such records. Could it be because such data could establish a definite link between cancer and parasites?

While at a health fair in Toronto, I enjoyed a fresh glass of juice made with tropical fruit made at a booth. Within two hours, I began to experience diarrhea and vomiting. I spent most of the next day in bed hoping to get better. Finally, I decided to take a large dose of the black walnut green-hull tincture used in the parasite cleanse products. Within minutes, I felt a warm feeling throughout my abdomen. It felt like it was glowing with heat. Within four hours, I was back to normal. I believe I destroyed the cause of my food poisoning before the parasite(s) invaded the membrane walls of my digestive tract, so that no long-term damage resulted. Food poisoning should be considered a major cause of cancer.

This experience reinforces what Dr. Clark teaches about the importance of thoroughly washing all fresh fruit and vegetables to remove chemicals and parasites. It also suggests that a purely natural anti-biotic can be made from herbal products such as the American black walnut green hull. These safe products can be taken as a preventative when we consume suspect food, while traveling to foreign countries and eating out.

Fundamentally, cancer is the result of normal cell division misdirected and mutated by microbial enzymes and proteins. Cancer does not modify or mutate DNA, but it does modify the cellular environment resulting in expression of dormant or repressed genes. Cancer modifies the cell-wall membrane and proteins in the cytoplasm of the cell. With each new generation, more and more normal genes are repressed, resulting in a cell with primitive life-form characteristics based on inherited genes.

A description of the cell-wall membrane can be found on the Internet at http://ernie.bgsu.edu/~midden/MITBCT/mem/s The cell-wall membrane is described as an ionic fluid 5 nanometers thick (5 billionths of a meter) "a spherical three-dimensional lipid-bilayer shell around the cell." In other texts, it is called an "ionic sieve" because it lets ions pass in and out like a sieve. It is called a "mosaic" because the cell-wall membrane contains numerous internal and external proteins that determine cell function. Different organs have different proteins and the quantity of receptors changes according to the needs of the cell. Human tissue cells are recognized by the mosaic of proteins in the cell wall; not by the expressed genes. It is easy to visualize how microbial cell components such as chitin can mutate a cell-wall membrane causing it to be rejected by adjacent cells although the DNA in the nucleus is normal.

Have you ever had goose bumps cover your arms due to some exciting moment in your life? I had this delightful experience when I first realized that cancer is a membrane disease and not a defective gene disease. Membranes carry and distribute ionic energy of the autonomic nervous system. There are no physical nerves used by the primitive autonomic nervous system and immune system (except in the balance mechanism of the middle ear). A break in the membrane wall is like a break in a primitive nerve. Ionic energy flows into the injured area, due to a break in the energy meridian. This is how the primitive body identified an injury and made repair of injury an autonomic function. This is also how the autonomic nervous system maintains the immune system defenses. These primal functions were developed in cells long before the first mammal walked upon the earth. They are still in use today as the autonomic system and immune system.

Mammalian cell-wall membranes contain high-energy phosphate groups connected to lipid molecules assembled in rows forming a plasma membrane. This construction allows a membrane flexibility and permeability. Just like DNA nucleotides are connected by deoxyribose-*phosphate,* and RNA is connected by ribose-*phosphate,* epithelial cells are connected by a lipid *phosphate.* If new cell-wall membranes contain chitin molecules, (lacking in phosphate) they will be lacking in the capacity to conduct energy. They fail to sustain the energy meridians. The immune system functions on ionic energy, and any chitin or processed fat in the cell wall will lead to a so-called autoimmune response. The immune system only attacks the cells that have a cell-wall deficiency due to nutritional deficiencies or pollutants.

Two major cancer specialists, who will be quoted later, Dr. Johanna Budwig and Udo Erasmus, describe why they believe that essential fatty acids with intact electrical properties are part of the cure for cancer. A loss of plasma fields disturbs the autonomic nerve system and disrupts communication of cells. I also believe that the lack of essential fatty acids in modern diets is one of the leading causes of cancer.

A hole in the plasma field, or lowered energy capacity, allows the cell to become parasitized. These parasites stop the oxidative process, which leads to a lack of energy for the cell.

Otto Warburg discovered that cancer cells produced energy by fermentation of glucose, and that a 35% reduction in cell respiration of normal embryonic cells would result in normal cells switching from oxidative metabolism to fermentation. For Warburg, the existence of cancer was based on the switch from oxidative glycolysis to fermentation. Microbial infection was not required. Nothing else was needed, except to reduce the oxygen levels so that respiration was reduced by 35%. According to Warburg, cancer occurred automatically, because these cells switched metabolism permanently from oxidative glycolysis to fermentation. According to Warburg, the cause of cancer was reduced respiration of oxygen.

Assuming the laboratory specimens that he used were not infected with microbes, the question then becomes, would these new cells have been rejected if their original purpose was to repair an injury in a membrane. Since they were embryonic cells in glass containers, Warburg would have had no way of knowing if these new cells would knit with normal membrane cells. There would be no way of knowing if these cells also had a mutated cell-wall membrane unless one could graft them to a group of normal membrane cells to observe if they were accepted or rejected. To my knowledge, this test was not done and there was no reason for the cell wall to have mutated during assembly.

Warburg concluded that cells were cancerous based solely on the switch in metabolism. I suggest that this conclusion, if based on in vitro laboratory research, is an error. Research shows that human cells can switch between oxidative metabolism and fermentation simply by expressing dormant genes, without becoming cancer cells. By reducing the oxygen levels, Warburg succeeded in changing the metabolism of cells. However, this method of research does not establish whether these cells would produce mutated cell-wall membranes incapable of repairing an injury.

This issue does not diminish Warburg's cancer research, because the only conditions in the body that will cause normal cells to switch metabolism are created by anaerobic microbes. Just as Warburg reduced respiration of cells by 35 percent mechanically, microbes reduce cell respiration by 35 percent chemically. This process will be discussed later.

Based on the theory that the current of injury causes cells to multiply, and repairing the injury stops cells from multiplying, the concept of destroying all rapidly growing cells with chemotherapy is fundamentally wrong. Stopping all replication and multiplication of all new cells ensures that the injury will not be healed, the current of injury will stay on, and out-of-control replication will continue. Taking toxic drugs to cure cancer is the worst possible treatment because it also destroys the immune system, allowing fungi and bacteria to proliferate as well as destroys essential new cells.

Based on this conclusion, no chemotherapy agents can cure cancer unless they are antifungal and antiparasitic. Amazingly, Dr. Costantini says exactly the same thing, based on his observations of effective cancer treatments. In his book, *Fungalbionics, The Etiology of Cancer,* he writes (Page 13):

> ... the series also documents that each and every dietary measure or drug found to be effective in treating these (degenerative) diseases share nothing in common except that they are all antifungal and/or antimycotoxic.

The word mycotoxin is derived from the Greek word "mkyes', meaning fungus, and "toxicum" meaning toxin or poison.

When you realize that chemotherapy aims to attack the new cells at the DNA level you understand why chemotherapy often fails. The letters ACT designate a base in DNA that specifies an end to a gene. The drug AZT used in treatment for AIDS, was originally designed as a cancer drug. I suspect that the letter Z, being the last letter of the alphabet, was taken to identify AZT as a gene terminator like ACT to stop DNA replication. Any toxic drug used to cure cancer by destroying replication of DNA is based on a false concept. There are no defective genes in the cancer process. Replication of DNA is required to heal the injury.

The effective cancer therapy drugs with a record of success in use today are just expensive antibiotics with horrendous side effects. Three people with leukemia found that their cancer was cured when doctors gave them antifungal drugs to cure their fungal problem. Antifungal herbs and vibrational medicine can do the same thing without side effects. Vibrational medicine uses electronic energy in the form of magnetic fields or electrical wave impulses.

When you realize that the 35 percent difference in respiration between normal cells and cancer cells is significant enough that drugs can be made to kill only the cancer cells, you realize that a magic-bullet cure for cancer is possible. Drugs that reduce respiration of all cells by say 50 percent, causes cancer cells to die from asphyxiation, but normal cells survive. CanCell, the magic bullet for treating cancer, has been suppressed for about 70 years.

When you realize that some bacteria produce enzymes to destroy fungi, you understand why effective vaccines can be made to cure cancer. My research discusses three such vaccines, one of which had better success with cancer patients fifty years ago than does any modern drug or combined treatment in use today. Vaccines are not used to treat cancer (at least publicly) because there is no way to explain how vaccines can cure defective genes.

When you realize that the difference of electromagnetic vibrations between normal cells and cancer cells is significant enough to locate cancer cells by their vibrational imprint on a meter, you understand why cancer can be detected long before tumors form and cancer becomes a death threat. Moreover, cancer cells can be selectively destroyed by appropriate vibrational frequencies that are harmless to normal cells. Cancer responds to electromagnetic therapy that destroys infectious microbes because cells must be infected before they can be made to mutate. We should have a choice between radiation that burns everything, and electromagnetic waves that destroy only cancer cells, but we don't.

When you realize the same hypocrisy that characterizes much of the cancer service industry is evident in other health care services, including heart and stroke problems as well as diabetes, you realize that conventional treatment for cancer is only the tip of the iceberg concerning medical fraud. That is why my thoughts about treatment for these other diseases are included in this research about cancer. The combination shows a pattern of wrong doing throughout the health care industry.

In his texts, Dr. Costantini groups all degenerative diseases, including cancer, as fungal related. The basic cause for all degenerative diseases is mutation of the cell-wall membrane that destroys cell function. Fungi and bacteria are the cause of most degenerative diseases. Hiding this truth from the public is creating a downward spiral in health care and the quality of life for humanity. Most health problems are not gene related; they are cell-wall membrane and function related. The significant difference between cells of one organ and another are in the cell-wall membrane, not the DNA. That is why any sample of DNA from your body or body fluids can be used to identify your body. DNA is not organ specific. Expressed genes are organ specific. Cell-wall membrane and cell components are organ specific and function specific. The primitive autoimmune system and the autonomic bodily functions rely on receptors and healthy plasma levels in cell-wall membranes. Minerals and vitamins forming enzymes and cell-wall membranes are the keys to understanding health and disease.

Skin tissue is a mosaic of attached proteins. For example, growth hormone receptors on the cell wall may or may not be present. Mainstream medicine claims the excessive number of growth receptors on the cell wall, due to defective genes, causes cancer. These defective genes are called HER1 and HER2 (Human Epidermal growth factor Receptors) and BRCA (Breast Cancer genes). I believe the excessive number of growth hormone receptors on the cell wall is a result of cell-wall membrane mutation due to availability of fungal and parasitic growth hormone in the blood stream or from enzymes produced by microbes resident in the cell. Defective genes have nothing to do with breast cancer. Breasts are storage vessels with membranes forming ducts and milk lobes. Cancer occurs in these membrane tissues due to mutation of the cell wall following a break in the membrane.

Researchers such as Dr. Costantini, author of *Fungalbionics*, have assumed that the fungal mycotoxins cause genetic mutations that lead to cancer. They have correctly identified the fungus by name and source, but cannot place all the rungs in the pathway leading to out-of-control replication. They have missed the fact that fungal mycelia invade the cells, cause injury, and the life-force initiates replication through the current of injury. Replication of DNA is a normal process following an injury. In order to find the cause in defective genes, as they were taught in medical classes, they have ignored the cell-wall membrane as a possible cause of cancer. They are looking past the problem without seeing it. Their education is getting in the way of observation and creative analysis.

With the mutated cell-wall membrane cause-of-cancer theory, all of the rungs are in place. Incorporation of primitive cell-wall chitin from fungi, like the skin of a mushroom, into human cell-wall membranes causes cancer. There is no need to look for a pathway in which mycotoxins, chemical toxins or virus cause defective genes, because defective genes are not involved. There is no need to assume defective genes cause excessive growth factor receptors on the cell wall. The mind can go from point A, a healthy cell, to point B, a cancer cell, with all rungs in place.

Cancer can be considered as a condition of molecule and nucleotide distribution errors in the cell-wall membrane due to infection. There are two ways to correct the problem.

1. Harvest protein molecules from yeast to produce costly drugs to block the receptor points or to supply the correct protein. This is the suggested value of Blobel's research discussed earlier.

2. Eliminate the microbes that produce enzymes and proteins that in turn disrupt the system and cause protein distribution errors. These

two approaches identify the essential difference between allopathic medicine based on use of pharmaceuticals, and alternative medicine, based on the use of natural health products and metabolic therapies.

We can control microbial enzyme production in our body through proper nutrition, effective metabolism, and cleansing our bodies of parasites. The first key to understanding cancer lies in recognizing that some of the enzymes for oxidative metabolism are interchangeable with enzymes for fermentation. That's why normal cells can switch to cancer cells and back to normal again and why microbial enzymes can take control of cellular metabolism. That's why a healthy immune system fails to recognize cancer cells as invaders and the first sign of cancer is often a large growth. The mutated cell-wall membranes are accepted by the immune system as self, allowing microbes to proliferate inside the tumor.

Let's now review important data on these enzymes that assist replication of DNA.

One billion years of replication with DNA polymerase

Doctors Varmus and Weinberg, describe how enzymes control normal growth and replication. As you read this passage, mentally substitute microbial enzymes for human enzymes, and you have the cancer process explained in full. The following reference can be found in the text *Genes and the Biology of Cancer,* (Page 16). *(My emphasis added in bold, explanation in italics.)*

How does a cell manage to choreograph these steps *[mitosis understood]* in precise order? Studies of a wide range of eukaryotic organisms *(having membrane-bound structures within the cell wall)* including yeast, clams, frogs, and mammals reveal a remarkably similar plan, executed by modular **components that experimenters can swap between organisms whose common ancestors existed more than a billion years ago. The exchangeability of parts shows that a master clocking mechanism governing the cell cycle developed long ago and has been preserved with great fidelity in all descendant organisms over a million millennia.**

In this plan, complex events like DNA replication and chromosomal segregation are triggered by centralized chemical regulators that are able to recruit the many components required for S and M phases. *(Please note this fundamental error claiming DNA replication is triggered by catalytic enzymes.)*

[Note: S and M phases are stages in replication of chromosomes. S for **synthesis** *refers to the 8-to10 hour period of synthetic activity when*

*DNA nucleotides or bases are formed from the base of free nucleotides in the cell. M refers to the stage of **mitosis** wherein the chromosomes divide and form two identical chromosomes by reorganizing the nucleotides assembled in the S phase]*

Each of these master regulators is now known to be an enzyme that can efficiently modify a wide range of proteins. These cell cycle regulators, like many other influential proteins to be described in this book, are protein kinases, enzymes designed to transfer phosphate groups from ATP *(adenosine triphosphate)* molecules *(the cellular energy source)* to specific amino acids in certain target proteins. The result of this phosphorlation process—the presence of a newly attached phosphate group—causes the target protein to gain or lose a function: to assemble or dissemble in the case of a structure-building molecule; to turn a biochemical reaction on or off in the case of a catalytic enzyme. Because each kinase may modify a variety of proteins, it can elicit a wide range of responses in the cell simultaneously.

The significant point in the above quotation is that enzymes that control replication can be swapped among "descendant organisms" that have existed for a billion years. This means that the enzyme that assists division and assembly on new cells can come from any "descendant" source that includes yeast, fungi, or bacteria. In the case of cancer, the enzyme does not have to come from human cells with defective genes. It follows that there is no requirement for defective genes in the cancer process. In addition, the proteins in the mosaic of the cell-wall membrane can be swapped from any life form. Cell-wall material called chitin can be swapped for phospho-lipid cell membrane material. The protein carrier delivers either one.

Only living things can deliver the products that can be swapped. Chemicals, toxins, pollutants, virus, fat, and injury cannot do so. It takes a living organism with DNA to transcribe DNA polymerase from genes. That is why only living things like microbes are capable of redirecting replication of human cells, modifying cell-wall membranes, and why life does not occur spontaneously from a batch of nucleotides. Living things are dependent on the energy bonds between phosphorus and oxygen. Increasing or reducing oxygen levels produces a corresponding increase or decrease in human energy. Utilizing energy or storing energy in phosphate bonds is called *phosphorylation.*

Note the statement: *"The result of this phosphorlation process—the presence of a newly attached phosphate group—causes the target protein to gain or lose a function...."* That's exactly what causes cancer. The lack of phosphate groups in the cell wall membrane due to the insertion of chitin cause replacement cells to be rejected in membranes or non-functional in leukemia, and liver cells. Without the normal phosphate molecule, cell-wall membranes are non-functional, deficient, and rejected. It is difficult to identify some cancer cells because the difference may be based on energy levels in the cell-wall membrane.

In the text *Biology, An Appreciation of Life,* we learn about three types of metabolism resulting in phosphorylation (Page 67):

In present-day living organisms, ATP (*adenosine tri-phosphate)* is formed as the result of three major metabolic processes. First, in organisms that live in oxygen-free environments, glucose is partially broken down in a process called *substrate-level phosphorylation.* Small amounts of ATP are formed, which are sufficient to support life. Secondly, in creatures able to carry out photosynthesis, light energy is used to convert ADP (adenosine diphosphate) to ATP by the addition of a phosphate group. This process is called photosynthetic phosphorylation. **Thirdly, in plant and animal organisms that live and thrive in an oxygen-containing environment, substrate-level phosphorylation is linked to oxidative phosphorylation. In this process oxygen is used and large amounts of ATP are produced.**

Allow me to rephrase this vital statement that explains the cancer process in human cells: *animal organisms that live and thrive in an oxygen-containing environment, link substrate-level phosphorylation to oxidative phosphorylation.* This means oxidative metabolism starts out the same as fermentation. The two processes are linked. When oxidative phosphorylation is stopped, the more primitive *substrate-level phosphorylation* process continues. That is all there is to normal cells switching and thriving as cancer cells. Defective genes are not involved.

Cancer is an ongoing battle within your body with human enzymes pitted against microbial enzymes. Your lifestyle and nutritional habits establish which side wins.

Ultimately, you are responsible for your cancer by failing to maintain control of parasites and effective respiration of your cells. Doctors, drugs or alternative therapies cannot stop cancer permanently if you continue to maintain the lifestyle that caused cancer in the first place. Surgery treats cancer by removing the tumor and the vessel capable of holding trapped blood sugars and proteins. You could also treat cancer by eliminating the cause while saving the vessel.

Maintaining conditions for oxidative metabolism of food nutrients is the key to preventing fermentation and cancer. Vital minerals and enzymes are required to function as *substrates* in order to complete breakdown of large molecules.

The meaning of 'substrate' in metabolism

Let's take a deeper look into the important function of substrates. In the digestion and assimilation of nutrients, chemical bonds in carbohydrates can be broken apart by removing hydrogen ions. However, a method is needed to keep the active hydrogen ions from recombining with each other or with other atoms. Special enzymes produced by the cell are required for this function and a *substrate* is needed to combine safely with hydrogen.

What is a substrate? Perhaps an analogy more specific than a blotter, as used in the introduction, would help clarify the concept of substrates. Imagine having a task in which you must remove a group of small magnets that have clumped together inside a bottle. The group of magnets is too large to pass through the neck of the bottle although small groups could get through. You must separate the magnets in order to remove them. As you pull magnets apart (with a suitable tool) within the limited space available within the bottle, they snap back together in another position due to magnetic attraction. Since space is limited, you can never achieve separation of the magnets and you cannot remove them from the bottle.

Suppose you introduce a strip of steel into the jar and position the magnets on it one by one as you pull them apart. The magnets would stay where you placed them. Your problem would be solved because you could stop the magnets from joining back together.

Your strip of steel would function much like a "substrate" does in metabolism. In metabolism, large molecules are broken down by removing hydrogen atoms from the molecule. Oxygen serves as a substrate in metabolism because two hydrogen ions can be chemically bonded to oxygen. Removal of the hydrogen ions separates phosphate molecules from carbohydrates allowing the production of ATP (adenosine triphosphate). Hydrogen atoms are controlled by an enzyme called *l-glutamate dehydrogenase*. *L-glutamate* is the protein portion (an amino acid) that serves as the postal-code for distribution. *De-hydrogen-ase* is the active enzyme portion that bonds with hydrogen and removes it from a molecule.

In later chapters, we will learn how **the loss of this enzyme function due to ammonia toxicity, shuts down the citric acid cycle in cells causing a cell to switch from aerobic metabolism to fermentation.**

Fungi consume only carbon in dead and living things, leaving nitrogen as a waste product. Nitrogen from protein serves as a substrate for fermentation in cancer cells because three hydrogen ions can be chemically bonded to a nitrogen atom to form ammonia (NH_3). Production of energy without oxygen requires enzymes that are different from those used for production of energy with oxygen. That is what is meant when it is said that a cell switches from the oxidative process to the fermentative process. The cell simply switches production of enzymes to suit the environment of the cell and adjusts to reduced oxygen levels.

Variations in acidity, and concentration of oxygen or carbon dioxide, are sensed by the DNA regulatory genes. Therefore, the DNA expresses genes to transcribe functional enzymes for the immediate needs of the cell. Fermentation starts the process. If oxygen is available, the oxidative process is linked to the fermentative process. If oxygen is not available, fermentation continues.

It is believed that enzymes function by serving as substrates to catalyze all chemical actions in living things. Complex multi-level pathways are used to break down large proteins and assemble new ones. Production of energy with oxygen as a substrate requires a series of steps called the citric acid cycle. Before cancer can spread, the oxidative process in adjacent cells must be stopped and oxygen levels reduced. The production of ammonia in cancer tumors serves to stop the oxidative process in adjacent cells.

Ammonia spreads to adjacent cells and shuts down the citric acid cycle by filling the capacity of oxidative enzymes to take on more hydrogen atoms. Cancer spreads, as a disease where microbes infect adjacent cells after ammonia interrupts the citric acid cycle and causes the cell to switch from oxidation to fermentation. Ammonia toxicity leads to loss of ATP, immune system dysfunction, infection, and cancer.

When oxygen is used as a substrate, two hydrogen atoms are combined with oxygen to make H_2O or water. This pure water formed inside the cell is used in other metabolic processes. Any excess flows out of the cell and transports waste to the kidneys. Exercise causes us to perspire, which is the result of excess water being produced inside cells. That is why an exercise level that achieves perspiration is so valuable and beneficial to health. Perspiration cleanses the cells of toxins and pollutants. That's why we must drink plenty of water and exercise regularly to stay healthy. A significant reason for the explosion in the frequency of cancer is due to the ease of modern living. We don't 'sweat it' often enough.

In a cancer cell, three atoms of hydrogen are combined with nitrogen to make NH_3 or ammonia. At body temperature, ammonia is a gas. Ammonia combines with water to form ammonium (NH_4) and circulates in lymphatic fluids and venous blood. The liver converts ammonia to urea but the process is limited by the loss of arginine and other essential amino acids—which incidentally are banned for sale as food supplements in Canada. Cancer is associated with liver dysfunction largely because ammonia cannot be expelled as fast as it is produced.

When fungi in cancer tumors consume protein, they use the carbon for energy and expel the nitrogen and hydrogen as ammonia. That is why cancer tumors become prolific users of protein, invade and mutate adjacent cells, and produce ammonia that enables cancer to spread throughout the body.

Anaerobic parasites cannot make enzymes to use oxygen

Microbes that cannot survive in oxygen are called obligatory anaerobes. *Obligatory* comes from a Latin word as used in obliged. *Anaerobes* is a word formed by combining the word anaerobic with microbes. *Obligatory anaerobes* cannot use oxygen because their genetic structure cannot produce the enzymes needed for oxidative glycolysis. Metabolism by obligatory anaerobes always results in production of lactate acid and ammonia as waste products. Anaerobic metabolism is fermentation. Waste products from anaerobic glycolysis lead to the spread of cancer and death of the person. Cancer is produced only by anaerobic parasites.

Obligatory anaerobes are destroyed by oxygen because they cannot produce enzymes to defend themselves from oxygen. That is why cancer can be cured by oxygen and ozone therapy.

Cancer cells ferment glycogen and produce lactate as a waste product, making cancer cells essentially the same as primitive anaerobic life forms that rely on fermentation of carbohydrates for energy. Carbohydrates convert to glucose and proteins contain a carbohydrate base. Proteins are carbohydrate molecules connected to nitrogen containing molecules. Proteins are subject to fermentation after the nitrogen molecules are removed as ammonia.

Genes dictate the capacity of our cells to produce enzymes because the enzymes are coded in the genetic structure and are transcribed from expressed genes to create the enzyme. Enzymes are assembled in the cytoplasm and mitochondria where the chemical actions take place to produce energy. Mitochondria are structures within cells that release energy from glycogen.

In the text, *Biology: An Appreciation of Life* we learn that mitochondria may actually be a form of bacteria (Page 107).

The evolutionary origin of mitochondria is controversial. They have about the same dimensions as bacteria; the functions of their membranes are similar to the energy-transforming functions of bacterial cell membranes; as self-reproducing bodies, they contain their own DNA, RNA, and ribosomes—all of which suggests they may represent symbiotic procaryotic microorganisms. *(Note: procaryotic means lacking a nucleus for the DNA structure. Symbiotic refers to a theory that traces the cellular ancestry of modern organisms to more than one ancient organism.)*

The fact that mitochondria contain their own special RNA and DNA supports the theory that human cells have evolved from an anaerobic life form as well as from an aerobic life form. Mitochondria produce enzymes that link the fermentative process to the oxidative process because they convert glycogen into energy with or without oxygen.

In summary, heredity and cellular environment dictate the type of genes that are available for the production of enzymes. Active genes are said to be **expressed**; inactive genes are said to be **repressed** or **dormant.** Genes come in groups called chromosomes. Human chromosomes have expressed genes for production of **enzymes for oxidation** of glycogen. In the presence of oxygen, these genes are always expressed. According to Dr. Warburg, the complete oxidation of glycogen requires about 30 different enzymes. This process is referred to as the citric acid cycle, or Krebs cycle.

The citric acid cycle can only occur within a cell, whereas fermentation can occur in the lymphatic system or in storage vessels and ducts. Fermentation occurs wherever fungi can feed on carbon in trapped blood sugars or proteins. Trapped blood in storage vessels and ducts leads to fermentation. The fungal process helps cleanse the body of dead tissue and pollutants. Normally, the process stops as soon as the nutrient base is depleted. Oxygen and amino acids serve to eliminate the waste products from fermentation before they accumulate enough to stop the citric acid cycle or damage adjacent cells. That is why cancer cannot start from the mutation of a single cell. A large number of cells, sufficient to support a colony of fungi are required.

Arginine is an amino acid that helps convert ammonia to urea for elimination from the body. Arginine supplements have been shown to prevent cancer. Ammonia toxicity drives the cancer process. Arginine is a cancer fighting amino acid banned for sale in Canada by an aggressive cancer industry.

There are two faces to the business of cancer care. One is the noble and valuable career of serving the public with treatments, which I refer to as the cancer service industry.

The other is the business goal to maximize profits, which I refer to as the cancer industry. An industry is a business run for profit. Suppression of competition is a common industrial practice and appears to be the only reason why some cancer cures are suppressed.

The enzyme *nicotinamide used to transfer hydrogen ions* is used in the first step of the fermentation process as well as in the first step of the oxidation process. An amide is a compound having a carbon-nitrogen group with oxygen joined in an unstable, double bond. Nicotinamide links the two metabolic processes as a substrate. When the citric acid cycle is stopped within a cell, due to lack of oxygen or lack of other enzymes required in the citric acid cycle, metabolism switches automatically to fermentation because nicotinamide is always present.

When the cell receives more oxygen or the oxidative enzymes are replaced, oxidation takes over and the cell returns to normal. Cancer cells do not have to be destroyed or removed to cure cancer. Cancer cells can be switched back to normal cells by changing the environment of the cell and establishing oxidative metabolism. This change can only occur after fungi and bacteria life forms are eliminated. Several generations with free oxygen may be required to return cancer cells to normal so that the microbial membrane component can be eliminated from the cell-wall membrane.

Let's now review some medical references to help verify and explain the above description of the cancer process.

Human cells have capacity for metabolism with or without oxygen

In Dr. Arthur Guyton's *Textbook of Medical Physiology*, we have a clear explanation of how human cells can switch energy production from aerobic to anaerobic glycolysis.

Dr. Guyton's textbook is available in seven languages and is used in medical universities around the world. Therefore, this medical knowledge is shared by the majority of medical doctors around the world. If Dr. Guyton makes a mistake, the entire medical universe makes a mistake. For example, in his text, the cause of ulcers was attributed to stress and too much acidity. That was an error accepted by all mainstream medicine. It is now known that bacteria cause ulcers.

Fortunately, he has not made many mistakes. He writes (Page 845):

> Occasionally, oxygen becomes either unavailable or insufficient so that oxidative phosphorlation cannot take place. Yet, even under these conditions, a small amount of energy can still be released to

the cells by glycolysis, for the chemical reactions in the glycolytic breakdown of glucose to pyruvic acid do not require oxygen. Unfortunately, this process is extremely wasteful of glucose because only 16,000 calories of energy are used to form ATP for each molecule of glucose utilized, which represents only a little over 2 per cent of the total energy in the glucose molecule. Nevertheless, this release of glycolytic energy to the cell can be a lifesaving measure for a few minutes when oxygen becomes unavailable.

Isn't that amazing? Only two per cent of the energy available in glucose is released through anaerobic metabolism. That leaves 98 per cent of the energy available for fungal metabolism, production of chitin, growth, and production of pollutants to inhibit oxygen from reaching the adjacent cells. Ammonia and carbon dioxide produced by fermentation play major roles in the cancer process.

Fermentation of trapped blood sugars in the lymphatic system, ducts, or vessels is the first step in the cancer process because fermentation pollutes the adjacent environment. When cells are deprived of oxygen, they switch to anaerobic metabolism, without any need for defective genes. That is why the immune system does not recognize early stage cancer cells as invaders. They are not foreign invaders or different from other cells.

Normal respiration is the process of breathing in oxygen and breathing out carbon dioxide. At the cellular level, normal respiration is the process of absorbing oxygen through the cell wall and expelling carbon dioxide. Otto Warburg established that all cancer cells have impaired respiration. He found that if he reduced respiration by 35%, cancer would develop. In other words, fermentation starts when respiration is impaired by 35%.

It is generally accepted that we do not have primary cancers developing in the heart, arteries, or veins. There are two main reasons. Fermentation cannot occur in flowing blood with high levels of oxygen, and the heart muscles are highly capable of rapidly converting lactic acid, a by-product of exercise and fermentation, into energy. Dr. Guyton writes (Page 846):

Use of lactic acid by the heart for energy

The heart muscle is especially capable of converting lactic acid to pyruvic acid and then utilizing this for energy. This occurs especially in heavy exercise, during which large amounts of lactic acid are released into the blood from the skeletal muscles.

Scientific basis for cancer lies in metabolism

We have the scientific basis for understanding cancer when we recognize that mammalian tissue cells have inherited both aerobic and anaerobic enzyme production capacities and can metabolize glycogen either aerobically or anaerobically because of inherited traits. Cancer is caused by the cellular environment. Genetic defects do not create the capacity for human cells to metabolize nutrients without oxygen. Limiting the oxygen supply or disrupting the citric acid cycle leads to fermentation. The capacity to ferment nutrients for energy has been inherited and is common to all energy-producing cells.

When we cut ourselves, we bleed externally (as opposed to internal bleeding). Normally, the blood clots and bleeding stops. If we take care to avoid infection, a scab will form, and the injury will heal. If infection occurs, it doesn't heal. Essentially the same process, occurring inside our body results in cancer.

Following internal bleeding, the blood clot is trapped and unable to return to the veins for a fresh supply of oxygen. The blood clot and the damaged cells with severed veins, arteries, and lymphatic drainage are no longer oxidized. Oxidative processes stop and fermentation begins. Simultaneously, the body produces a current of injury that causes adjacent cells to divide and heal the injury. With fermentation, 98% of the available energy is maintained by the cells for new growth. Fermentation of glucose in blood clots, after an injury, serves as the mechanism for repair and renewal. Cancer does not occur following all injuries because all cells are not infected with microbes.

As soon as oxygen reaches the cells, the citric acid cycle can be re-established, fermentation stops, and microbial life destroyed. The complete repair process is driven by the cellular environment and responses to electrical and chemical stimulants. Genes do not make the decision to replicate. Replication occurs by default if energy meridians carrying the current of injury are broken by membrane damage. Replication stops as soon as the energy meridians are reconnected. **Cancer occurs in membranes because cancer requires a large number of cells, replicating simultaneously to start a cancer tumor. Membrane integrity is vital to life, so membranes receive an extensive current of injury to replicate a large number of cells simultaneously.**

When we supply more oxygen to the cells, fermentation ceases and oxidative glycolysis takes over, thereby reversing the fermentation process and reducing the capacity of microbial enzymes to control cellular replication cycles. Cancer can be cured by increasing the oxygen levels of the cells. Cancers have been cured by taking amino acids that convert ammonia to urea and revive the citric acid cycle. Cancer cannot exist in cells where the oxidative process can function. There are many simple ways to cure cancer. Reviving the oxidative process or stopping the fermentative process is the basis for these cures. All cancer cures based on oxygen illustrate that cancer cells are mutated by anaerobic bacteria or fungi. Otherwise, oxygen would not harm them.

Destroying the source of microbial enzymes and toxins is the only way to permanently cure cancer. Any drug, herb, or process that eliminates fungi and toxins can be used to cure cancer. We do not need radiation, toxic drugs with horrific side effects or surgery if tumors are not life threatening.

Does all this seem too simple to be true? Have we donated billions of dollars to finding the genetic cause of cancer even though defective genes are not the cause of cancer? I believe we have. Have we also destroyed millions of lives, disrupted families, and caused the loss of loved ones? I believe we have.

Oxygen supply controls metabolism and cancer

On June 30, 1966, at a meeting of Nobel-Laureates at Lindau, Lake Constance, Germany, Dr. Warburg gave a series of lectures on the "Prime Cause and Prevention of Cancer" *(See www.o3zone.com)*. In this lecture, he established the simple and irrefutable proof that cancer is only a switch in metabolism due to oxygen levels in the cell. In this experiment, he starts out with embryonic cells in a growth media. The embryonic cells do not require an additional source of DNA polymerase or a current of injury to initiate DNA replication. In this experiment, by reducing the oxygen levels, Dr. Warburg created a low oxygen microsphere for these cells. His mechanical control of oxygen levels corresponded to the function of fungal mycotoxins produced by fermentation. The reduced oxygen level leads to fermentation of glucose, increased rate of replication, and cancer.

Dr. Warburg gave humanity a simple method to avoid and cure cancer by using oxygen to stop fermentation. In a speech he gave to the cancer establishment he said as follows:

> If one puts embryonic mouse cells into a suitable culture medium saturated with physiological oxygen pressures, they will grow outside the mouse body, in vitro, and indeed as pure aerobes, with pure oxygen respiration, without a trace of fermentation. However, if during the growth one provides an oxygen pressure so reduced that the oxygen respiration is partially inhibited, the purely aerobic metabolism of the mouse embryonic cells is quantitatively

altered within 48 hours, in the course of two cell divisions, into the metabolism characteristic of fermenting cancer cells.

Later in the speech, he made it clear that cancer cells require some oxygen in order to function. This reference appears as a note following his speech.

These experiments show that it is more correct to designate tumor cells as "partial anaerobes" rather than "facultative anaerobes." A body cell is transformed into a tumor cell if only a part of the respiration is replaced by fermentation.

The fact that cancer cells are partial anaerobes provides a cure for cancer. One of the most amazing cures for cancer is based on this feature of cancer cells. By further reducing the respiration of cancer cells, cancer growth is stopped. Since cancer cells use different enzymes and oxygen levels than normal cells, cancer cell respiration can be specifically targeted and stopped. The important enzyme discovered by Warburg called nicotinamide provides the oxygen microbes use to produce ATP for their needs. CanCell, as already mentioned, probably disturbs this enzyme and reduces cancer cell respiration causing cancer cells to die. Perhaps other formulas could be developed to achieve the same thing.

CanCell illustrates that effective cancer cures are possible but are suppressed. CanCell has been suppressed for about seventy years. More details will be presented in the chapter on suppressed cancer cures.

The English edition of Dr. Warburg's speech is attributed to Dean Burk of the National Cancer Institute, Bethesda, Maryland, U.S.A. There is no doubt in my mind that the cancer establishment has known about the true cause of cancer since at least 1966. If oxygen levels are reduced and maintained at a low level for a period of two cell divisions, the embryonic mouse cells develop the "metabolic characteristics of fermenting cancer cells." Without microbial infection, these cells would not produce chitin to mutate cell walls until after dormant genes are expressed for this purpose.

There is nothing in mainstream medicine to prove this research is false and that the true cause of cancer is to be found elsewhere. Indeed, just the opposite is true. Instead of researching the capacity of increased oxygen or ozone, for example, to cure cancer, ozone therapy is banned in North America.

Two generations of mutation leads to fermenting cancer cells because genes expressed for producing enzymes to use oxygen are no longer expressed. Consequently, Dr. Warburg concluded that cancer cells couldn't be returned to normal cells. More recent experiments with salamanders have shown that tumor cells will return to normal cells if the primary tumor is removed.

Similarly, women who have cured themselves of breast cancer by using essiac have observed tumors shrink and disappear. Surgery of tumors is not compulsory to cure cancer.

Dr. Guyton has devoted Chapter 67 of the *Textbook of Medical Physiology* to *Metabolism and Temperature Regulation*. The following statement describes how easily cells switch from one form of metabolism to the other. The reference to NADH and H+ identifies molecules called *nicotinamide adenine dinucleotide* derived from niacin and used as a substrate for hydrogen atoms in the oxidative citric acid cycle. On page 845 and 846 on *Anaerobic Glycolysis* we read:

> When a person **begins to breathe oxygen again after a period of anaerobic metabolism,** the extra NADH and H+ as well as the extra pyruvic acid that have built up in the body fluids are rapidly oxidized, thereby greatly reducing their concentrations. As a result, the chemical reaction for formation of lactic acid immediately reverses itself, the lactic acid once again becoming pyruvic acid. Large portions of this are immediately utilized by the citric acid cycle to provide additional oxidative energy, and large quantities of ATP are formed. This excess ATP then causes as much as three-fourths of the remaining excess pyruvic acid to be converted back into glucose.

Saying, *"when a person begins to breathe oxygen again"* is the same as saying, "when a cell receives oxygen again" because the events that follow occur within cells. Switching back and forth between oxygenation and fermentation is a perfectly normal function. Some of the enzymes that support oxidation will also support fermentation. The oxidative process supports animal life and enzyme production; the fermentation process supports microbial life and enzyme production. If the cell does not receive oxygen, the fermentation process continues indefinitely resulting in microbial enzymes taking control of replication cycles. Continued fermentation results in cancer through the process of infection followed by mitosis.

Cancer can be considered a metabolic disease because the switch in metabolic processes from oxidative metabolism to fermentation allows microbes to thrive and deprives the human immune system of ATP. Without ATP and oxygen, human cells cannot assemble cell-wall components, defensive enzymes, or produce hydrogen peroxide to destroy anaerobic life forms, thereby allowing anaerobic microbes to proliferate.

Alternately, cancer can also be considered a parasitic disease because parasites thriving in ducts and storage areas damage the cell walls, thereby allowing internal bleeding or lymphatic fluid seepage to occur. Bleeding into ducts and liquid storage vessels leads to trapped blood sugars and proteins in quantities sufficient to cause a microsphere of fermentative cells. The process is similar to repair of damaged skin tissue below a scab and is perfectly normal. The problem of out-of-control replication (cancer) only occurs when microbes take over the general area and exclude oxygen from getting into the new growth and thereby direct new-cell growth towards a non-knitting single-celled or primitive chitin cell-wall membrane. Benign growths of infected cells that are ruptured become cancer growths due to an increase in the current of injury.

The direct relationship between cancer and tissue damage in storage vessels and ducts is obvious in the description of many cancer-causing conditions. Let's look at several examples.

Fermentation within ducts and vessels starts the cancer process

There is a common denominator to most cancers. Epithelial tissue, infected with microbes, and damaged sufficiently to allow internal bleeding, creates a sphere of influence that converts a fairly large mass of cells into cancer cells. The following references can be found alphabetically by type of cancer in *Everyone's Guide to Cancer Therapy. (Italics are mine and have been added for emphasis.)*

1. In the section on bile duct cancer we find typical medical descriptions such as the following: "people with chronic inflammatory processes, such as *ulcerative colitis* or *parasitic infections* of the bile ducts, are at higher risk for developing this cancer."

2. On breast cancer we read: *"lobular cancers start in the many small sacs* in the breasts that produce milk. The much more common *ductal cancers start in the tubes that carry milk* from the lobules to the nipple."

3. On colon cancer, which accounts for 13% of cancers, we read: "About *90% of colorectal cancers are thought to arise from these polyps"* —(mushroom-like growths protruding from the inner layer of the colon or rectum).

4. On bladder cancer, we read: "*chronic bladder infections*…can cause cell changes that may turn into cancer."

5. On childhood brain tumors we read: "About half the brain tumors in children occur below the tentorium, most being in the cerebellum or *the nearby cavity* called the fourth ventricle. "

6. On cervical cancer we read: "Over 90% of cervical *carcinomas start in the surface cells lining the cervix* and are called squamous cell carcinoma."

It soon becomes obvious that the great majority of cancers start where a significant amount of fermentable products become trapped in a storage vessel or ducts and ferment. Others start in membrane tissue consisting of several layers of cells. It takes a large number of cells, multiplying simultaneously to start a cancer tumor.

The fact that cancer is known to spread by cancer cells breaking off from the tumor and drifting in the bloodstream or lymphatic system arises because cancer cells do not knit together to form membrane tissue.

Cancer can also start within a group of damaged bone cells or connective tissue (*a sarcoma*) due to trapped blood. Bones contain mast cells that produce new red and white blood cells. That's why bone marrow transplants serve as a cancer treatment. Why not just destroy the fungus and bacteria that are infecting the cells and mutating the cell-wall membrane during mitosis? Wouldn't that be less painful and costly?

After a physical injury, blood can flow into cartilage tissue and start to ferment just as it would in a storage vessel or duct. Fermentation of blood in connective tissue can lead to cancer of connective tissue, known medically as a sarcoma

Skin cells contain oil and sweat glands with ducts leading to the surface. Skin cancer can start in these storage vessels and ducts. Sunburn and excess ultra-violet rays can damage skin tissue leading to loss of function. Kaposi's sarcoma with blotches of blue and red nodules produced in skin sweat glands and ducts illustrates how skin cancer grows within skin storage vessels and ducts.

Fermentation controlled by fungal enzyme results in growth of mycelia. Mycelia (root-like structures) of fungi grow in storage vessels or along ducts and cavities and invade cells. Mycelia penetrate epithelial cell walls, invade the cell and bring ready-to-use DNA nucleotides into the cell. Fungal mycelia become the source of nucleotides or DNA bases required for DNA replication. Without fungal mycelia producing this 'yeast artificial chromosome', growth of cancer cells would not be as rapid.

In Canada and USA, the frequency of occurrence of types of cancer, in descending order, is lung, colon, breast, and prostate. The overall size of these organs and capacity to trap blood sugars and proteins, in descending order, is also lung, colon, breast and prostrate. The close correspondence is not coincidental.

Large masses of muscle tissue as in the legs, buttocks and thighs, or fat around the waist and hips do not initiate cancer often, if at all. The limited frequency of primary cancer in these areas can be explained by the fact that there is a corresponding limited opportunity for blood sugars to become trapped in fat or active muscle tissue. In addition, no parasites produce growth factors for fat or human muscle tissue and bone. Without these contaminants, cancer cannot occur. I believe all human cancers are directly related to injury of epithelial tissue even though mainstream medicine admits up to 96% occur in these tissues.

Up to 96% of cancers occur in lymphatic, ductal or storage vessel tissue.

According to medical data, up to 96% of cancers occur in epithelial or skin tissue. Cancer of epithelial cells is called a 'carcinoma' and carcinomas can occur anywhere in the body, as all organs have membrane tissue and are nourished by the arterial and lymphatic system.

According to mainstream medicine, cancer occurs most frequently in epithelial membrane walls because the DNA in these cells replicate the most often and are therefore the most susceptible to error during replication. Dr. Joseph Levine and author David Suzuki summarize this concept in the text *The Secrets of Life* (Page 93):

> But some cells keep growing and dividing throughout life, including one large and important class of cells that form both the skin that covers our bodies and the lining of many internal organs, including the colon, uterus, lungs, and milk ducts in the breast. These are called epithelial cells, and the tissues they make are called either epithelium or epidermis. The fact that some of them keep growing throughout life is of special interest, because from them spring the vast majority of human cancers—up to 96 per cent, according to some estimates. Several other type cells keep growing during adult life; these too, are candidates to become cancerous. Two prominent examples are stem cells in the bone marrow that churn out blood cells throughout life and liver cells.

The error in conventional thinking on epithelial cancer

The medical explanation for the abundance of epithelial cancers is that skin tissue cells are continually being replaced and hence are more subject to defective replication. Cells go through various stages of growth and cells *'differentiate'* into specific types of cells with specific functions. The problem with the defective-replication concept is that the vast majority of these epithelial cancer-cells are identifiable because of recognizable cell traits by the time cancer forms.

Cells with normal specialized traits are said to be *differentiated*. If cells are normal in function and appearance, cancer occurred after replication and differentiation. If defects occurred during replication, cells would appear bizarre or embryonic and not similar to corresponding tissue cells. Membrane cells would not have knitted to form a membrane if they were already mutated. The inability of cancer cells to knit with human cells is the major significant difference in structure between normal cells and cancer cells. The error only occurs during mitosis due to infection of the cell.

The theory that defective genes cause cancer during replication cannot be mathematically or scientifically correct if 96% of cancers start in cells that are functionally normal and formed normal membrane tissue. There were no defects in the genes during replication. Defects occurred after replication of DNA but during assembly of the cell-wall membrane.

Skin tissue cells in surrounding muscles should experience the same frequency of cancer as any other rapidly replicating tissues. Obviously, that is not the case. Microbes do not produce these contaminants in muscle tissue and storage areas are not available.

In the introduction, I requested that you compare the logic of the medical dogma to the research being presented. The microbial-cause-of-cancer theory says that parasites damage membrane tissue that form cavities and ducts within the body. Tissue damage leads to bleeding with trapped blood proteins and sugars, thereby allowing fermentation to occur. The current of injury initiates replication of cells through ionic-field energy. Fermentation leads to cancer of adjacent cells and this explains why up to 96% of cancers occur in epithelial cells. That's why women have three types of breast cancer: ductal, lobular and outer skin. There are epithelial cells forming the lobular cavities, milk ducts, and outer skin. Storage areas and ducts do not receive sufficient oxygen to stop fermentation should internal bleeding occur. Breast cancer in men is very rare because milk lobes and ducts do not develop to trap blood proteins.

Can you think of anything you know about cancer that cannot be explained by the theory that *'replication of infected cells causes cancer*? There are many references in books that support the theory.

Author and speaker Jan De Vries in his book *Cancer and Leukemia* confirms how cancer spreads or *metastasizes* in the body due to trapped blood sugars (Page 20) *(Emphasis added.)*:

> *Metastasis* or a secondary cancer is formed of cells out of the primary growths, detaching and grouping together elsewhere in the

body. **The circulating cancer cells do not survive.** For such cells to establish a secondary growth, contact with tissue is necessary in a location which is favorable and, for example, **a blocked vessel, a stationary blood clot or a trauma somewhere provides a perfect place for them to settle.**

We can explain all the mysteries about cancer by reference to natural phenomenon. We do not experience cancer of the heart, arteries or veins, and cancer cells do not survive in the blood stream because there is too much oxygen and too rapid a rate of blood flow. Blood clots, stationary blood and trapped blood sugars are essential for cancer to start. Cancer cells do not knit to one another nor do they knit to normal human cells. That's why they metastasize so readily. The toxins that cause cancer can also flow in the lymphatic system and start cancer in other areas where they can collect as in lymphatic nodes, and start the cancer process. That is why cancers spread to the lungs from distant points in the body.

Cancer is out-of-control replication due to microbial proteins for cell-wall membranes causing human cells to mutate. Giving cancer 200 different names based on physical properties, appearance, and where it occurs, serves only to confuse the public.

There is only one primary cause of cancer and one cure for cancer. Microbial infection causes cancer. Eliminate all microbial proteins from the cell and cancer must stop.

There are many different methods by which to do this, but there is still only one cure for cancer. The cure requires two steps. Eliminate the source of microbial enzymes and proteins that cause mutation during normal cell replication, and prevent further contamination.

Eliminate the fermentation of trapped blood sugars and proteins that feed microbes allowing them to take over cellular functions. Proper nutrition is the fundamental method to stop parasites, fungi and bacteria from thriving in our bodies.

In the invasive stage, cancer cells or microbes in the tumor produce special enzymes to metabolize protein and amino acids anaerobically. These enzymes also metabolize blood proteins in the lymphatic system causing rapid weight loss of the cancer victim. Cancer can remain active in the storage-vessel ducts and sacs as long as nutrients are available.

Does all this make sense to you? Normal growth or an injury causes cells to multiply. Parasites cause injury to tissue. The repair mechanism creates a current of injury, and initiates cell division, but microbial growth factors mutate the cell-wall membranes so that new cells are rejected by the body. Repairs fail and replication continues.

Is it possible that this simple explanation for cancer has been overlooked by all the dedicated researchers? Could thousands of researchers spending billions of dollars in cancer research not have connected these individual discoveries? I don't think so.

The cause of cancer is well known because all the data in this text to support the concepts comes from existing publications. A person with the name of Royal Rife was curing cancer 50 years ago by selectively destroying the cancer cells with a device called the Rife generator. It functioned by radiating the cell-wall membrane of cancer cells with ultra violet light and causing the membrane to disintegrate. There is no reason why the process cannot be used today in all hospitals.

Although it is difficult to believe that effective cancer cures are suppressed, the facts cannot be denied. It is mentally easier for me to deny the holocaust, which I have not seen, than to deny suppression of cancer cures, which I have seen. It is similarly impossible for me to believe that intelligent cancer researchers cannot connect the obvious close relationship between cancer, infection and cell-wall mutation. The appearance of cancer tumors to primitive life form chitin membranes is obvious. Why have we never heard of chitin, fungi, or storage-vessel cancers in mainstream cancer information?

Perhaps there is a middle road that says cancer cures are suppressed but the cause of cancer is not known. Scientists were looking past the membrane wall problem, and mistakenly assumed enzymes to be the cause of DNA replication. Infection caused mutant DNA. The original error was made before they realized the DNA nucleotides are bonded by a weak ionic hydrogen bond that is released by an ionic field with energy from the cell-wall membrane. If that is the case, I have discovered the cause of cancer as the combination of the current of injury to initiate replication of DNA and the influence of microbial enzymes and proteins causing mutation of cell-wall membranes during mitosis.

Since Dr. Robert Becker's research on the current of injury has been well publicized, and Becker nominated for a Nobel prize for his research, it is obvious that this information is well known. Due to the obvious simplicity of the solution, the concept that I discovered the cause of cancer, is a concept, which in my opinion, is far more difficult to believe than a worldwide cover-up of the true cause of cancer.

Consider these issues which will be described more fully later in the text.

1. DNA is routinely replicated in test tubes, in the DNA polymerase chain reaction, and repair of fractured bone is stimulated by approved electromagnetic devices.

2. The current of injury has been studied for over 200 years and Dr. Becker proved the current of injury causes cells to divide and multiply.

3. Microbes are always associated with cancer cells, and microbes have a cell-wall membrane closely similar in structure to human cell-wall membranes and cancer cells.

4. Bacterial enzymes are used in the DNA polymerase chain reaction.

5. Up to 96% of cancers occur in epithelial tissue because microbes have the genetic capacity to mutate the cell-wall membrane.

6. Cancers are known to occur with growths, polyps, and infections that do not heal.

In addition to the above points, there is far more profit in researching the cause of cancer, and treating it, than there is in preventing or curing it quickly. Billions of dollars in profits are being taken from tax revenue and private funds to maintain the cancer industry. Due to the suppression of cancer cures and information on them, it is impossible for an individual researcher to benefit by announcing the cause of cancer.

In a series of notes regarding Otto Warburg's speech at Landau in 1966, we find this statement condemning the cancer establishment of the 1960's era for inhibiting the application of his scientific research. See Internet www.o3zone.com. The statement reads as follows:

> But nobody today can say that one does not know what cancer and its prime cause be. On the contrary, there is no disease whose prime cause is better known, so that today ignorance is no longer an excuse that one cannot do more about prevention. That prevention of cancer will come there is no doubt, for man wishes to survive. **But how long prevention will be avoided depends on how long the prophets of agnosticism will succeed in inhibiting the application of scientific knowledge in the cancer field. In the meantime millions of men must die of cancer unnecessarily.**

The failure to use oxygen and ozone to cure cancer is an obvious illustration that effective cancer cures are suppressed in North America. If cures are being suppressed, knowledge of the true cause of cancer is also being suppressed along with knowledge gained through modern research.

2. Why mainstream medicine rejects the cancer microbe theory

The critical error in the germ theory

A critical error in a theory establishes that the theory is wrong. The critical error in the germ theory is that all diseases are divided into two main categories, infectious and non-infectious. If there are three or more main categories of disease, the main theory is false.

The protocol for establishing an infectious disease is based on four postulates set forth by Dr. William Frederick Koch, about 1905. Dr. Koch received a Nobel Prize in 1905 for his outstanding research into tuberculoses. According to these postulates, an infectious disease must pass four tests before it can be classed as microbial.

1. Microbes must be found in an animal or person with the disease;

2. Microbes must be isolated and grown in a culture;

3. Microbes must be capable of producing the disease **when injected into a healthy experimental animal;** and

4. Microbes must be recoverable from the experimental animal.

Some biologists now recognize a serious error in the germ theory diagnostic protocol. The use of healthy animals with a strong immune system should not be used as the sole criterion for proving the capacity of microbes to cause a disease. No consideration is given to evaluating the capacity of a healthy immune system to destroy injected microbes and no consideration is given for microbes to survive for years in a latent or non-infectious mode. Further, there is no consideration that microbes may live as parasites in the body without causing any health problems until the microbes mutate or take on new life forms due to environmental changes.

The cancer microbe theory lost favor because it could not pass test three. Injecting suspected cancer-microbes into healthy experimental animals could not cause cancer. Apparently, no one thought to consider that the oxidative process of healthy animals could destroy the microbes and their enzymes before cancer could be initiated.

Research to the contrary was simply ignored. In 1913, Dr. J. Fibiger of Denmark developed cancer in laboratory animals by feeding them parasitic worms from horses. Fibiger proved that cancer was a microbial disease and received a Nobel Prize for his work. Fibiger found mice with cancer in a sugar warehouse and discovered that cancer could be initiated in immune suppressed animals. High sugar levels in the body suppress the immune system and allow fungus to thrive.

Many other so-called degenerative diseases were also classified as not being microbial, without taking into account that parasites can reside in hosts and contaminate cells with microbial enzymes and proteins. These unwanted microbial guests generate disease in many different ways, depending on the organs in which they reside and the enzymes and toxins they produce. The germ theory needs a category of disease based on the presence of microbial enzymes, protein, and cell-wall membrane material such as chitin in the cells.

The fatal flaw in the germ theory of disease flows from having only two categories, microbial or non-microbial. There should be a third category identified as *non-infectious microbial*. A healthy test animal or human person cannot 'catch' most microbial diseases because of a strong immune system. Some diseases are *genetic,* relating to genetic faults at the DNA level, but all genetic diseases produce defective human parts. Some diseases qualify as *infectious microbial* based on the germ theory of disease. Some diseases are caused by nutritional deficiencies.

The great majority of diseases should be classified as *non-infectious microbial*. Virus, yeast, and fungi cause disease due to immune system dysfunction, following a period of nutritional and metabolic deficiencies or ingestion of toxic chemicals and drugs. These diseases cannot be treated successfully by more drugs that are toxic because they are deficiency diseases. Deficiencies in essential fatty acids, essential minerals and trace minerals, essential amino acids, and essential sugars account for the immune system dysfunction. The polluted environment, farming methods, and food processing are creating the plague of non-infectious microbial diseases facing humankind. The medical mindset that drugs must be used to cure all diseases is the reason why so many millions of people now die from microbial diseases. A new type of drug—better classified as functional foods —are needed to support the immune system.

U.S. National Cancer Institute creates false cancer dogma

Why does the cancer industry continue to reject the theory that cancer microbes cause cancer? The only reference I could find from the cancer establishment *(which dictates what we are told about cancer)* comes from the U.S. National Cancer Institute publication *Science and Cancer*, Chapter 10, *Biological Carcinogens*. Oddly, it is in a chapter promoting viruses as a cause of cancer. The author states that it is theorized that viruses cause cancer but not through the mechanism of an infectious disease. Viruses can only cause defective genes. Defective genes cause cancer. Bacteria and fungi are not involved in the cancer process, although numerous researchers have observed and photographed them in cancer cells. Viruses must gum up the cell machinery causing mutations that somehow lead to cancer. The pathway has never been proven.

Viruses that produce cancer surmised by indirect reference

Here is what the National Cancer Institute writes in the publication *"Science and Cancer."* by Michael Shimkin, M.D. N.I.H. Publication 80-568. This publication was revised in 1969, 1973, 1978 and 1980, so it represents the fundamental view of the U.S. cancer specialists as of that time. Recent publications such as the 1998 *One Renegade Cell* by Robert A. Weinberg repeats and maintains the basic concepts.

The reasons for rejecting the microbial cause of cancer are expressed as follows (Page 51):

> Toward the end of the Pasteur era of bacteriology and infectious diseases, cancer, too, received attention. Many bacteria, fungi, and other microorganisms were observed, isolated and claimed as causes of cancer. None of these reports were substantiated, and more careful work that avoided incidental contamination was always negative. By 1910, scientists became quite sure that cancer was not caused by microorganisms of any kind. From this was derived the dictum that cancer was not infectious. Even today, *some stubborn workers* continue to claim that fungi, usually with complex life cycles including filterable phases, produce cancer, but their demonstrations are unconvincing.

> The period that closed with the disappointing bacteriological chapter in cancer research coincided with the earliest descriptions of diseases caused by viruses.

The reason for rejecting "bacteria, fungi and other organisms" was that "more careful work that avoided incidental contamination was always negative."

From this point forward in the text, the writer goes on to review and support the viral cause of cancer. Numerous examples are given, but all statements are carefully guarded. For example, he writes (*Italics are mine for emphasis*):

- The role of RNA **viruses in human cancers** *is surmised* **by indirect reference.**

- Oncogenic *viruses appear to become* part of the genetic material of cells where they can exist in latent or repressed state.

- At least **some cancers** *eventually* **will be found** to be produced by viruses, and this implies transmission.

Statements like these, repeated over and over, have created myths and medical dogma that cancer is caused by viruses and defective genes. There is no proof of the validity of the theories. Nevertheless, these theories are now used as medical dogma and repeated as fact in definitions.

For example, the definition of oncogene in The Canadian Medical Association, *Home Medical Encyclopedia* reads as follows:

> **Oncogenes: Genes, found in all cells, that are involved in the control of normal cell proliferation. Abnormalities of these genes have shown to be one of the steps responsible for cells becoming cancerous. Of the full human complement of 50,000 genes, fewer than 100 are probably oncogenes.**

The definition is not expressed as a theory. It is expressed as a factual statement. *"Abnormalities of these genes have shown to be one of the steps leading to cancer."* The simple truth is that no one has ever identified these genetic abnormalities that cause cancer and proven that they do. Defective genes are identified by chromosome and type of error in the base structure. Saying fewer than 100 are "probably oncogenes" tells us they do not know for sure. It has never been proven.

If someone discovered, even one gene that controls replication of cells wouldn't that be newsworthy? We would know the cause of cancer. The person who discovered it would be famous and should have received a Nobel Prize.

Who discovered this abnormality and when? It is certainly not mentioned in any books I have researched.

Look at the previous statement from the National Cancer Institute: "*...some stubborn workers continue to claim that fungi, usually with complex life cycles including filterable phases, produce cancer.*"

Why are the workers who say fungus in cancer cells described as "stubborn" rather than as dedicated or persistent? Why have we never heard of cancer-causing fungi in cancer research information published in the media? Why have we never heard of microbial cell-wall chitin? Why have we never heard of Dr. Fibiger's cancer research causing cancer with parasitic worms? Why is this research ignored and suppressed from the public?

Cancer is not infectious, "except in dogs and chickens"

NCI's *Science and Cancer* publication first establishes that cancer is not infectious in humans but the chapter ends by stating that cancer is infectious in other animals. The author implies that cancer is microbial in dogs and chickens but not in man (Page 56):

> In dogs, there does exist a cancer entity known as veneral sarcoma that is transmitted by direct contact. In chickens, the virus complex that causes several forms of leukemia and other cancers is communicable from infected to young non-infected fowl.

Cancer can be microbial and still not appear infectious because the cancer microbe needs anaerobic conditions in which to survive. Attempts to create cancer by infecting healthy animals with microbes will result in failure because high oxygen levels destroy the microbes, DNA polymerase, and other microbial enzymes. In order to initiate cancer, cells must be replicating, due to an embryonic stage, natural growth, or a current of injury and be infected. The environment of the cells must also support anaerobic life forms and inhibit the oxidative process of metabolism.

The medical conclusion that cancer is not a microbial disease has no basis in science or logic. It is based on the simple concept that 'infection' in healthy animals cannot be made to occur. Therefore, cancer is not an infectious disease. The influence of microbial proteins on human cell and cell-wall membrane is not considered. In addition, the influence of microbial toxins and enzymes on human cell metabolism is not considered.

The observation referred to earlier from NCI that *"more careful work that avoided incidental contamination was always negative"* comes to the wrong conclusion. The contamination and pollutants are needed to duplicate real-life situations. You can avoid contamination in a test tube but you cannot avoid contamination from parasites in your body. If more careful work that avoided contamination was always negative, or did not cause cancer, it follows that contamination causes cancer. The only problem left to solve is what contaminants cause cancer.

Medical professors maintain defective gene theory

A second reference explaining why mainstream medicine rejects the microbial cause of cancer can be found in Dr. Allan Cantwell's book *The Cancer Microbe* (Page 107).

To summarize Dr. Cantwell's point, because researchers at the turn of the century could not initiate cancer using parasites and microbes, they concluded that microbes did not cause cancer. This conclusion was adopted as fact, published, and taught in medical schools so that it soon became medical dogma. Once established as dogma, it could not be retracted without embarrassing a host of respected researchers and doctors. A concerted effort was made to dissuade researchers from proving microbes cause cancer.

Dr. Cantwell's book is printed with 19 full-page microphotographs of cancer microbes (Pages 234-272). I have listed some of the different types of cancers and summarized the appearance of microbes in these cells. The point being is that in every case, bacteria are visible and have been photographed. This is solid evidence that infection leads to cancer.

Figure 1: Scleroderma; rod-shaped bacteria in skin smear

Figure 7: Lymphoma; coccoid (circular) bacteria in skin

Figure 8: Hodgkin's Disease; coccoid bacteria in skin

Figure 11: Breast cancer; coccoid bacteria in breast

Figure 12: *Staphylococcus epidermidis* coccoid bacteria cultured from breast cancer

Figure 13: *Interstitial Pheumonitis* (AIDS); coccoid bacteria in lung

Figure 19: Basel Cell Carcinoma; coccoid bacteria in skin

The use of dark-field and bright-field microscopes now allows researchers to observe and videotape cancer microbes in living tissue. A fresh blood smear is used most often. The fact that mainstream medical check-ups for cancer still rely on mammograms and biopsies is unforgivable. Cancer microbes have been observed and photographed far too often to justify denial of the fact that microbes cause cancer. The knowledge that benign growths lead to cancer is universal. What causes these growths? Cancer can be detected through the observation and study of cancer microbes long before tumors form and operations are required.

3. Cancer is a microbial disease in the New Germ Theory

In this chapter, I would like to establish credibility in the concept that cell walls mutated with microbial cell-wall proteins such as chitin cause new cells to be rejected by the body. Since microbes are the only possible source of these primitive life cell-wall components, microbes cause cancer.

In chapter 5, *Cell Structure and Cell Division*, of the text *Molecules and Cells*, by D.A. Dent, we read (Page 61):

> Some fungal members of the plant kingdom appear to secrete chitin rather than cellulose in their walls, and chitin is a compound which is much more characteristic of animals than plants. In the bacteria, a wall is secreted outside the cell membranes which is a compound made up of a complex mixture of polymers in widely varying proportions. The polymers are based upon fundamental building units which may include hexoses, the derived hexosamines and various amino-acids. . . *(sugars and proteins)*
>
> *One of the many problems which still face cancer research workers is the inability of some cancer cells to adhere to one another in an organized manner.*

Dent tells us that fungal and bacterial cell walls are made up of sugars and proteins, with chitin being largely protein. In Harper's Review of Biochemistry (Page 150) we can review the molecular structures of chitin. Four distinct compounds are described, with varying similarities to compounds found in human cell walls. One of these, called heparin, contains sulfur molecules. Such sulfur containing molecules would be highly irregular for human cell membranes and would lead to rejection by basement membrane cells in injured epithelial layers.

Human cell walls are made of a lipid or fat-like molecules combined with phosphate to produce a plasma field in the membrane. Numerous protein elements are woven into the lipid layer to serve as receptors for nutrients and bioactive chemicals such as growth hormone or insulin.

The "inability of cancer cells to adhere to one another" is a direct result of microbial cell-wall contaminants in the membrane. Single celled life forms do not connect their cell walls to form membranes or bodies. Mentally connect this phenomenon with the current of injury causing cells to replicate to repair a broken membrane and you have the cause of cancer. Remove the current of injury, but allow microbes to mutate the cell wall during normal cell replication and you have the cause of degenerative diseases. Allow a defect in the plasma field of individual cells to occur from heavy-metal contaminants or other pollutants and you have the cause for chronic fatigue or autoimmune diseases in which the immune system appears to attack normal cells.

The amazing thing about these theories is that they correspond with reality. We do not have to assume the DNA of human cells to be mutated or defective. We do not have to assume existence of an oncogene or assume the lack of suppressor genes. How can you prove the lack of something such as a suppressor gene? If microbial infection or other conditions inside a cell mutates the cell wall during assembly of new cells, the cell function is mutated. If the cell wall is mutated, we have a disease. If the cell is rejected by adjacent cells, we have a tumor. If the current of injury is not shut down, we have out-of-control multiplication of cells in that area. All the rungs are in the pathway explaining how cancer occurs.

We have been wrong about infectious diseases

The following information is from an article in the Atlantic Monthly, February 1999, by Judith Hooper. Biologist Paul Ewald, author of *Evolution of Infectious Diseases* is quoted as follows: *(My emphasis added in bold italics)*.

> The infectious age is, we now know, far from over. Furthermore, it appears that many diseases we didn't think were infectious may be caused by infectious agents after all. By guiding researchers down one path, Koch's postulates directed them away from alternate ones. Researchers were guided away from diseases that might have been infectious but had little chance of fulfilling the postulates. That is, just because we couldn't discover their cause, we rather arbitrarily decided that the so-called chronic diseases of the late twentieth century must be hereditary, environmental, or "multifactorial." *And, we have been wrong.*

Cancer is now recognized as a microbial disease by this eminent American biologist. The tide of public opinion is changing. How long will it take for the accepted treatment of disease to catch up to the new theory of disease?

Some biologists and doctors are beginning to accept the fact that conditions in the body can lead to disease. They are rejecting Koch's postulates for the germ theory. They now believe cellular environment causes disease. Microbes are a secondary cause. Cures for disease follow from correcting the cause of disease. Toxic drugs are not the answer because drugs do not cleanse the cellular environment. Indeed, drugs just add toxins and further deplete minerals and upset the mineral balance, leading to numerous adverse side effects.

Prof. Paul Ewald creates Germ Theory, Part II

In his book, *Evolution of Infectious Diseases,* Paul Ewald concludes that only microbes can account for the majority of diseases that are now classed as genetic, of unknown origin or as autoimmune diseases. He proposes a new germ theory to take into account the effect of non-inflammatory parasitic infection and a weakened immune system.

The term *autoimmunity* and *immunity* are somewhat confusing. Autoimmunity occurs when the body builds defense mechanisms that recognize and destroy invaders. For example, resistance to a second infection of measles illustrates immunity or acquired immunity.

Autoimmune diseases, in theory, occur when the body's defense mechanism attacks the body's healthy cells in error. Autoimmune diseases are a type of defective gene disease. The theory of autoimmune diseases developed because Koch's postulates prevented many conditions from being classed as microbial diseases. The theory has never been proven factual even though over 80 conditions are now being treated as autoimmune diseases.

Paul Ewald used statistics to prove that Koch's Germ theory is wrong and that the majority of diseases, including cancer are not caused by genetic defects. By comparing the death rate of people with 'so-called' defective genes and other hereditary diseases with their life span and reproductive rate, he saw a statistical problem. Statistics indicated the frequency of these diseases was rising far faster than the rate of known genetic defects. He concluded that old diseases that continue to thrive must be infectious. Survival of the fittest should have resulted in reduced populations of these diseased people.

As a result of Ewald 's theories, there is now a movement to create the Germ Theory, Part II. Paul Ewald now classifies the following diseases as microbial and has removed them from the list of autoimmune diseases. This microbial disease list now includes:

> sarcoidosis, inflammatory bowel, rheumatoid arthritis, lupus, Wegener's granulomatosis, diabetes mellitus, cirrhosis, heart disease, arteriosclerosis, Alzheimer's, cancer, multiple sclerosis, psychiatric diseases, and cerebral palsy.

Another prominent American doctor, A.V. Costantini has come to a similar conclusion but for different reasons. Dr. Costantini's research identifies fungi and fungal mycotoxins in all 'so-called' autoimmune diseases and cancer.

What Dr. Costantini has to say about the true cause of cancer cannot be taken lightly or easily discarded. His self-funded research is totally independent of outside influences.

His medical credentials and accomplishments speak for themselves: *Head, World Health Organization* (WHO), *Collaborating Center for Mycotoxins in Food.* Professor, School of Medicine, Albert Ludwig University, Freiburg, Germany and, Clinical Professorial Faculty (Retired), University of California, School of Medicine, San Francisco, California, USA.

Dr. Costantini was the keynote speaker at a two-day "Fungalbionics" conference held in Toronto in 1994. In my opinion, and that of most attendees, Dr. Costantini destroyed the credibility of the defective gene theory of cancer and established credibility of his belief that fungi are the primary cause of cancer.

Dr. Costantini has published his research in books filled with charts and references. His research based on worldwide statistics and information collected by the World Health Organization establish cancer as a fungal disease.

The major proof that cancer is a fungal disease is that all known cancer cures have only one thing in common. All effective cancer cures are antifungal.

The introduction to the first edition of his book *Fungalbionics, Book II, Cancer*, provides this significant statement:

> The Fungalbionic Series of books present data documentary evidence that fungi and their biological metabolites, the mycotoxins, are the silent and relentless attackers of human

health by causing the major "degenerative" and "cancerous" diseases which plague mankind.

Dr. Costantini, using the resources of the World Health Organization, has access to information that is in complete support of Germ Theory Part II. For example, many crops harvested during a rainy season create regional epidemics of 'autoimmune' disease through mycotoxins in the grains or produce. Obviously, you cannot create epidemics of autoimmune diseases, so the theory of autoimmune disease must be wrong.

Dr. Costantini describes the autoimmune disease concept as just another unproven medical postulate. It is totally illogical that the human species would have survived and improved over millions of years, if life were subject to autoimmune diseases. According to Dr. Costantini, the following diseases are caused by fungal mycotoxins ingested in food or mycotoxins produced in our body from fungal infections:

AIDS, gout, Crohn's disease, multiple sclerosis, hyperactivity syndrome, infertility, psoriasis, Alzheimer's, scleroderma, Raynaud's disease, sarcoidosis, kidney stones, amyloids, vasculitis, arthritis, Cushing's disease

If we were to calculate the billions of dollars spent on drugs to continually treat people with all of the above 'so-called' non-microbial diseases, we would quickly recognize why this false medical dogma is maintained. Treating children for hyperactivity with drugs to slow them down is sheer nonsense. Treating people with mineral deficiencies and parasites for allergies does not make sense. The treatment of cancer and misinformation about defective genes as the cause of cancer is only one disease of many that the drug-focused medical establishment controls as a business profit center. The Heart and Stroke Foundation (read industry) is another.

Textbooks must be rewritten and mindsets changed

In spite of all this evidence of a relationship between cancer and microbes, publications such as the *Scientific American Science Desk Reference,* 1999 edition, list cancer in the non-infectious diseases section and make no reference to fungi and bacteria in the cancer process. Suggestions are given on how to avoid the 8 most frequent cancers, but not one word promotes a parasite cleanse. This modern desk reference tells us cancer now kills about 6 million people a year worldwide. Over 16,000 people will die of cancer—today!

The fact that Dr. J. Fibiger initiated cancer in the laboratory using parasites is never mentioned. Virtually all research and evidence that cancer is a microbial disease is never mentioned in the media, not even to discredit it. Why is that? I believe it is because there is no way to discredit the fact that microbes cause cancer. It is far easier to confuse the issue with oncogenes and suppressor genes, cell-clocks and the like.

Judith Hooper ends her report in *Atlantic Monthly* on the New Germ Theory with a statement that should make every medical professional and politician take note:

> The textbooks say, in 1900 most people died of infectious diseases and today most people die of cancer and heart disease and Alzheimer's and all these things. Well, in ten years, I think the textbooks will have to be rewritten to say: 'Throughout history most people have died of infectious disease, and most people continue to die of infectious disease.'

In my opinion, most people continue to die of infectious diseases because they believe in medical propaganda that cholesterol, defective genes, or autoimmune problems cause illness and because they ingest toxic drugs for therapy. In most cases, these drugs do not treat the real problem such as nutritional deficiencies, pollutants, fungal infections, mycotoxins, and parasites. Treatments are designed to sell drugs, not to cure the patient.

The Dec. 6, 1999 issue of the Hamilton Spectator quoted a news report from the Miami Herald quoting these U.S. medical statistics:

> The National Academy of Sciences says that more people die of medical mistakes each year (at least 44,000) than die from automobile accidents (43,500), breast cancer (42,300) or AIDS (16,500), and that $8.8 billion is spent on medical costs associated with medical errors.

The report goes on to suggest a system be put in place to record and analyzes these deaths, not to lay blame, but to "track medical errors and recommend fixes... Devising a system for determining what goes wrong, when and why in hospitals—just as the National Transportation Board vets airline, train, and highway accidents—is the right approach."

The reason given for not having such a useful public service is that: "Federal regulatory agencies become bloated and inefficient, losing sight of their missions."

The monopoly on health care does not serve the public interests. It serves the agencies that have the "*mine*opoly".

4. Cancers originate in storage vessels and ducts after injury

Let's now turn to reviewing how fermentation of trapped blood sugars causes up to 96% of human cancers.

In this chapter, we will apply the 'mutated cell-wall membrane' theory of cancer to the four most common cancers. If the theory is correct, the frequency of cancer by type should relate directly to the capacity of these organs to maintain fermentation of trapped blood sugars and proteins.

The common denominator of all cancers appears to be that they are located in cells the body considers vital for life. The liver, for example, is capable of replacing itself because it is so essential to life. Liver cancer results when these cells are infected and cell function is mutated by microbial infection during replication.

Similarly, mast cells for production of white, and red blood cells remain reproductive throughout life. These important cells are protected within bones because they are so vital. When mast cells become infected, we end up with leukemia. Bone cancer begins with bone fractures that do not heal or simply invasion of bone marrow due to fermentation in adjacent areas. Prostate cancer uncured frequently becomes bone cancer.

Membranes are also considered essential for life and are capable of rapid repair. For example, following a colon operation, new cells repair the colon membrane within days. It is this capacity to reproduce rapidly that enables these cells to become cancer cells. That is why the large majority of cancers, up to 96% according to medical publications, are membrane cell cancers.

It is no accident that the four most common cancers —lung, colon, breast, and prostate —occur in organs that are essentially storage vessels for body fluids or gases. Less frequent cancers, such as bile duct, bladder, ovary and testicular cancer also illustrate this phenomenon. Lymphomas are another obvious example.

What's the connection? An injury in the cell wall that allows internal bleeding leads to trapped blood nutrients that ferment and support fungal growth. The fungal mycelium nourished by the nutrients in the blood clot, invades adjacent cells, and causes a break in the cell-wall membrane of more cells. Secondary products of fermentation modify the cellular environment of adjacent cells, disrupting production of ATP, and thereby allowing further microbial infection. Microbial infection follows contamination of cells and loss of energy. Here's how I see the cancer process at work.

1. Injury to epithelial cells, from parasites, accident, chemical toxins, or nutritional deficiencies, result in blood or lymph fluids flowing from circulating to non-circulating areas and becoming trapped.

2. Trapped blood leads to fermentation, a fungal process, with fungal mycelia invading adjacent cells and byproducts of fermentation modifying the cellular environment so as to stop the oxidative process and production of ATP.

3. Cells become infected with bacteria that have a cell wall closely similar to the corresponding human cell but do not knit one to another. In order to repair the injury that allowed blood to flow out of the normal circulation route, the body produces a current of injury to initiate replication of cells and repair the damage.

4. During the assembly process of new cells, and specifically during the process of assembly of phospholipids to form the cell wall, bacteria produce chitin cell-wall proteins that are assembled into the new cells as contaminants. Life and function of cells are controlled by the cell wall, and the mutation of the cell mutates the function. New cells do not bond to existing cells to repair the injury. Consequently, the current of injury stays on, replication of mutated cells continues out-of-control, and cancer results in these storage vessels and ducts.

Lung cancer from fermentation in adjacent tissue

Lung cancer presents an interesting problem regarding microbial enzymes as the cause of cancer, as one might think there would be too much oxygen available for anaerobic microbes to develop cancer in lung tissue. However, lungs are filled with air ducts and spaces where blood can accumulate from injury or internal bleeding. In addition, the lymphatic system contains numerous lymph nodes throughout the lung cavity that can lead to trapped industrial fumes, gases, cigarette toxins and ammonia.

According to the text, *Everyone's Guide to Cancer Therapy*, lung cancer is divided into two groups: small cell, and non-small cell. Small cell cancer does not always develop in lung tissue. The chapter on lung cancer tells us (Page 458):

Small cell cancer does not always originate from the lung. Occasionally it may arise in other organs such as the esophagus or cervix, and sometimes may occur without the primary site of origin being identified.

We also learn that small cell lung cancer can spread via the lymphatic vessels to the lymph nodes in the center of the lung, the center of the chest, in the neck and above the collarbone and in the abdominal cavity. It is likely to spread through the bloodstream to the liver, to the opposite lung, the brain and to bones.

Non-small cell cancer consists of three types: squamous cell, large cell, and adenocarcinoma. Squamous cells are flattened cells used to form layers of skin tissue. An adenoma is a growth or cyst and an adenocarcinoma is cancer that develops in a growth or cyst due to the repair process staying in high gear. We read as follows (Also page 458):

> Squamous cell carcinoma is the most common and is referred to as an **epidermoid type of cancer associated with the lymphatic system and lymph nodes.** Adenocarcinoma occur in peripheral portions of the lung (near the edge) and therefore may invade the lining of the chest and produce fluid in the chest cavity more commonly than in other types.

Production of fluid in the chest cavity leads to loss of lung function, as in drowning. What produces the fluid? Is this fluid the same as the fluid in a blister? Cells produce hydrogen peroxide to destroy anaerobic life forms and to fight infections. Hydrogen peroxide is a molecule of water with an additional atom of oxygen. When an atom of oxygen is removed to help destroy an anaerobic life form, the molecule of peroxide becomes a molecule of water. The normal process of the body to fight infection results in production of fluids commonly referred to as pus. Pus contains millions of dead white blood cells, dead and living bacteria, and other substances. A collection of puss within solid tissue is called an abscess. When an abscess breaks, epithelial tissue is damaged, and the body tries to repair the injury. Cancer spreads rapidly in lung tissue through the process of microbial infection, abscesses, and blisters.

As you can see, lung cancers occur in the lung area, but inside epithelial cells of the lymphatic system, or abnormal growths within the periphery of the lung cavity. Lung cancer often occurs when lung tissue is invaded from outside of the lung. The various locations of lung cancer do not invalidate the theory that trapped blood fermenting in a low oxygen environment leads to cancer. The presence of oxygen in the lung sacs does not equate with the presence of oxygen in the cells. Enzymes are required to clear the lungs of carbon dioxide and ammonia or industrial gases so that oxygen can be absorbed. Smoking coats lung tissue with tar and fills lung tissue cells with gases that the body is not equipped to handle. But most of all, ammonia from smoking, parasitic waste, personal care products and household cleansers damages enzymes in these delicate tissues so that cellular damage occurs. Cellular damage leads to replication and repair of cell walls.

Smoking is closely associated with cancer, but smoking does not cause DNA to replicate out of control. Smoking only leads to lung cancer by polluting the lymphatic system and lung tissue with ammonia and other toxins. Smoking causes cell wall damage of lung tissue. Cell wall damage causes cancer, if cells are also infected.

Dr. A. Costantini has found that smoking rolled cigars does not cause cancer.

Smoking sugar-cured tobacco containing ammonia and fungal mycotoxins provides the elements needed for cancer. Lung cancers occur mainly in ducts, cavities, and surrounding tissue. Smoke contaminates cell walls causing reduced respiration of tissues in the throat, airways, and lungs. Reduced respiration is all that is needed to stop the citric acid cycle. Ammonia toxicity is probably the leading cause of lung cancer. Ammonia toxicity will be discussed more fully later in Chapter 15, *Using amino acids to stop cancer.*

Intestinal cancers of the colon and rectum

Colon cancer is second in frequency only to lung cancer. The colon and rectum, or large bowel is about seven feet long and is the permanent home for most parasites in the body. The opportunity for parasites to damage cell walls, and for microbial enzymes to cause replication, is self-evident. The colon wall is also subject to ammonia from fermentation of food in the gut.

The colon wall consists of four layers of tissues: a mucous lining, a submucous coat of connective tissue in which are embedded the main blood vessels of the tract, a muscular coat, and a fibrous coat. The muscular coat propels food from the stomach to the rectum. The large bowel differs from the small intestine in width and shape. The small intestine is essentially a long muscular tube whereas the colon has numerous small sacks (*called haustra*) giving the large bowel and rectum a puckered appearance. The small intestine serves as a container for making sausage.

The colon is prone to developing small pouchlike areas called diverticula, which protrude from the colon into the abdominal cavity. A low-fiber diet leading to constipation and hard-to-pass stools is suspected as the cause. When the colon wall is stretched to form a pouch, the blood vessels in the colon wall are also stretched and become subject to internal bleeding. A common sign of diverticula problems is blood in the stool. These pouchlike vessels rising from the small sacks (the haustra) provide numerous vessels for trapping blood sugars and proteins. Extended periods of fermentation with the subsequent invasion of the colon wall by fungal mycelia leads to colon cancer. As with other cancers, the first sign is an abnormal growth or lump.

In *Everyone's Guide to Cancer Therapy (Page 367)*, on colon cancer we read:

> The colon is also subject to abnormal growths called *polyps* starting in the colon wall.

> These tumors may be common because about half the population over forty is thought to have clumps of tissues protruding from the inner layer (mucosa) of the colon or rectum. These mushroom-like growths are called polyps, and while most are benign, at least one type, adenomatous polyps, may be a precursor to cancer. About 90 per cent of colorectal cancers are thought to arise from these polyps and a person with colorectal adenoma runs three times the risk of developing colorectal cancer.

It is obvious that the cause of replication of colon cells in colon cancer is the normal process of tissue repair. These "mushroom like growths" are epithelial cells mutated with chitin, the same material as found forming mushroom skin. Cysts and polyps lead to cancer following injury because the current of injury does not shut down due to rejection of mutated cells.

The frequency of colon cancer also increases with age as people tend to have fewer bowel movements and therefore store body wastes for longer periods of time. Passing a hard stool through the colon containing polyps results in damage to polyps and torn tissue. Nutritional factors are also involved as well as tape worms and parasites that damage the colon wall causing internal bleeding.

Breast cancer from fermentation in milk lobes and ducts

The third most common cancer is breast cancer in women. *(Breast cancer in men is very rare because men's breasts do not develop milk lobes, storage vessels and ducts. There is a limited capacity to trap blood sugars and proteins in male breast tissue.)*

Breast cancer is classified into three types based on where it occurs. The most frequent type of breast cancer begins in the ducts (the tubes that carry milk) and is called ductal cancer. When cancer reaches an invasive stage and starts to spread, it is called "infiltrating ductal breast cancer."

Lobular breast cancer, the second most frequent, arises in the glands that produce milk. These glands are formed by membrane tissue that line the milk glands and milk storage areas.

The least common type is inflammatory breast cancer, which involves the skin over the breast as well as the tissues underneath. These cancers may be related to toxins in synthetic material in brassieres that cause irritation of the skin. Breast cancer in men may also occur in skin tissue. All of these cancers are related to epithelial layers where fermentation of blood sugars may occur in the lymphatic system or storage vessels.

The most common causes of breast cancer result from internal bleeding, with blood sugars and proteins becoming trapped in milk ducts and glands. Bleeding may be caused by physical injury, parasites or due to weakened epithelial tissue from excess hydrogenated oils, lack of minerals such as silica, or lack of natural Vitamin C containing bioflavanoids required for proper skin tone.

Varicose veins in legs and thighs are a visible sign of blood proteins outside of veins and arteries caused by weak skin tissue. However, cancer does not occur in varicose veins due to the rapid circulation of blood and lymphatic fluids that occurs as we walk or exercise. Cancer requires reduced circulation as in storage vessels and ducts. Breast lobes and ducts are low-volume blood circulation areas ideal for fermentation of trapped blood and other chemicals or hormones. It is well known that breast milk may contain toxins such as DDT. It follows that breast ducts and lobes can accumulate toxins and parasites after menopause.

It may be that the body deposits unwanted toxic material and excess hormones in these convenient and empty storage areas in order to isolate them from the rest of the body.

Frequency of cancer by type parallels capacity for storage

The frequency of the occurrence of each type of breast cancer (ductal, lobular, and epidermal) is also in direct proportion to the amount of volume or space available for trapping fermentable products in one place. The larger the storage area, the more frequent the cancer.

One woman who experienced breast cancer related to me how her left breast would not release milk following the birth of her son. A nurse at the hospital tried to induce release of milk with a breast pump and drew blood through the nipple. That breast bled on and off for about forty years. Shortly after bleeding stopped, cancer developed.

After we discussed the concept of trapped blood proteins and fermentation causing her cancer, she agreed that it made sense. She remarked that her cancer began six months after bleeding from the nipple stopped. As we discussed the microbial cause of cancer, she agreed that all the circumstances she experienced correspond to the theory. We believe trapped blood proteins in her milk ducts and lobes, without periodic cleansing through the nipple, fermented and caused cancer. I wonder how many other women have had a similar experience.

She experienced breast cancer and had her breast and several lymph nodes removed. A few years later she experienced cancer of the backbone. This woman, now in her eighties, has recovered from her bone cancer through a combination of chemotherapy and parasite cleansing based on Dr. Hulda Clark's program. She now relies on a daily program of herbal parasite cleansing, zapping and exercise (mainly walking) to maintain her good health. Interestingly, her older brother experienced prostate cancer at age 82 and recovered by following the same program but without the chemotherapy or radiation. They both use essiac on a regular basis as a maintenance program to prevent microbial infection.

The reason I know so much about these people and am willing to mention them is that one is my sister, and the other is, of course, my brother. They are living testimony that cancer can be cured and beaten using methods described in books by Dr. Hulda Clark and others.

Prostate cancer follows from fermentation in prostate

Prostate cancer is the fourth most common type of cancer. The prostate gland accounts for a huge majority of cancers in men. The prostate gland produces and stores semen, which is ejected through the seminal duct during ejaculation. As men age, and frequency of intercourse reduces or stops, there is a corresponding opportunity for these storage vessels to accumulate toxins. In addition, bladder infection and sexual intercourse can lead to parasitic infection of the male reproductive organs.

Just as the breast has lobes and ducts for the production, storage and delivery of milk, the prostate gland has lobes and ducts for the storage and delivery of semen. If these storage areas become filled with fermentable products, fermentation will take place and all of the essentials for the conditions of cancer are available. The organ doesn't have to be large to cause cancer; it is the total capacity to trap blood sugars and proteins in an environment of poor oxidation that is the important factor.

The outer skin of the prostate is an epithelial layer surrounded by lymph fluids. Microbial infection in the surrounding lymphatic channels can also cause prostate cancer if parasitic infection damages tissue. The general area of the prostate gland is outside of main arteries and veins carrying oxygenated blood as well as outside of lymphatic system veins—compared to arms and legs—so toxins can accumulate quite readily. Exercise and physical activity are important to help keep this area of the body well oxidized. Being a couch potato is not recommended.

Internal bleeding or the flow of lymphatic fluids into liquid storage vessels, with the subsequent fermentation, can account for the high rate of cancers in prostate and breast tissue. Swelling of the prostate in benign prostatic hypertrophy non-cancerous lumps in breast, and polyps in the colon wall indicate that fermentation and growth are in progress but that all of the conditions necessary for cancer are not in place. Several generations of progressive mutation are necessary for cells to mutate into aggressive protein-hungry invasive cancer cells.

Bile duct cancer follows from fermentation in bile duct

If we can visualize the cause of cancer arising from fermentation in liquid storage areas or ducts, we can see why cancers are almost entirely related to epithelial layers or skin tissue. Bile ducts, for example, may become clogged with bile stones that rupture the bile duct wall, cause bleeding, trapped blood proteins and fermentation. In addition, chronic inflammation, parasites, and ulcers can lead to internal bleeding. Ductal tubes account for cancer of the liver and bile ducts leading from the liver. Cancer does not occur where cells enjoy a rapid blood flow or high oxidative levels. Ducts provide the shelter necessary to trap blood sugars and for fermentation to occur.

In *"Everyone's Guide to Cancer Therapy"* on bile duct cancer we read (Page 271):

> **What Causes It?** The cause is unknown. *People with chronic inflammatory processes, such as ulcerative colitis or parasitic infections of the bile ducts, are at higher risk for developing this cancer.* But no one cause has been clearly demonstrated.

I believe the obvious connection between most human cancers and storage vessels must be explained. The only theory that makes any sense is the fungal process of fermentation of nutrients trapped in the vessels or ducts. Fermentation produces toxins that pollute adjacent cells, causing loss of the oxidative process. Dr. Otto Warburg gave us the true cause of cancer long ago. This valuable information is just not being used.

Let's move on now to other forms of cancer that are more difficult to explain such as leukemia and cancer in children.

Childhood cancer explained by microbial theory

Most mainstream medical information on cancer states that cancer tumors take many years to develop based on the capacity for cells to double. The obvious fact that children only a few months old develop cancer tumors defies the slow-development theory of cancer. The fact that that cancer-free mothers give birth to healthy babies who get cancer within a few months after birth suggests that childhood cancer is not inherited.

The cause of childhood cancer, if microbial, could be fungi or yeast ingested in baby food, mother's milk, or through environmental factors that lead to infection of the fetus or infant.

The Nobel Prize in Medicine in 1960 was awarded to Sir Macfarlane Burnet and Dr. Peter. B. Medawar for their outstanding research in infection and immunology. They proved that full immunological maturity is reached weeks or months after birth. They illustrated that the developing embryos inoculated with foreign tissue would accept the foreign tissue as 'self' and not develop an immune response to it. The embryos develop an *immunological tolerance* to the virus or other microbial life form. For more information see http://nobel .se/laureates/medicine   The mystery of childhood cancer can be explained through the immune system development stages. According to Dr. Costantini, mycotoxins have been found in the umbilical cords of pregnant women, aflatoxin in breast milk and formula, and in contaminated baby food. In addition, some childhood cancers could be an unfortunate result of vaccinations.

AIDS in infants follows this pattern. It is generally believed that mothers with HIV can transmit infection by breast feeding, and that the chances that a child will have HIV is 25 per cent for a vaginal birth, but only 10 per cent for a Cesarean birth. Obviously, the viral population resident in the vagina could infect the child during birth or viruses in the milk could infect the child. Burnet's research suggests that fungi and bacteria that infect a developing fetus or newborn child will be recognized as 'self' rather than as 'intruder'. Consequently, these microbes will continue to thrive in the infant after birth and multiply freely.

The research by Gunther Blobel, winner of the 1999 Nobel Prize in Medicine, for research on how proteins are located in cells, is very significant in understanding hereditary childhood diseases. The disease may actually be caused by fungal proteins being accepted as self and incorporated into cell walls and organelles (*structures within cells*). Since the immune system does not recognize these cells as invaders, cells are assembled with fungal and parasitic proteins in place of human proteins. Without the immune system recognition of these microbial parasites, infants are prone to birth defects, sudden death syndrome, mental retardation, cancer, and so on.

Whatever the source, immune system dysfunction due to immunological tolerance can explain why children get cancer tumors and leukemia. It can also explain why only 25 per cent of children born to mothers infected with HIV, are similarly infected. We must remember that the letter S in AIDS stands for *syndrome*. A syndrome is not a disease, and no one dies of AIDS. They die of opportunistic infections. The HIV virus is secondary. The increased incidences of HIV in infants born by way of the vagina, as compared to Cesarean, follows from an increased opportunity for fungal or yeast infection from contact with the vaginal canal. The immune system is undeveloped or dysfunctional allowing virus to thrive in human cells. HIV in infants is another opportunistic parasite that the body accepts as self rather than intruder. HIV is probably no stronger or more dangerous than any other virus that has been around for years.

Leukemia forms cancer cells without forming tumors

Leukemia is defined as cancer of the blood-forming organs and the bone marrow and is characterized by an abnormal increase of white blood cells (*leukocytes*) in the blood.

The influence of chitin microbial growth factors on the cell-wall membrane is not evident because these cells do not normally knit to existing cells. The defect probably reduces the flexibility in the membrane wall, making it difficult for white blood cells to engulf an invader.

White blood cells are produced in the bone marrow as normal, and are mutated during the assembly process. Leukemia continues to survive in flowing blood although the oxygen level is adequate to destroy anaerobic life forms because the defect is in the cell-wall membrane.

Leukemia is a viral or fungal infection of white blood cells as they are assembled in the bone marrow and the cell wall is mutated in the same manner as cancer that forms tumors.

Three leukemia patients have recently been cured by application of anti-fungal drugs. A brief article in the Hamilton Spectator, Sept. 29, 1999 reads as follows:

Leukemia patients recover after treatment for fungal infections

Three leukemia patients who received a cocktail of antifungal drugs are alive and apparently recovered from their cancer, much to the surprise of their physician . . . In addition to the conventional antifungal drug amphotericin B, the patients received high doses of two other antifungal treatments: fluconazole and liposomal amhotericin

Dr. A.V. Costantini of the World Health Organization and author of several books identifying fungi as the cause of all cancer, tells us that all cures for cancer have only one thing in common. They are antifungal. He also claims that if an antifungal drug cures a disease of unknown cause, the disease is of fungal origin. On that basis, leukemia is a fungal disease.

The Oct. 29, 1999 Hamilton Spectator had another reference to the possible fungal cause of childhood leukemia as being fungal related.

Scientists trace origins of childhood leukemia to womb

Scientists have discovered that most cases of childhood leukemia start in the womb and are caused by a genetic defect that is not inherited...The researchers found that the leukemia cells taken from the children with ALL (Acute Lymphoblastic Leukemia) had an altered or mutated gene...Previous research, conducted by the same team, has shown only 5 per cent of twins both develop the illness, so the researchers concluded that the mutation was not enough to lead to full-blown leukemia and that some post-natal event or exposure was also necessary.

The writer speculates that radiation, chemical pollution and infection are possible causes of leukemia because radiation, pollutants, and viral infection are considered capable of causing defective genes. Obviously, fungal infection and immune tolerance would be a better explanation since antifungal drugs have cured leukemia in adults.

The word "fungi" is never mentioned when it comes to speculation on the cause of cancer by mainstream medicine. In the previous reference to antifungal drugs curing leukemia, the doctors are "surprised." There was no mention of their researching antifungal drugs as a cure for leukemia.

Even the 1988 book *Cancer and Leukemia, An Alternative Approach* by an alternative health specialist, Jan de Vries, does not mention fungi as a possible cause of leukemia. Virus in listed in the index in several places but fungi not at all.

Fungi invade cells lacking in high plasma energy and white blood cells engulf virus and fungi. Perhaps lack of minerals and vitamins reduces the ability of white blood cells to create enzymes necessary to destroy the fungi they engulf. These microbes thrive in the bone marrow and produce proteins to disturb defense mechanism function in white blood cells. They overload the receptor cites or block the enzyme production pathway as a defense mechanism. Perhaps too, the immune system does not recognize these fungal cells as invaders and allows them to proliferate freely because they infected the body before the immune system developed.

The research of Sir Macfarlane Burnet and Dr. Peter. B. Medawar reveals that embryos develop an *immunological tolerance* to virus or other microbial life form. The research of Dr. A.V. Costantini identifies fungi in placentas and mother's milk. Any yeast infection in the womb during pregnancy or birth as well as contamination from hospital staff diseases could result in childhood leukemia.

In addition, the lack of natural oils and fats in the mother's diet could lead to 'hydrogenated' cell walls that fail to function normally. This concept will be developed more fully in discussion of the dangers from hydrogenated oils (Chapter 18, *Why fats appear to cause cancer*).

I have not researched leukemia fully and this text applies mainly to cancers of epithelial origin or *carcinomas*. Since fermentation within or adjacent to epithelial cells leads to cancer, it is very likely that fermentation of blood in bone marrow causes defective white blood cells. Anaerobic bacteria have been photographed in numerous types of cancer, but I have not seen any references to bacteria in leukemia.

Both epithelial cancer and leukemia cancer in children may also be the result of sleeping in areas where magnetic energies interfere with their enzymes and create havoc with their digestion and cellular respiration. Trace minerals, known as electrolytes, are required for cells to function and the lack of these minerals limits metabolism and leads to fermentation of food nutrients. Fermentation leads to cancer. Leukemia could be a mineral deficiency disease.

Ammonia in the air from household cleansers, carpets, and bedding could lead to ammonia toxicity and loss of metabolic enzymes. Second-hand smoke is a major source of ammonia. Toxic food additives such as aspartame ingested by the mother could cause enzyme damage, or lead to fermentation of proteins and cancer shortly after birth. There are many ways for yeast and fungi to contaminate infants lacking fully developed immune systems, liver function, respiration, and metabolism.

Conditions that lead to extended periods of fermentation in children or adults will lead to cancer. Cancer does not take years to develop in children or adults. The cancer process starts as soon as the cellular environment stops the oxidative process and supports fermentation. A change back to an oxidative metabolism is required to switch cells back to aerobic metabolism and stop the cancer process. It takes several replication cycles to convert a normal human cell to an invasive cancer cell, and it takes a corresponding number to revert a cancer cell back into a normal cell. Spontaneous remissions illustrate the capacity for cancer cells to revert to normal.

Let's move on to a discussion of defective genes causing breast cancer and prove that the concept has no scientific basis.

Excessive growth factor receptors are not the cause of breast cancer

The medically stated cause for about 30% of breast cancers is defective genes producing excessive growth factor receptors. This condition supposedly results in rapid growth and breast cancer. It is important that we deal with this misinformation to stop the practice of preventative mastectomies *(removal of healthy breasts)* to prevent cancer.

When I first heard about this medical treatment from a speech by Harvey Diamond, I thought he must be mistaken. Harvey Diamond is co-author of the best seller *Fit for Life* as well as sole author of *You Can Prevent Breast Cancer.*

Further research showed he is not mistaken about preventative mastectomies. Researchers at the Mayo Clinic in Rochester, Minn. studied the cases of 639 women who underwent the procedure (removal of healthy breasts) at the clinic between 1960 and 1993. Doctors at the Mayo Clinic rely on genetic screening to prevent cancer. Women who are carriers of BRCA1 or BRCA2 (genes that can lead to breast cancer) are at greater risk of developing the cancer. Removal of the healthy breasts is recommended and used as a means to prevent breast cancer.

Information promoting use of Herceptin, a drug used to treat breast cancer, reveals how the cancer industry slants information to support the theory that defective genes cause breast cancer. This misinformation also serves to maintain public confidence in surgery, chemotherapy and costly gene therapy. Now that Herceptin has been approved for widespread use in other genetic diseases, we should take a close look at one of the typical applications. An article was published in the Hamilton Spectator (Oct. 19, 1998) on the use of the drug. *(My emphasis added in bold print.)* The report reads as follows:

> Herceptin is part of a novel approach to fighting cancer. Rather than the scorched-earth policy of traditional chemotherapy, which kills all rapidly dividing cells cancerous or not, biologic treatments

such as Herceptin are programmed to attack only the **genetically haywire** cancer cells.

About a decade ago, scientists learned that about 30% of all breast cancers are the result of a mutation in a specific gene called HER2 – *H*uman *E*pidermal growth factor *R*eceptor 2.

It is important to note that this mutation is not hereditary but the result of an environmental cause of unknown origin.

Clinically, with people who express this, what we typically see is a pattern of breast cancer that is much more aggressive than the other types. It can spread rapidly.

Normally, the HER2 gene tells a cell to produce a protein that acts as a growth factor receptor on the cell surface. In breast cancer with the HER2 mutation, a damaged cell will continue to multiply copies of the gene, sometimes as many as 30 copies.

This causes a dangerous chain reaction: the cancerous cell overproduces the protein, which leads to excessive growth factor receptors on the cell surface, which leads to increased cell division, which means a high rate of tumor growth.

The balance of the article goes on to describe how the drug Herceptin plugs the receptor cites, blocks the growth factor and stops cell division.

The treatment is not a cure. Weekly injections are required to maintain the person in that condition. No further mention is made of the *"environmental cause of unknown origin."* No further mention is made as to how the excessive growth factor receptors result in cancer. No mention is made of what the receptors receive although growth factors are assumed. Obviously, cancer is caused by what they receive, not because they are receptors. The problem is **not hereditary** but the *"result of an environmental cause of unknown origin."*

Wouldn't it make sense to analyze the cellular environment to find out what is causing the so-called defective gene? Is there any reason to ignore the possibility of enzymes from fungi and bacteria as being the environmental cause of unknown origin?

There is no discussion as to what causes the cell to produce more receptors. We are left to assume it must be defective genes by references within the article to "genetically haywire" cells.

A reader is led to conclude cancer is caused because genetically haywire cells express excessive duplication of proteins. If the protein is a growth factor receptor, it leads to increased rate of cell division.

Let's list the major concepts concerning genes and breast cancer as described by this article on Herceptin:

1. Cancer results from an excessive amount of "human growth factor receptors" and these receptors can be found "on the cell's surface." The defective gene is only implied by saying "genetically haywire".

2. The gene creates up to 30 copies of the growth receptor protein on each cell wall.

3. Mutation is not hereditary but is the result of an environmental cause of unknown origin.

It is obvious that the genes are not defective in their DNA genetic structure or in the expression of receptors. The gene is assumed defective because it produces too many repetitions of standard and functional parts on the cell surface. The DNA in the nucleus is normal and functional. Only the regulatory genes are defective. Regulatory genes overdo the job of producing growth factor receptors and position them on the cell's surface in direct contact with the intracellular nutrients and hormones where they normally occur. Where is the defect in that?

Perhaps the regulatory genes are not defective. Perhaps the regulatory genes are responding, as they should, to an abundance of growth factors in the intracellular environment. Perhaps parasites are mutating the cell wall with additional growth factor receptors for a purpose.

The abundance of cell-wall receptors creates a problem similar to the problem of which came first, the chicken or the egg. Did defective genes produce far too many growth factor receptors first or did regulatory genes sense an abundance of growth hormone and express additional receptors? Without scientific data to indicate why excessive growth factor receptors are produced, there is no reason to conclude they are due to defective genes. The medical conclusion simply does not make sense.

There is considerable evidence to indicate that an increase in growth factor receptors is a result of an increase in growth hormone. In growth hormone therapy, for example, a therapeutic increase in growth hormone is known to cause a corresponding increase in growth hormone receptors on the cell wall. Regulatory genes sense the environment and respond with additional growth receptors. No defective genes are involved or required to explain this phenomenon.

Growth hormone therapy increases growth hormone receptors

Dr. Ronald Klatz is considered America's leading authority on anti-aging medicine and has written several books on the use of human growth hormone to stop or slow the aging process. During an appearance on an American talk show with host Debbie Day, Dr. Klatz related the following significant finding about growth factor receptors on cell walls. An audiocassette of this interview is available to promote use of growth hormones for health purposes and this information is taken from that source.

Dr. Klatz said that he compared cells from a young person to cells from an older person and found them very similar except for one major difference. The cell from the young person had far more growth factor receptors on the cell wall than did cells from the older person. However, after providing growth hormone therapy with human growth hormone for the older person, the cells from the older person had a significant increase in the number of growth factor receptors.

The significant point is that increased receptors in the cell wall emerged AFTER the known therapeutic increase in levels of growth hormone in the cell nutrients. The genes were not defective. Cancer did not result simply because cells had an abundance of growth factor receptors. Since the cellular environment contained oxygen, and only genes for aerobic metabolism were expressed, fermentation and cancer did not occur.

Dr. Klatz's growth hormone research shows that an increase in the quantity of growth factor receptors on the cell wall follows from signals in the environment. Genes are not defective. They are responding as nature intended.

In establishing the cause of cancer without an analysis of the cellular environment for microbial growth hormone, there is no scientific reason to assert that genes are defective. If microbial DNA polymerase will cause human DNA to replicate, it is safe to assume that microbial growth factors would also cause an increase in the number of growth factor receptors on the cell wall.

Estrogen therapy increases estrogen receptors in cell wall

In *Harper's Review of Biochemistry* (Page 533), we find a direct reference to a similar increase of cell-wall receptors *following* estrogen therapy.

> Both uterine and mammary gland tissues contain membrane receptors for oxytocin. The number of these receptors is increased by estrogens and decreased by progesterone.

Estrogen increases and progesterone decreases the number of receptors for oxytocin. Genes do not make excessive repeats of perfectly normal hormone receptors without just cause. The increase in the quantity of receptors is a response to increased signals in the cellular environment. The increase in receptors indicates that an increase in hormone levels has occurred and the regulatory genes are functioning normally.

Let's look at the names for these defective genes. Some women have defective genes BRCA1 and BRCA2 (*BR*east *CA*ncer genes 1 and 2). The name for these defective genes is simply based on function because no one can identify the location of them.

Let's look at how true defective genes are identified. Known defective genes are numbered according to their location in chromosome and by the type of genetic disorder. For example, myotonic dystrophy is a disease in which the muscles fail to relax after use, due to a genetic fault. For this disease, researchers found that myotonic dystrophy was worsening with each generation because the gene was expanding. The gene for the disorder, in chromosome 19, has an area rich in the DNA trinucleotide CTG, which is repeated over and over, like a molecular stutter. (The explanation for all this medical terminology will be found in Chapter 7, *Defective Genes Produce Defective Human Parts, Not Cancer.*)

The important issue is how the defective genes that supposedly cause breast cancer are identified and named. There are many defective gene conditions in which the defective gene has not been isolated and recognized precisely. Genetic researchers have devised a mapping guide to locate defective genes on a chromosome. The method is called an *ideogram* and enables defective gene locations to be identified by chromosome number, arm location, relative position in major regions already identified, and finally the specific location or loci.

However, the so-called defective genes causing breast cancer through excessive growth factors have not been identified by chromosome location and genetic fault. Instead, they are simply identified by their apparent dysfunction and classified as "genetically haywire."

Even the names suggest they do not know anything about the genetic fault. BRCA stands for "BReast CAncer". The letters do not refer to any genetic code relating to defective genes. The name is just made up to describe the observed result. Do the numerals 1 and 2 in BRCA 1 and BRCA 2 designate different genetic faults or are these simply left and right breasts? I really do not know. I have not been able to find any scientific description of the defects based on chromosome location or structural fault in these so-called defective genes. Another pair of breast cancer genes is called HER1 and HER2 (*H*uman *E*pidermal growth factor *R*eceptor genes 1 and 2). Human Epidermal Receptor does nothing to identify the gene's location or structural defect.

In the book *Biotechnology Unzipped*, by Eric Grace, we find reference to regulatory genes controlling gene expression. He explains how the bacteria

Escherichia coli can metabolize either lactose or glucose sugars for energy depending on the sugar in the environment of the cell (Page 44):

> In bacteria, we now know that certain genes are turned on or off according to the conditions in which the microorganisms are growing. By tying gene expression to environmental cues, the bacteria don't waste energy and materials making products they don't need.

In the case of this bacteria, it has been shown that the cellular environment signals the cell to turn specific genes on or off. It is highly possible that the same process occurs with so-called breast cancer genes. The concept that defective regulatory genes cause an excess number of growth hormone receptors has not been proven and the genetic defects have not been identified. Moreover, several similar conditions are known to be caused by the cellular environment such as growth hormone therapy and estrogen therapy.

Why are the receptors normal and functional if produced by defective genes? If regulatory genes in bacteria produce different enzymes according to the slight difference between lactose and glucose sugars, isn't it reasonable to assume that growth hormone receptors in human cells are a result of regulatory genes recognizing excess growth factor in the cellular environment? The unknown environmental factor must be from a living thing with DNA and DNA polymerase in order to control or speed replication. In my opinion, all indicators point to low-level microbial parasites as the cause of too many growth factor receptors.

This important point is very significant to women with so-called defective genes. There is a biological reason for the increased expression or abundance of growth factor receptors beyond genes and heredity. This biological reason—growth factors from parasites—can be controlled or eliminated. Your genes are not defective. There is simply an excessive amount of growth hormone available.

If the environmental factors that caused the genes to over-express the number of receptors were of human origin in an aerobic environment, the growth would result in cells dependent on oxygen for metabolism. Large but not cancerous breasts would result. There is no scientific reason for these cells to switch from oxidation to fermentation simply because there is an abundance of growth factor.

Research has not proven that defective genes cause any type of cancer. The whole concept that defective genes cause an excess quantity of growth factor receptors that cause cancer is without scientific validity. This is one of the areas of misinformation that must be dealt with as soon as possible. Every woman in North America should fight to eliminate this form of cancer treatment. Chapter 22 in this book, *Ruthless ongoing suppression of effective cancer cures* lists several better options.

Essiac and other proven herbal remedies for cancer

There are hundreds of case histories in which women have eliminated lumps and cancer in their breasts by taking the herbal formula called essiac. Essiac has herbs that are antifungal and antiparasitic. When these herbs are brewed for twelve hours as a tea, the tea appears to develop essential enzymes needed to kill fungi and cancer cells. The tea also contains essential trace minerals such as potassium that helps revive the oxygenation process.

People without cancers, who drink this tea, report a large increase in energy, better sleep, and improved digestion. These qualities can account for the beneficial effects of essiac and other herbal remedies. By combining essiac with other cancer treatments designed to stop fermentation and kill parasites electronically, you can stop cancer and prevent the reoccurrence. By taking essiac as a cancer preventative, one can help avoid cancer. In the story of Rene Caisse called *I Was Canada's Cancer Nurse*, Rene Caisse reports that none of her relatives died of cancer, if they took essiac to prevent cancer.

Anyone wishing more information on essiac should read *The Essence of Essiac* written by Sheila Snow. Mrs. Snow worked with Rene Caisse in the Bracebridge Cancer clinic before the clinic was shut down by the Canadian Medical Association. Mrs. Snow is probably the world's best source of information on essiac. Her book describes the chemical constituents of the four herbs used by Rene Caisse and explains how to identify quality herbs for making your own tea. These four herbs are sheep sorrel, burdock root, slippery elm bark, and Turkey rhubarb root. The exact formula used by Rene Caisse is well known and there is no such thing as a "counterfeit formula" on the market. Some companies have trademarked the essiac name, and this provides them with exclusive use of the name, but not of the product.

I find that the best that can be said of essiac is that it works for some of the people but not everyone. It also works for some people for some of the time and appears to lose its effectiveness. The fungi and bacteria may become immune to it, just as they do with other antibiotics. In addition, the problem may be in the herbs, processing, or storage. If the herbs are finely powdered the nutrients may be oxidized and lost long before the tea is made.

If you are making your own essiac from purchased herbs, your tea should have a strong aroma and should give you a lift. There are many good suppliers of these herbs but some supplies are too old by the time they are used. No one has a patent on the formula and anyone can assemble these herbs effectively when they know what to look for and what to avoid. Sheila Snow's book is ideal for this purpose.

Most cancers (if not all), start with precancerous growths in the forms of lumps, ulcers, polyps and the like. Upon diagnoses of these growths as benign tumors, if mainstream medicine would advise a series of colonics (colon cleansing), a parasite-cleansing program along with mineral supplements and balanced nutrition, these pre-cancerous conditions could be eliminated. Medical check-ups should focus on identifying mineral deficiencies, pollutants, and parasites, with recommendations to correct the cellular environmental causes that lead to cancer.

Instead, cancer tumors are allowed to develop. The focus then moves to 'gene therapy' drugs to block the growth factor receptors, or chemotherapy to poison all rapidly growing cells. If suitable the tumors are radiated or removed surgically along with the organ or body part.

Cancer victims are advised that modern medicine is *scientific*, and we are warned to be wary of *quacks* in the alternative health fields or clinics in Mexico. Warning people to stay away from unapproved therapies automatically includes warning them to stay away from effective therapies that are not approved for economic or other reasons.

Successful cancer operations are ones that remove the infected organ, tissue, or bone so that infection cannot spread or return. This is a costly way to eliminate an infection. When you review the success rate of mainstream medicine for various types of cancer, if we rejected those that deformed the body or removed essential parts, what would the success rate be?

Alternative cancer therapies are available to eliminate the infection that causes cancer while saving the body parts. Why not use them?

5. How microbial enzymes cause mutation of cell-wall membranes

The purpose of this chapter is to review the function of growth enzymes or growth hormones in the process of cancer. Textbooks claim that enzymes control all chemical functions in the body, and therefore enzymes must control replication of DNA. Mainstream cancer researchers are looking for the elusive oncogene that produces the chemical signal for DNA to replicate. I believe I can prove that the chemical signal does not exist because replication of DNA is controlled by an electrical stimulus.

There is a fundamental misconception in mainstream medicine that enzymes initiate DNA replication. This error leads to the search for drugs to control the enzymes and genes that cause out-of-control replication of DNA. Viruses are assumed to cause defective genes or excessive replication of normal genes is assumed to lead to out-of-control replication of cells.

Dr. Hulda Clark believes that the growth hormone from parasites contaminates human cells and causes DNA to replicate. This conclusion seems so logical, that I wrote most of this book while believing that growth hormones from parasites caused human cells to replicate. Further research shows that this concept needs revision, although the error has no bearing on the cure for cancer. The cure for cancer remains the same whether microbes cause cells to replicate and mutate, or just cause cells to mutate.

The current of injury or normal growth—an electrical stimulant—causes DNA to replicate. Growth hormones control only the assembly of new cells, and microbial growth hormones and proteins mutate the cell-wall membrane during the assembly process. Mitosis of infected cells, whether through injury or normal growth, leads to mutated cell-wall membranes and cancer.

Benign growths occur if the growth is due to normal growth or replication of cells following a small injury. Cancer occurs if the current of injury is large and stays on because an injury is not repaired with suitable new cells. The current of injury is required to initiate replication because an ionic energy field is required to break the weak ionic hydrogen bonds the form the DNA bases and genes.

Cancer is the continuous multiplication, mutation, and rejection of cells. In fully grown adults, multiplication is initiated by the autonomic nervous system to repair a membrane injury. Mutation is initiated by microbial infection during the assembly of the new cell-wall membrane. Rejection of muted cells is initiated by the immune system because cells with mutated cell walls cannot bond to normal cells and repair the membrane injury. Tumors form from the continued growth and multiplication of mutated cells. The amazing feature about cancer is that neither virus nor defective genes are the primary cause of cancer.

Viruses are a secondary cause of cancer in two major ways. Virus cause 'so called' benign growths that create a current of injury when the growth is torn or damaged, and virus overload the immune system allowing bacterial, fungal, and parasitic infection to occur. Viruses create the conditions for infection and membrane injury; bacterial and fungal infection cause mutated cell-wall membranes. Mainstream medicine holds that viruses do not cause cancer directly, viruses only cause mutated genes that cause cancer. In reality, viruses cause benign growths such as warts. Rupture of benign growths causes cancer.

For example, the *Home Medical Encyclopedia* in reference to cervical cancer states:

> Cancer of the cervix (neck of the uterus) is one of the most common cancers affecting women worldwide, and in many areas is becoming more common... Cervical cancer has well-defined precancerous stages. Before any cancer appears, abnormal changes in cells on the surface of the cervix, referred to as dysplasia, can be detected by a cervical smear test. (Dysplasia is defined as any abnormal growth with cell features including abnormal size, shape, and rate of multiplication of cells.)

Obviously, intercourse could rupture benign growths in the uterus. The relationship between virus and cancer is similar to the relationship between influenza and opportunistic bacterial infections. The viral influenza infection, in the weak and elderly, further weakens the immune system allowing bacterial and fungal infections to occur. The flu virus does not kill directly. Opportunistic infections of larger parasites lead to illness and death such as from fungal and bacterial toxins.

The current of injury initiates cellular replication

Robert O. Becker, M.D. and Gary Seldon have written one of the most provocative books available today. It is called *The Body Electric* and deals with *Electromagnetism and the Foundation of Life*. Life is an electromagnetic phenomenon with its foundation in the electromagnetic spectrum.

Electromagnetism is normally a study of physics, not biology. Replication of DNA, however, is an electromagnetic phenomenon driven by electric energy produced in and by the body.

The fundamental cause for replication of damaged epithelial tissue as well as the cause for replication of cancer cells is the same. Research shows that the electrical energies around damaged skin tissue is significantly higher than that around normal tissue. The following three points can be found on pages 64 to 67 of Becker's book. I have summarized the major points here for convenience.

Study of the current of injury goes back to the time of Luigi Galvani who in 1794 observed that the muscles of a frog's leg contracted when an electrical device in the room made sparks. The muscles would only contract when an assistant held a steel scalpel against the nerve of the frog he was dissecting while the machine produced sparks. Further research showed that there was a high energy level around an injury and this energy became known as the 'current of injury'.

About 1868, after development of the galvanometer to measure an electric current, Julius Bernstein determined that the energy was not in the nerves. The energy was a property of membranes and consisted not of a current but a disturbance in the ionic properties within a field of energy surrounding the membrane cells.

In the late 1950's a Russian researcher (A.V. Shirmunski of the Institute of Cytology in Leningrad) studied the mechanism for new cell growth and discovered that the current of injury was responsible for stimulating new growth at the point of injury. He observed that the current of injury is proportional to the extent of injury and that regeneration is proportional to the current of injury. Healthy people heal faster than worn and feeble people heal due to a stronger current of injury.

The ionic properties of membrane cells have become a major field of interest for alternative health specialists. It is used for testing the health of an individual and the alignment of the body. Many mysteries need to be answered. For example, if you store credit cards in a wallet made of eel skin, the ionic properties of the skin will destroy your credit card magnetic imprint, even though the eel is long since dead. How is this energy stored in dead cells that have been preserved through the leather making process?

Membrane walls contain rows of phosphate molecules that form energy meridians. The term 'plasma membrane' is now used to identify these membranes because of the high energy levels. Mitochondria, the energy producing organelles within the cell, also have a two-layered membrane with membrane panels proceeding into the cell. What is it about mitochondria that make them the powerhouse of the cell? Research also shows that the cell nucleus has a continuous two-layered membrane with numerous openings to allow passage of RNA.

Cell-wall membranes are diploid layers of phosphate molecules and with two lipid layers and proteins dissolved in the lipids. Membrane walls have electrical properties that serve as electrical conduits called meridians and store ionic energy for emergencies. Healthy individuals have a higher energy reserve than unhealthy people because they have more ionic energy in storage and can produce energy quickly if needed.

The immune system is an ionic energy system. The field of alternative medicine, with measurement of energy systems in the body using muscle testing or electro-dermal devices is largely based on this phenomenon. Energy testing and balance will become the medicine of the future because most physical diseases result from disturbances to the primitive ionic energy storage and distribution system of the body. This phenomenon is largely ignored by mainstream medicine. Licensed medical doctors who treat patients with ionic energy devices tend to lose their medical license rather quickly. One of the charges by the Ontario Medical Association against Dr. Joseph Krop is the use of an electro-dermal testing device. Not only is electomedicine ignored by mainstream medicine. It is openly suppressed.

The nervous system of primitive life forms (parasites) runs on ionic energy. Single celled life forms do not develop nerves and ganglions, which are a special type of cell for controlled currents of energy to signal desired changes such as movement in large bodies.

Animals with billions of cells have two major nervous systems. The first to be developed was the primitive, direct current membrane and invisible meridian system that connects every cell in the body to the primitive brain stem. This autonomic connection is made through the electrical properties of phosphate molecules in membrane walls connected through the electrolytes in the body fluids. The cell-wall membranes are the nerves because energy travels along the outside of the phosphate molecules. It is similar to having an FM radio signal travel along the wires that conduct electricity throughout the home.

The second more visible energy pathway connects every cell in the body to the brain. This nervous system relates to the human person and his or her control of human actions. The visible nerves for this system use alternating current that is easily measured by modern electronic devices.

Some primitive functions, such as orientation of the body, equilibrium and balance have developed visible neurons for this essential function, but these nerves are not part of the main system. These nerves are called the 'vestibular apparatus' (see Guyton, pages 641-643) because they conduct the 'vestibular ionic energy' from the 'vestibular hydrogen bond'. All of these terms will be developed later in the text. The point is that all this information about ionic energy distribution in the body is well known but ignored by mainstream medicine. The Chinese acupuncturists have used this knowledge for over 5000 years with great success.

Millions of people who suffer from ringing in the ears and loss of balance (Meniere's Syndrome) are suffering from a disturbance to the vestibular apparatus. The problem is considered incurable by mainstream medicine because drugs cannot be found to solve the problem. Many side effects of toxic drugs such as dizziness are related to damage of the autonomic functions such as balance. Check the side effects of any prescription drug and note how many side effects destroy essential, life-giving autonomic functions or cause dizziness.

Meniere's Syndrome and psychotic illnesses have been cured by improved nutrition. Orthomolecular physicians such as Dr. Abram Hoffer have made significant advances in curing mental illnesses, but these gains are also ignored and suppressed in favor of drugs.

How the current of injury specifically initiates replication is not known. It is known that salamanders, for example, can grow a new foot or tail. The blood of salamanders is different from mammals because the red blood cells have DNA molecules within their membrane wall. Mammalian red blood cells do not. It has been found that the red blood cells of salamanders, when placed in an ionic field, start to multiply. Red blood cells containing DNA will replicate and the red blood cells will become the new tissue, including flesh, bone and cartilage. Precisely how this is accomplished is not known, especially if one refuses to consider the part the life-force has in controlling replication. Something must exist that controls all new growth so that it corresponds to the needs of the body. If the life-force or spirit is considered as an ionic or wave field with intelligence, communication through the ionic hydrogen bonds in DNA would provide a feasible concept. Without the influence of the life-force, there is no logical way to contain the growth so that body parts are replaced correctly. Assuming the existence of controller genes only places the problem at a different level as we need something to control the controller genes.

In the text, *Magnetism and its Effects on the Living System* by authors Albert Davis and Walter Rawls, Jr., we have a possible explanation to describe how a current of injury causes DNA to replicate. Magnets can give iron in red blood cells a polarity, or make atoms containing iron more magnetic by organizing or polarizing the atomic forces within cells. Perhaps the DNA in a current of injury ionic field becomes more highly energized through polarization, which leads to replication. Polarization patterns are governed by the pattern inherent in the life-force. Here is what is written (Page 7):

> Taking whole blood, then spinning off the fluids and plasmas, leaving the red cells, presents a very remarkable piece of evidence as to the effect of magnetism on life fluids. Take some of the resultant red blood and place on a microscope slide in a good powered microscope, focus, bring up under the slide's bottom one end of a magnet. Note that the red blood cells all spin around in the same direction. *This is polarization of the red blood cells.*

Perhaps the hidden force that causes genes and DNA to replicate in red blood cells arises from polarization of the red blood cells. Similarly, polarization of the DNA crystalloid molecules could increase the energy level to initiate the process of gene expression, RNA production and DNA replication. If the combination of nucleotides in a DNA base is polarized, the weak hydrogen bonds holding them together are not strong enough to resist the increased magnetic forces of repulsion. Polarization of DNA molecules causes genes to separate because the ionic bond would be cancelled out. The increased ionic field would cause the DNA nucleotides to separate. DNA polymerase and other enzymes would then control assembly of cell components.

In a cancer cell, if the dominant protein for cell-wall membrane assembly is chitin produced by fungi, for example, the dominant traits of the new cell will have membrane traits of a fungal, mushroom-like growth. In order to prove or disprove this speculation, one need only compare the electrical characteristics of normal human cells-wall membrane to that of the bacteria or fungi found to be infecting the cancer cell. If cell wall molecules are found in both the microbial cell wall and the human cell-wall membrane of the rejected cells, we will have proof of the precise cause of cancer.

Combining these observations into a single theory, cancer starts in epithelial tissue when injury (normally from parasites or nutritional imbalance) causes internal bleeding. The injury causes a current of injury or an ionic field of energy that initiates replication of DNA in adjacent cells and microbes. Cancer starts in conjunction with trapped blood sugar because fermentation of glucose allows fungi and bacteria to deprive adjacent cells of vital oxygen sufficient for oxidative metabolism. The current of injury is the driving force that causes DNA to replicate but fungi and bacteria cause the cell wall to mutate. Fermentation of protein creates low oxygen levels in adjacent cells allowing anaerobic microbes to spread and cells to function on fermentation of glycogen, instead of oxidation of glycogen. The fermentation process also produces high-energy molecules that are used to convert glucose to chitin to build primitive cell-wall membranes.

In the book *Life, The Unfinished Experiment*, by Nobel Prize winner Salvador E. Luria, we find reference to the crystalloid structure of membranes such as skin, and the importance of cells to form crystal-like structures. Cell-wall membranes must be fluid enough to provide cell function and flexibly, but solid enough to contain the cell contents and give it form. The cell wall determines cell function, and expressed genes determine cell-wall structure. That is why a single fertilized egg cell can differentiate into all the different cells making up the human body. That is why a cancer-microbe can mutate the assembly of a cell and cause cancer. The assembly process of a cell membrane is based on the mechanical, crystal-forming laws of magnetic attraction. The mutated cell membrane is rejected, like an attempt by a surgeon to replace an organ or repair skin damage with skin from any other life-form or person. Although organs can be transplanted, skin cells must come from another part of the body, or an identical twin with the identical skin cell-wall membranes. Even a minute invisible change in the cell wall relating to ionic energy fields will cause the new cells to be rejected.

In *Life, The Unfinished Experiment* (Page 97, my italics added for emphasis), we read:

A survey of the assembly processes within cells—to produce enzyme molecules, complexes of enzymes, tubes, filaments, shells, and membranes—reveals no directive mechanism for creating them other than the play of the molecules themselves. Like the growth of a crystal, the sculptural work of the cell is fully automatic. But unlike crystal growth, the outcomes of the assembly process are wonderfully diverse because they reflect the enormous diversity of the molecules that take part in it. The assembled products—even the geometrical shells of viruses—resemble not crystals but works of art…. *The crystals of the inorganic world stem from the workings of immutable physical forces of attraction upon a limited variety of atoms and molecules. The sculptural features of living organisms are created by the same physical forces acting on the innumerable molecular species made available by the genes.*

An understanding of the disease process for all microbial diseases, and fungal mycotoxins ingested or inhaled, rests on this one vital statement: "…the crystals of the inorganic (and organic) world, stem from the immutable physical forces of attraction within molecules". The contamination of human cell parts with microbial structural equivalents results in disease. It follows that the cure for all diseases is to stop the exchange of microbial proteins and enzymes for human cellular proteins and enzymes. The cure for disease lies within repair to the autonomic nervous system through metabolism, trace minerals, essential fatty acids, and elimination of toxins. Increased oxygen is one of the most significant contributions to better health.

Getting back to the previous text, Lauria goes on to say (Page 112):

...Slightly different versions of a gene will produce slightly different proteins, which are often equal or nearly so in effectiveness of function....A few hundred molecules of a foreign protein on the surface of a cell can cause the production of enough antibodies to destroy all cells of that alien type.

Please note the point: "a few hundred molecules on the surface of a cell" can lead to an autoimmune attack. The error in the medical concept of autoimmune diseases, now accounting for about 80 diseases, is evident in the above quotation. The immune system is not attacking healthy cells. The body's defense mechanism is attacking mutated cells, perhaps these cells have small gaps in the ionic energy fields due to missing phosphate molecules. Such gaps are identified as genetic defects in order to support defective gene theories. The substitution of primitive chitin molecules in cell-wall membranes is all that is needed to create an apparent autoimmune disease. The problem is not one of defective genes. The 30 per cent of breast cancers caused by defective genes HER1 or 2, and BRCA1 or 2 are good examples. As we shall see later, these genetic defects do not exist.

The cancer cell traits and function can be totally understood as a replacement of human proteins by microbial proteins in the cell-wall membrane. Indeed, all so-called autoimmune diseases can also be understood in this way. The greater simplicity of bacterial DNA, unencumbered by a nucleus and long chains of genes, allows for production of proteins, such as membrane wall proteins, at a rate ten times faster than that of the human cell. In the roughly nine-hour period of production and assembly of a new daughter cell, the bacterial components have a significant quantitative advantage to mutate the cell-wall membrane, or other functional proteins, during assembly. The body produces a current of injury that causes replication of DNA, in both human cells and parasites infecting the cell. Enzymes from the human cell may control assembly, but these enzymes may also select microbial molecules in place of normal molecules. The resultant defect would appear to be a defective gene problem. In truth, it is only a microbial induced fault due to microbial infection.

Cancer is a perfectly natural process of replication altered by microbial infection and contamination during cell division. With each succeeding division, more of the human traits are lost and more of the primitive repressed genes are expressed. Cells dedifferentiate into aggressive cancer cells capable of replicating faster and faster, as more and more unnecessary DNA strings are abandoned.

In *Asimov's New Guide to Science* (Page 575), in a chapter on proteins, we learn how proteins that are similar in form can replace one-another. The process is called *competitive inhibition,* and describes, for example, how malonic acid inhibits citric-acid cycle enzymes by filling in the position meant for another protein. For cancer to develop, all that is needed is for bacteria or fungi to produce a cell-wall protein that replaces the position of the human protein designed for the enzyme that builds the cell membrane. Since bacteria have cell-wall membranes similar to human cells, the proteins they produce are enzymatically compatible for cell wall growth. The problem of out-of-control replication develops later when these hybrid cells are rejected by normal cells and the injury does not heal. Due to some retained similarities in cell wall construction, the immune system does not recognize the mutated cells as invaders. They are allowed to multiply freely providing they are in a low-oxygen environment. If oxygen levels are increased, oxygen attacks the cell-wall membranes where the ionic field is absent. That is why anaerobic microbes are destroyed by oxygen and why increased oxygen or ozone kills cancer cells.

Do not underestimate the importance of this observation that enzymes do not cause replication of DNA. This observation explains why all people with parasites do not get cancer, and why cancer cannot be initiated by inoculating healthy tissue with cancer microbes. Cancer occurs only when the current of injury and infection of cells combine to mutate the normal process. This observation also explains how large parasites, such as flukes, cause cancer by creating holes or injury in epithelial cells. This observation also destroys the major pillar in the false theory that defective genes cause cancer. There is no longer any need to assume existence of an oncogene that signals DNA to replicate out of control. Financial support of research on the cause of cancer, relating to genes, enzymes, and DNA is a waste of money.

Enzymes only control chemical actions between atoms and molecules in which electrons are exchanged or electron orbits are shared. The sphere of influence of an enzyme is far too limited to cause a large gene to divide. The DNA nucleotide *ionic hydrogen bonds,* do not fall within the function of enzymes because genes are too large. Enzyme function is limited to controlling bonds between atoms and molecules.

The purines to pyrimidine bonds in DNA are long strings of *ionic hydrogen bonds* in which no electrons are shared. The ionic hydrogen bond is about $1/20^{th}$ as strong as a normal chemical bond. This weak bond disintegrates in the presence of an ionic field. Control of the energy field provides the life-force of the body with control of DNA replication and maintains the integrity of the body.

Injury to epithelial tissue breaks the ionic-energy field of the cell-wall membranes, and creates a current of injury that polarizes molecules in DNA crystals. This is nature's signal to repair the injury by multiplying adjacent cells. The ionic hydrogen bonds in DNA are broken by an ionic field, not enzymes. The ionic current of injury is the only natural force that will initiate out-of-control division of the DNA nucleotides.

Research by Robert Becker shows that batteries implanted in tissue will also initiate replication of DNA. This research will be reviewed in the next chapter.

Once the hydrogen bonds between the pyrimidine and purine molecules of DNA are broken, the growth hormones and growth factors commence to assemble new nucleotides from the pool of atoms and molecules in the cytoplasm. After separation of DNA molecules, the process switches to chemical bonding controlled by enzymes and driven by the electromagnetic forces within atoms and molecules.

DNA will not replicate without a growth hormone

One of the more important facts concerning multiplication of cancer cells is that cancer tissue cells in cultures will not multiply without a growth hormone in the nutrients. This proves that cancer is dependent on growth hormone from an external source. The cause of cell replication cannot be found within the DNA structure of cells if an external growth factor is required to manage replication. The DNA polymerase enzyme is called a polymerase because it helps build strings of molecules. This vital step cannot occur in the absence of this enzyme.

Dr. Alexis Carrel, a French physiologist, kept cells from a chicken in a petri dish alive for 28 years. Since he maintained the conditions required for oxidation of glycogen by adding fresh blood every day, these cells did not die nor did fermentation occur. Without the addition of a growth hormone, these cells did not replicate and grow into larger masses. Even after 20 years, much longer than the normal life span of chickens, these cells did not die or multiply. Carrel concluded that life of a cell is eternal providing conditions for life are maintained. These cells did not have a cell-clock or cell-cycle that initiated replication from time to time.

Replication is always dependent upon enzymes that cause DNA to assemble new strands. Life does not arise spontaneously from chemicals and food nutrients, because chemicals do not contain DNA polymerase enzyme. Only living things have DNA. Therefore, only living things can produce DNA polymerase enzyme to cause cancer or other growths.

Calf serum used to cause cancer replication in petri dishes

In the text on cancer by Drs. Varmus and Weinberg, *Genes and the Biology of Cancer (Page 41)*, the authors state:

... All mammalian cells, normal or cancerous, require a common set of nutrients, including glucose, vitamins and amino acids. But these alone usually do not suffice in culture, and calf serum is almost always required to complete the cocktail. Calf serum does not contain nutrients but instead supplies so-called growth factors that stimulate the cells to divide in culture. As we shall see in chapter 6, these serum growth factors mimic similar factors used by cells in normal tissues to stimulate each other's growth. In their absence, cells will be viable, with an active metabolism, but will not proliferate.

Pause for a moment to reflect on the above statement: *"Cancer cells will be viable...but will not proliferate."* If you were a cancer researcher, and you knew all cancerous cells, in vitro or in bodies, require growth hormones in order to proliferate, you would know that growth hormones are required to cause cancer. If you simply connected this knowledge with the knowledge that bacterial DNA polymerase is used to cause human DNA to replicate in a test tube, you would theorize that microbial enzymes could cause cancer. How could cancer researchers not connect the two observations?

It is possible that both bacteria or fungi provide the DNA polymerase enzyme, but I cannot find any direct references to researchers using DNA polymerase from fungi to support replication of DNA in test tubes. Bacterial life forms are always present in cancer cells. In either case, microbes and parasites are the only logical source for growth factors of unknown origin. I have never read one statement in medical literature that microbial growth hormones could be related to the cause of cancer. Have you? How could this have happened without a direct and purposeful effort to avoid such speculation?

Why haven't cancer researchers discovered microbial growth hormones in cancer patients? Cancer research is filled with terms such as "growth factor of an unknown source" or "insulin-like growth factor" or "growth factor receptors" in recognition of a growth factor being present in most types of cancer. Why are there so many cancers with growth factors of unknown origin? Let's consider these two main reasons.

(1) All living things use the same or very similar DNA polymerase enzyme for DNA replication. It is not easy to identify the source by viewing the enzyme for specific features. If DNA is in the process of replicating, we must assume the enzyme is present. Any source will do.

(2) The cellular environment causes cancer. The source of the growth hormone is not the cause of cancer. Calf serum is used in laboratories to cause cancer growth in glass containers. Bacterial growth factors are used for growth hormone therapy in humans. Growth hormones only support replication. For mainstream medicine to publicly acknowledge that microbial growth hormone plays a part in cancer would destroy the mystery about cancer.

In the future, when you read "growth factor of unknown origin" in cancer information, consider the unknown source to be from an "unknown species" of fungi or bacteria.

Past generations followed a routine spring and fall parasites cleanse program but our present generation does not. In the past meat was always well cooked and cloves or garlic was inserted into pork roasts. Cloves and garlic were two herbs most often associated with parasite cleansing. Most people are not aware of the cancer-parasite connection because mainstream medicine refuses to publicize this vital information. The same issue applies to all degenerative diseases caused by fungi and mycotoxins in our body. Mycotoxins are microbial enzymes that interfere with human cell functions. They are the cause of degenerative diseases. Parasites thrive for years in host bodies without causing an infection or death because it is in their interest not to destroy their host. Nevertheless, they continue to mutate cell wall membranes and cell functions.

Growth hormones and insulin serve as active transport mechanisms to carry amino acid proteins through the cell wall. The proteins transported by insulin are different than those transported by growth hormone. In Guyton's *Textbook of Medical Physiology* we can see diagrams illustrating that the growth rate of rats was near zero when either insulin or growth hormone was deprived. Growth only occurred when both insulin and growth hormone was available in adequate amounts.

We also learn that the control of insulin is regulated not only by the level of glucose in the blood, but also by other factors such as the level of lipids and proteins. Guyton writes (Page 965):

Formerly, it was believed that insulin secretion is controlled almost entirely by the blood glucose concentration. However, as more has been learned about the metabolic functions of insulin for protein and fat metabolism, it has been learned that blood amino acids and other factors also play important roles in controlling insulin secretion.

Amazingly, since my copy of the above textbook was printed in 1981, this information is more than 20 years old and I have never seen it mentioned in any publication for public knowledge. Have you? The significance of this information is that IGF (*Insulin Like Growth Factor)* is probably normal insulin transporting proteins to the cell wall of cancer cells.

One of the most effective diet books available today is called *Enter The Zone* by Barry Sears and Bill Lawren. The basic concept behind this nutritional advice is to maintain a balanced diet consisting of 40 percent carbohydrates, 30 percent fat and 30 per cent protein. If you have an excess of any one of these, you cannot metabolize these nutrients as well and you disturb enzyme balance in your body. In addition, excess nutrients are converted to fat. It is not only the quantity of food you consume that makes you fat, it is the ratio of fats, proteins and carbohydrates.

The importance of this information should not be overlooked as part of the cure for cancer as well as many other diseases. Here's what Sears has to say about a retired IBM executive named Chris (Page 6):

> But Chris's "golden years" weren't so golden. Not only had he developed diabetes, but he had high blood pressure; he'd already had a heart attack and was stricken with kidney cancer. "In 1992" he wrote me later, "my weight was 265 pounds, my blood pressure without medication was 220/120, my blood sugar was over 200 mg/dl, my right kidney had been removed because of cancer, and my left kidney showed signs of abnormal cells."

> Today, after two years on a Zone-favorable diet, Chris writes: "My weight is 176 pounds, my blood pressure is 70-90 mg/dl, I have no sign of my previous diabetic retinopathy, and my remaining kidney is free of any sign of cancer.

How can a single switch in dietary habits result in so many health benefits? The answer lies in normalizing the hormone levels in the body by eating the proper balance of carbohydrates, proteins and fats. The fact that insulin levels are controlled by protein levels as well as glucose levels, and that insulin carries proteins into cell walls is critically important information. Instead, the heart and stroke industry tells patients to increase carbohydrate intake and reduce fats and proteins to control cholesterol. Diabetics are advised to eat a high-complex-carbohydrate diet. This advice is wrong.

The fact that both insulin and growth hormones serve as protein transport mechanisms essential for treating cancer is not public knowledge. The use of hormone therapy and insulin therapy for cancer makes sense. Instead, important hormone precursors, such as DHEA, are banned from the market place. Cancer patients are advised that mineral supplements will not help them to have more energy, when they should be advised to take mineral supplements for hormone production. Proper nutrition is essential for curing and preventing cancer. Much of this information is contradictory to what mainstream medicine recommends. People are confused about what to do for better health so they often end up doing nothing.

Normal cells respond to non-human growth factors

In the book by Scott Chinery (1983) *Human Growth Hormones, Bodybuilding's Perfect Drug.* (Page 14), we learn that the human growth hormone (HGH) is produced in the pituitary gland in amounts not exceeding 500 micrograms per day. Mature adults produce far less.

According to Chinery, the characteristics of human growth hormone are well known. It is a "single-chain peptide containing 190 amino acids: its molecular weight is 21,500." HGH as a supplement is valuable for helping midgets grow to normal height. It is very costly, as extraction from human pituitaries after death is the only source (in the 1980s). Alternate sources have been evaluated. Scott Chinery writes:

> Research has looked into the possibility of using animal glands as a source of growth hormone, but due to what is called "species specificity," the substances do not have the same effect. Recently, Rhesus monkey hormone has been considered as an alternative, but since its use is accompanied by a variety of skeletal abnormalities, it cannot be used safely.

Here we have documentation that growth hormones from different animal species will support replication of human bone cells, but such replication follows the biological pathway of the source. Rhesus monkey DNA polymerase and coenzymes produced Rhesus monkey bone structure in humans. The coenzymes are "species specific" because the growth factors for bone growth from Rhesus monkeys reproduce the bone structure of Rhesus monkeys. You cannot develop human bone structure from Rhesus monkey bone-growth factors because they are different. Some of the 190 proteins in growth hormone are species specific. The same principle applies to epithelial cells in humans. You cannot develop normal human epithelial cells with microbial growth factors. Microbial DNA polymerase will regulate and control replication of cells, but the cells will mutate toward single-cell, non-knitting, independent life forms functioning on fermentation of glucose. Cells that replicate due to primitive life form contaminants will dedifferentiate with each new generation into a more primitive embryonic life form.

The reason why I believe that 100 percent of cancers are of epithelial cell-wall type is that human and microbial cells have a common ancestry in which parts can be switched in cell-wall membranes. Liver cancer and leukemia are cell-wall membrane cancers as well. We do not have a common ancestry for growths of muscle tissue because microbes do not have muscles. We do not have tumors formed of brain, nerve, bone, ligaments, arteries, heart, eye balls or teeth. Cancers do not initiate in these non-microbial tissues because microbes do not have competitive growth hormones to produce cell parts that mimic these cell types. All cancers initiate where there is a common ancestry between human cell parts and microbial cell parts. In addition, the current of injury or natural growth has to be active to initiate replication of DNA.

The modern source for growth hormone supplements comes from bacteria. The following reference is taken from the Grolier Interactive Encyclopedia.

Today, however, genetically engineered HGH is produced in bacteria, providing a continuous supply to those children needing injections to enhance skeletal growth.

Obviously, microbial growth hormone can increase human cell growth but growth hormone supplements cannot cause cancer. Growth hormone from another mammal or bacteria can only maintain normal growth rates because the current of injury is not active. Cancer only occurs when environmental conditions, infection, and injury combine.

Microbial growth factors only cause cancer when cells are restricted from oxygen. Out of control replication occurs only when the current of injury is left on as the body tries to repair damage to skin tissue or injuries that do not heal. Broken bones that are not set properly may lead to cancer, just as membrane injury and blood clots in connective tissue does.

Growth is a two-step process: (1) DNA division due to an ionic field, and (2) molecular duplication due to electrostatic forces found in atoms and molecules. If the cellular environment is suitable for oxidative metabolism, with high oxidative levels, normal human cells will develop. It may well be that giants are the result of excessive microbial growth hormone in an aerobic environment. There is reason to believe that the increased stature of today's children is a direct result of bovine growth hormone ingested from meat and dairy products. Rapid growth and replication of normal cells is different from cancer because the high oxidative environment of the cell prevents microbial infection.

What causes benign growths? Klaus Kaufmann tells us "**The organism of cancer patients often presents mineral imbalance**.... benign tumors such as warts are known to develop mainly during periods of bodily demineralization or shortage of these minerals, and sometimes disappear spontaneously when the mineral imbalance has been corrected." Obviously, one of the ways to prevent cancer is to prevent 'benign' growths. We should also recognize that these growths are only 'benign' to the cancer service industry.

The growth and spread of cancer requires conditions suitable for anaerobic life forms to survive and multiply. **Conditions and growth factors combine to produce a cancer cell only in anaerobic conditions found in an injury that will not heal due to microbial infection of the cells.**

The phenomenon of benign tumors becoming invasive can be explained as the result of a break in the membrane wall due to physical damage or successive generations of dedifferentiation,. Warts, for example, are caused by a virus that modifies cell-wall membranes but viruses lack the capacity to produce sufficient DNA polymerase, growth hormones, and competitive cell components to mutate a cell wall.

The powerful chemical company known as Monsanto has succeeded in producing genetically engineered Bovine Growth Hormone (rBGH or rBST). Shots are given to milking cows on a two-week basis to increase production of milk and thereby increase profits for dairy farmers.

The growth hormone available in serum made from the blood of calves has been used for years to initiate growth of cancer cells in laboratories. Without the serum, cells in a growth media will be viable but will not multiply. Does that not suggest that the bovine growth hormone residue found in milk products and flesh from animals fed bovine growth hormone would stimulate growth of human cells? It is therefore conceivable that beef and milk products would support rapid growth of cancer cells as well. The growth hormone residue would not cause cancer of healthy well-oxidized cells, but the residual growth factors would increase the growth rate of existing cancer cells and possibly increase the chances of initiating cancer from a minor infection. Numerous books on cancer diets advise cancer patients not to eat red meat. It would certainly seem wise for cancer patients to avoid products with bovine growth hormone residue and young animals such as veal (calf flesh) and baby-beef liver.

In the USA, reporters Jane Akre and Steve Wilson lost their jobs with Fox TV because they refused to cover up disease-related data in a report on Bovine Growth Hormone. The true facts were never made public. What news could have been so significant that reporters were fired for refusing to cover up the truth? It must have been significant to cause these reporters to fight the issue and risk being fired. This issue tells us we are not being told all there is to know about growth hormones. We will read more about this later in Chapter 26.

Growth hormone contains a variety of growth factors

In *Genes and the Biology of Cancer*, Drs. Varmus and Weinberg tell us about nerve growth factors in growth hormone research by Nobel prize winner Rita Levi-Montalcini (Page 122)(Emphasis added):

> Rita Levi-Montalcini observed in 1950 in St. Louis, Missouri, that mouse sarcoma cells, implanted into developing chicken embryos, could dramatically stimulate the outgrowth of nerve fibers toward the engrafted tumors.

> While attempting to purify this nerve growth factor (NGF) from an alternative source – *normal salivary glands* – her co-worker, Stanley Cohen, uncovered another strange phenomenon: his extracts could hasten the opening of the eyelids of newborn mice. In time, he ascertained that the opening was due not to nerve growth factor (NGF) but to epidermal growth factor (EGF). **We now recognize that NGF provokes the differentiation rather than the growth of nerve cells, whereas EGF (and its receptor) regulates the growth of many kinds of normal and cancerous cells of epithelial origin.**

Here again is Nobel Award medical research proving growth hormone regulates cancer cell growth and that mainstream medicine knows it. If we remove the details about nerve growth factor from the above statement, Drs. Weinberg and Varmus are saying:

We now recognize that EGF (*epithelial growth factor*) regulates the growth of cancer cells of epithelial origin.

The above statement is in direct conflict with cancer information that states defective genes cause cancer and signals from defective genes control cancer growth. The EGF that regulates cancer growth was from the normal growth hormone source in human saliva. Oncogenes, lack of suppressor genes, or defective genes were not involved.

If they had of said: "**We now recognize that microbial EGF and chitin are the cause of mutated cell walls that lead to cell rejection and cancer tumors**", they would have given the world the true cause of cancer in the 1950's.

It is interesting that we cannot find reference to any other growth factors in human saliva that cause abnormal growth such as cancer. Insulin-like growth factor (IGF) is probably just normal insulin transporting protein or glucose across the cell-wall membrane of cancer cells.

All new cells go through stages of development starting with the embryonic stage and developing into one of the more than 200 types of cells. For each type, there must be a number of special growth factors. Skin cells contain nerves for sensing the environment. Consequently, epidermal (skin) growth factor also contains nerve growth factor. The nerve growth factor provokes the differentiation or specialization of nerve cells that are very different from epithelial tissue cells. Since growth of one is dependent on the other, growth factors for both are in the growth hormone. Microbial growth factors are like a co-enzyme. When microbes contaminate the replicating cells with divergent growth proteins and signals, human cells are no longer capable of functioning like normal human cells. We have diseases which mainstream medicine mistakenly ascribes to genetic liabilities, aging, autoimmunity, and free-radical damage.

Dr. Cohen used nerve growth hormone, taken from human salivary glands, and found it *"provoked differentiation"* of nerve cells. Similar differentiation may be an important clue to the traits of brain tissue in Alzheimer's disease. Nerve growth, which differentiates according to a primitive microbial pathway, would explain why people with Alzheimer's disease grow memory tissue not suitable for short-term human memory. (See Chapter 26, *Unlimited power through control of Medicare and the media,* on Alzheimer's for more details.)

One of the important traits concerning growth hormone and cancer is how little is needed to have a profound effect.

Rapid growth stimulated by one billionth of a gram/milliliter

OMNI Magazine, in an interview with Dr. Rita Levi-Montalcine, reports as follows:

> In Rio she put mice tumor cells near a single nerve ganglion in a culture dish full of solution. Within ten hours the nerve ganglion gave rise, she said, 'to a dense halo of nerve fibers, radiating out like rays from the sun. *So powerful was the substance that one billionth of a gram in a milliliter of culture solution produced the effect'.*

It is not possible to easily identify growth hormone measuring one billionth of a gram per milliliter. She knew the ratio only because she concocted it. We must remember too, that growth hormone produced by microbes multiplying within ducts or closed vessels is retained within that vessel and affects only the adjacent epithelial cells. You would not find these same levels circulating in blood or lymph fluids. Microbial growth hormone is also trapped in the storage vessel or duct. Consequently, its effect is highly concentrated in the immediate area.

With such a small amount capable of having such a profound growth effect, it is easy to see why cancer researchers, not looking for external growth factors caused by fungi or parasites, would not accidentally find such minute amounts located only in the tumor area. We must remember that enzymes are protein catalysts that control chemical reactions in biological systems. Catalysts control the reaction but are not consumed or destroyed by the chemical action. That's why a tiny amount of microbial DNA polymerase enzyme can cause cancer and escape detection. Such small levels can also be dismissed, because human growth hormone is also present in human blood, and because parasites and microbes occur naturally in the body without causing cancer.

It is heartbreaking to consider the waste of millions of dollars donated by the public to cancer societies to fund research in university and pharmaceutical company laboratories. Researchers do not want to put themselves out of a job by finding a cancer cure or the cause of cancer. The fact that known cancer cures are suppressed eliminates any possibility of financial gain by finding another cure.

A major failing of cancer research is that cells cultured from cancer cell lines and carefully nourished in incubators are in an artificial environment. With all ingredients in the nutrients carefully controlled and monitored, they cannot be accidentally contaminated, as is the case with cells in human bodies infected with parasites and mycotoxins from food.

Another significant failing is that cancer research is mainly limited to finding drugs to solve the problem. Research does not strive to eliminate the problem by identifying the cause and removing it. All of these problems are a direct result of a medical monopoly on health care and tax revenues for health care controlled by pharmaceutical interests. These problems will be discussed at length in later chapters.

Let's move on to review genes and the defective-gene theory as the cause of cancer.

6. The fatal flaw in the defective-gene theory of cancer

The defective gene theory of cancer helps maintain the mystery of cancer and serves as an excuse to justify more fundraising for research. If you still believe defective genes cause cancer, you must face the issue with an open mind and be prepared to evaluate what you have been taught. Belief in one theory excludes belief in the others.

In this chapter, I will show that the defective gene theory as the cause of cancer is based on a fatal flaw that renders the theory illogical. In addition, I will lay the foundation for an understanding of why effective cancer cures can by made with electromagnetic devices as well as explain how the current of injury initiates replication of DNA. Even if you already know defective genes do not cause cancer, read this chapter for an understanding of genes in order to have confidence in alternative therapies based on electromagnetic devices.

The fatal flaw in the defective gene theory of cancer comes from assuming and saying genes CAUSE production of enzymes and functional products. The fatal flaw is based on a chemical-mechanistic philosophy in which life itself is no more than a series of chemical actions initiated and controlled by a combination of atoms in crystals of DNA.

The fatal flaw is indoctrinated into medical students from day one at medical universities. Few students, if any, question this fundamental concept. In Dr. Guyton's *Textbook of Medical Physiology, Chapter 3, Genetic control of Cell Function —Protein Synthesis and Cell Reproduction,* we read:

> Almost everyone knows that the genes control heredity from parents to children, but most persons do not realize that the same genes control reproduction of and the day-to-day function of cells. The genes control function of the cell by determining what substances will be synthesized within the cell—what structures, what enzymes, what chemicals.

By agreeing with the professor that "genes control reproduction" and "*genes control function of the cell by determining what substances will be synthesized*", it follows that defective genes cause cancer. For medical students this is probably the turning point in their mindset concerning the cause of cancer. If you have been taught to believe that genes control all functions of the cell, can you recall when and where you first accepted this dogma?

According to the 1997 textbook, *Human Genetics*, Francis H. Crick, one of the scientists who unraveled the structure of DNA, is quoted as saying (Page 140. My emphasis added in bold italics):

A genetic material must carry out two jobs: duplicate itself and *control the development* of the rest of the cell in a specific way.

The text goes on to say:

At the molecular level, reproduction depends upon a biochemical that has the dual abilities: *to direct the specific activities of the cell* and to manufacture an exact replica of itself so that the instructions can be perpetuated.

Crick is probably the original source of this error. *Direct* and *control* are the key words. If genes do not actually direct the activities and control reproduction, it follows that cancer is not necessarily caused by defective genes. Genes did not control replication that gave life to the original body. The genes did not exist with the capacity to do anything until life gave them the capacity. Life came first, and life directs the activities of genes.

That mysterious thing, which I will refer to as the *spirit* or *life-force* had control of genes to form the body. Life only comes from living things. Genes exist without life, and life exists, as a waveform of energy, without genes. Genes connect the life-force to atoms and molecules making up the body. Genes are only tools controlled by the life-force.

What if genes serve only as a template to control how replication will turn out, but the life-force controls if and when genes will replicate? What if the life-force controls when and if genes replicate through an electrical stimulus that gives the life-force control of replication? If this is the case, genes do not determine what substances will be synthesized, and defective genes do not cause out-of-control DNA replication and cancer.

The human body began with a male sperm cell, a living cell, capable of a swimming motion, but not capable of replication on its own, and a female egg cell, a living cell not capable of replicating on its own. The fact that sperm cells with DNA do not replicate individually indicates that DNA is not capable of replication on its own. The fact that an unfertilized egg cell, with DNA, cannot replicate on its own, just as unfertilized bird's eggs do not hatch, indicates there is more to the control of replication then the presence of DNA nucleotides. DNA must exist as two parallel strands, one from the male, one from the female, in a bipolar combination with a *vestigal ionic bond* between the two strands. It is this ionic bond, called a vestigal ionic bond that connects the life-force within the body to DNA nucleotides. Vestigal ionic bonds will be explained later.

Life is still a mystery but we do know it exists. There is a life-force that controls the body. This life-force initiates replication of the available genes to produce a new body. Life only rises from life, and genes cannot create life without a life-force. Replication is controlled by the life-force.

The fatal-flaw in the defective gene theory is to deny the life-force that initiated replication of the fertilized egg to have the capacity to initiate replication later in life. To do so is obviously wrong. The life-force strives to maintain the integrity of the body. An injury to the body results in immediate replication of cells to repair the injury and the replication stops as soon as the injury is repaired. A sudden fright causes the heart to beat faster, for fight or flight, to save one's life. The autonomic nervous system using direct current energy initiates these instant responses.

Cancer occurs when a group of cells which are already replicating DNA nucleotides initiated by the life-force, are taken over by growth factors from another living thing, (a parasite) and the new cells are mutated to become a hybrid cell, part human, part parasite. The fatal flaw in the defective gene theory also denies the capacity of parasites, resident inside or adjacent to a replicating cell, the capacity to produce enzymes and proteins that can mutate the cell during replication. That too, is wrong.

As I said earlier, it is a serious error to assume that either human or microbial growth hormones initiate replication of DNA. If genes had the capacity to initiate DNA division, there would be no controlling mechanism in place to maintain the integrity of the body. Human growth hormones and microbial growth hormones only facilitate growth and differentiation of the cell during assembly. All that is needed to understand the cancer process is to recognize the universality of DNA in all living things, that all living things produce growth factors as enzymes, and that enzymes from one life form can mutate the replication of a cell of another life form. That is what genetic engineering is all about. DNA replication is initiated only by the normal processes of growth or repair controlled by the life-force through wave energy. Defective genes have nothing to do with cancer. Genes have control of cell traits incorporated into the cell and cell-wall membrane during assembly of cell components and cell-wall membranes but genes do not initiate this action without instructions from the life-force or spirit that animates the body. Upon death, the life-force or spirit leaves the body, and the genes, still intact, cannot continue to multiply Genes cannot initiate replication after the life-force departs.

According to Guyton (Page 36): "The DNA begins to be reproduced about 5 hours before mitosis (*separation*) takes place, and the duration of DNA replication is about four hours." Replication of DNA occurs in the cytoplasm of the cell. Parasites resident in the cell are capable of producing growth factors that contaminate the pool of nucleotides from which the new cell forms the outer phospho-lipid layer of the cell. Bacteria and fungi, being primitive life-forms, produce a membrane wall that has resonant traits different from the bipolar lipid layer forming the membrane of normal human cells. The cell walls of a single-celled life form do not knit together to form layers of skin or membranes and these cells to not knit to existing epithelial cells to heal the injury. Proteins on the exterior of the cell wall probably account for this lack of knitting as well as the resonance of the lipid layer forming the membrane. Primitive life form cell walls are formed of a protein material, similar in structure to cellulose, (much like the structure of a honey comb) called chitin.

If the new growth does not knit to form new tissue, or fails to repair an injury, the current of injury, which stimulates replication, stays on. Cancer is no longer a mystery. Cancer is a microbial disease. Infection of replicating cells causes cancer by mutating the cell wall during mitosis.

The defective gene theory as a cause of cancer demands belief in a mechanistic-chemical force that controls life in which the genes initiate replication. People who adhere to this belief are said to have a mechanistic philosophy and millions of people have this belief. The one major problem with it comes in explaining life and death, thought processes, mental concepts, creative ideas, as well as the emotional and spiritual aspects of life. The major philosophical problem is that it denies the existence of a life-force activating and controlling the body. In this regard, it fails to account for observations in the real world.

Even if you adhere to the mechanistic-chemical theory of life, cancer can still be explained without reference to defective genes. The current of injury is delivered to the injured area by special meridians that release this energy only when the cell-wall membranes are broken. The cell components produced by bacteria, through a similar mechanistic-chemical process, are incorporated into the cell wall during the mechanistic-chemical process of cell division and cell-wall membrane assembly. Contamination of the cytoplasm of the cell during stages of normal cell growth for repair result in cancer, whether the process is considered a mechanical-chemical phenomenon or a life-force driven phenomenon. The end result is the same. Defective genes are not required because the initial division of DNA is a mechanistic force based on electromagnetic energy and weak ionic bonds holding DNA nucleotides together. If you wish to deny the existence of a life-force, you must find something else to explain the production of the current of injury which can be measured in the immediate area of an injury. You must also explain why the damage of a heart attack is measured by the current of injury using an electrocardiogram device (ECG). The current of injury is not a chemical.

Proteins that form skin tissue, for example, are crystals, or more properly *crystalloids*. Crystalloids are combinations of atoms of carbon, hydrogen, oxygen, nitrogen, and minerals in a crystal-like formation. A fundamental law of crystals recognizes that bodies of the same crystalline composition have the same crystalline form; bodies of different crystalline composition have a different crystalline form. The form of crystals gives rise to its physical properties, one of which is its capacity to conduct electrical currents. Phospholipids have a high capacity to carry an electric current so that membrane cells are highly conductive. Electric eels, for example, demonstrate the conductivity of membrane tissue and the capacity of living things to produce electrical currents.

Cancer, expressed in mechanical terms, is the failure of the crystalline composition of human cells to combine chemically with the crystalline composition of hybrid cells. Defective genes are not required. Contamination of microbial enzymes and proteins produces cancer through chemical modification of the crystalline composition of membrane cell protein.

There is a lot to say in favor of the mechanistic-chemical theory of life. Most, if not all of the automatic processes that go on in the body, can be accounted for by the mechanistic-chemical theory. DNA is assembled by the electromagnetic forces in the atoms. The crystalloid structures of proteins resonate to the vibrational frequency of the earth, and life is the result of resonance with the earth. Life is a resonant frequency of crystalloids made up of carbon, hydrogen, oxygen, nitrogen, and essential minerals. Every nucleotide or base in DNA contains a phosphate crystal that resonates with the life force to energize the DNA nucleotide. It follows that every crystalline structure, or every protein, and enzyme, will resonate differently than any other crystalline structure, protein, or enzyme. The base around which an enzyme is built is a mineral. Cobalt and iron are minerals that hold a permanent magnetic charge, and all mineral oxides have a north and south magnetic polarity. The introduction or loss of one atom of a mineral, for example, will change the resonant frequency of that protein. The lack of one essential mineral will eliminate the possibility of making an essential enzyme. Crystalloid form is the fundamental basis for systems within living things such as kidney function, and circulation and digestion. A lack of minerals can interfere with all parts of the body. A specific crystalloid structure and resulting vibrational frequency give physical properties such as function and form to a specific protein.

A physical property of a substance is that which can be specified without reference to a specific component of that substance, for example, specific gravity, vibrational frequency, conductivity, color, or form.

Kidney tissue and all of the urinary system, for example, is a functional unit due to compatible resonance of these proteins. Other organs and systems operate at a different resonant frequency. Pollutants are organ specific in the body, meaning you will normally find certain chemical toxins lodged in specific organs due to a compatible resonant frequency. That is why cancers occur in different organs, depending on the type of pollutant in your body.

There is no limit to how many combinations of DNA nucleotide bases can be formed, which accounts for the variety of living things. The human body has resonant frequencies covering a range of 7,900 KHz, from 1520 KHz to 9460 KHz. For sake of comparison, the complete AM radio station dial covers a range of only 1060 KHz, from 535 KHz to 1605 KHz. There are approximately 200 identifiably different tissues in the human body, because of different crystalloid structures and resonance.

It is precisely the unique range in resonant frequency of cancer cells that explains why benign growths and cancer cells can be identified electronically and destroyed with electromagnetic energy. Dr. Clark states that wart frequency, for example, range from 402 KHz to 464 KHz. Royal Rife states that cancer cells have eight frequencies ranging from 666 KHz to 2128 KHz. This also explains why the most effective way to identify cancer tumors, toxins, parasites, and pollutants in the body is to look for and measure the resonant frequencies. That is why cancer can be identified before tumors form and be treated at a fraction of the cost of modern approved methods. These issues will be discussed later in suppressed cancer cures.

Dr. Hulda Clark bases her research on the resonance of living things, which she calls bioradiation. She measures resonance with a device she invented called a syncrometer. All living and dead things have a specific bioradiation or resonant frequency that can be measured, and dead tissue of microbes and bodily parts have the same frequency as living ones. Bioradiation is not a function of life, but a function of the crystalloid form creating a unique resonance of the crystalloid proteins in cells. In using the syncrometer, a sample of organ tissue, such as the kidney or liver, is placed on one of two plates connected electronically, and a sample of a parasite or toxin is placed on the second plate. By running a current through the two plates, the current picks up the resonance of the two samples. By conducting this same current through your body, if you have that contaminant in that organ, the syncrometer will signal resonance. Resonance tells you that you have that pollutant or parasite in that organ. Doing a tissue and parasite cleanse and checking for resonance later will tell you if the cleansing process worked. Removing the toxins and parasites returns the cells to normal.

Imagine how easy it could be to diagnose cancer, accurately, and without significant cost by measuring for the specific frequency of cancer cells. Several of the suppressed cancer cures are based on this scientific principle of resonance. Cell Specific Therapy and Royal Rife are two well-established cures. We will study these in Chapter 20, *Historical documents on suppressed cancer cures.*

Dr. Clark was awarded the prestigious U.S. Scientist of the Year Award in October of 1999. With book sales more than a million copies, it is safe to say more than one million people now subscribe to her theory that microbes and pollutants cause cancer.

In order to attend the award presentation she had to interrupt work in preparing a legal defense to avoid being jailed for practicing medicine without a license in the State of Indiana. Charges relate back six years to 1993 when she was a student. The U.S. medical syndicate is now in action to suppress her research and potential benefit to humankind. Court appearances are set for January and February of the year 2000.

Hopefully, her case will polarize public opinion against the medical establishment so that the world can advance into a new era of vibrational or electromedicine. Dr. Clark is so far ahead of mainstream medicine in the study of cancer parasites and pollutants, they cannot even comprehend what she has accomplished. As I mentioned earlier, one of the purposes of this book is to inform people with information that will make alternative therapies more credible. This chapter helps explain the connection between the autonomic nervous system, energy fields, and cancer.

Genes are only crystalloid forms to store and transfer information. The crystalloid composition of a gene made up in units of three bases gives rise to a unique crystalloid form with a resonant frequency of its own. Only three bases are required to produce a unique functional crystalloid enzyme or functional product. Stimulation of the life-force through emotions of fear (flight or fight), or desire, or thought processes, leads to production of functional products, just as the perceived need to replicate and repair an injury causes replication of cells.

Amazingly, DNA resonates the same whether it is in dead or living tissue and the resonance of the liver, for example, from any mammal, resonates the same as the liver from any other mammal. In using a syncrometer, one must purchase laboratory supplies or collect tissue samples from a butcher such as beef or pork at meat markets. DNA does not give life to tissue. A living thing is capable of causing duplication of the DNA crystalloid forms using only the natural valences of atoms and molecules to form crystals. By duplicating the resonant composition in DNA, duplicates can be formed for replication of cells. Life is almost a mechanistic-chemical phenomenon, based on resonance with the earth. However, the fact that the human mind can conceptualize and create is far beyond the capacity of genes. Living things use genes as templates. Genes do not control living things entirely.

By duplicating the resonant composition of a gene in mRNA, functional products can be formed in the cytoplasm of the cell having the same resonant pattern or waveform. Parasites resident in the cell introduce closely similar proteins during the assembly process that alter the resonant frequency of the skin tissue. That's cancer. All other microbial diseases, autoimmune diseases, and degenerative diseases can be accounted for by this principle of protein substitution. Defective genes are capable of producing defective human parts only because the proteins they produce are structurally interchangeable with products from normal genes.

Genes are reliable tools, accounting for the stability of life, because they resonate at a specific frequency, and only one frequency. Genes do not mutate and deform. Genes exist as chemical combinations. Genes do not initiate replication on their own. Life begets life because the energies inherent in living things modulate or polarize crystals in DNA strands, causing DNA to replicate. The concept that life began in water, possibly following a bolt of lightning, pays tribute to the need of an energy source to start life.

The concept of polarized atoms explains how one makes a magnet by stroking a steel bar with another magnet. The magnetic field of the magnet polarizes atoms in the steel bar, giving the bar a magnetic quality. Something quite similar happens when the current of injury causes DNA to replicate. Polarization of atoms in crystals and an increase in the volume of resonance causes replication of DNA crystalloid bases. DNA cannot replicate without breaking the ionic hydrogen bonds. An increase in the strength of the resonant frequency by the current of injury does that.

DNA only functions as a template to guide production of identical crystalloid forms to serve as enzymes and functional products for living things.

Let's use an analogy for the template concept. We use a ruler, as a template to draw a straight line, and we use a circular template to draw a circle. If a person draws a circle using a pencil and a template, it is the person who decides if the circle will be drawn, not the template. It is not the template or the pencil that make decisions. In much the same way, genes serve as templates to guide the production of enzymes and replication of DNA. Genes do not decide if and when replication will occur. Genes are only templates; genes do not make decisions. Claiming that genes cause replication based on a mechanistic concept of life gives rise to the fatal-flaw in the defective gene theory of cancer. Looking for the cause of cancer in genes is a mistake. They should be looking for the cause of cancer in the cell wall to find out why the normal membrane cells reject the mutated cells and fail to knit with them. Cancer cells are cell wall defective, not gene defective.

Any injury that results in loss of skin cells, for example, initiates an immediate replication and growth response to repair the injury. This growth response is initiated and controlled by the current of injury, which is, itself, controlled by the life-force that gives structure and form to the body. The resonance inherent in crystalloid DNA molecules allows the current of injury to modify this resonant frequency and cause DNA replication. The signal to replicate is the current of injury and this has been proven beyond any reasonable doubt. It is well known that bone fractures will heal faster with the proper electromagnetic stimulus. Salamanders have been made to grow new parts with a current of injury, and rats have grown new leg tissue with an artificial current of injury. The current of injury also affects the function of genes.

Let's return to more research on genes and how they function.

Genes have only two functions: store and provide information

In *Harper's Review of Biochemistry* genes are recognized for having only two functions. First is to store information, and second is to provide the information that is stored (Page 363):

Function of DNA

The genetic information stored in the nucleotide sequences of DNA serves two purposes. It is the source of information for the synthesis of all protein molecules of the cell and the organism, and it provides the information inherited by daughter cells or offspring. Both of these functions require that the DNA molecule serve as a template—in the first case for transcription of the information into RNA and in the second case for the replication of the information into daughter DNA molecules.

In *Harper's Review of Biochemistry*, genes are only templates for the storage and transfer of information.

The fatal error in the defective gene theory is found only in medical texts and mainstream medical propaganda on the cause of cancer. It is, without question, the most significant piece of *misinformation* responsible for the ongoing success of the cancer industry. It is vitally important that people come to recognize this dogma as false.

The following three references show that the cancer establishment want us to believe defective genes or defective cells cause cancer, not as a template, —but directly, and in conflict with normal wishes of the body. To do so, genes would have to be classed as living things with considerable power for a relatively simple crystalloid molecule.

There is a vast difference between the two functions of storing energy and dictating its use. The distance is equal to that between living and non-living things. The issue is evident in computer information storage systems. Computers do not dictate use of stored information. IBM is still working on computers that will repair themselves, but this goal has not been accomplished. Perhaps they should duplicate life by energizing the complete system with a form of wave energy that senses lack of function. In this way, lack of function initiates repair.

Psychologists tell us that only two things motivate human action: desire and fear. Knowledge on its own does not influence the will. Knowledge influences desire and fear. Addiction to drugs, habit, and prejudices are also powerful motivators of human choices, but these too, influence our desires or fears. In order for genes to dictate control of the information stored in the genetic structure, genes would have to be independent living things capable of desire and fear.

Think about it. Why would genes give the wrong message? How could they give the wrong message? Where is the proof that genes control life? Why should I believe you?

Misinformation on the function of genes

Let's look at some of the medical misinformation that claims that genes dictate life functions in our bodies. Robert A. Weinburg is one of the leading cancer specialists in the world. He was co-author of the text, *Genes and the Biology of Cancer* as published by Scientific American Books in 1993. In this 200-page book on cancer, fungi and parasites are not mentioned as a possible cause. Ninety years of cancer research during this century is totally ignored, if it does not support the defective gene theory as the cause of cancer.

In the 1998 book, *One Renegade Cell* by Robert Weinberg we read (Page 7) (My emphasis added in bold type):

Genes act directly to control the behavior of individual cells. Each cell, operating under the control of its genes, collaborates with all the others to create the body's form and function. Hence, the complexity of an entire organism represents nothing more than the aggregate behavior of all of its individual cells. This means that the set of genes governing the cell and the set of genes controlling the shape and behavior of the body are one and the same.

The author has assigned a third function to genes. Genes control the cell. *"Each cell, operating under control of its genes."* The author believes that life is nothing more than a chemical-mechanistic force within atoms and molecules. Genes control life.

What is life? What is the life-force doing if not controlling the cells that make up its body? He concludes by saying: *"...genes controlling the shape and behavior of the body are one and the same."*

He claims genes control the *behavior* of one's body. Are your genes responsible for your behavior? How ridiculous! If you go out and rob a bank, are you not guilty of a crime? You might get off with claims of insanity, but not because your genes made you do it.

Life is not caused by a specific arrangement of atoms. If it were, life could come from non-living things, and death as we know it would not be possible. When death occurs, the life-force leaves the body with all the genes intact. The polymerase chain reaction establishes the profile of genes years after death. Stable genes don't suddenly fall apart causing death. Due to modern medical procedures, thousands of people have had a near-death experience in which they experienced life outside of their bodies before being revived. One cannot deny existence of a life-force or spirit that animates the body and controls replication of cells.

The conclusion that genes control behavior of living things denies freedom of choice in human actions. Human behavior is not controlled by genes, nor is the shape of the body controlled by genes.

All living things share the genetic structure. Why is there so much variety in living things? The life-force gives shape to the body and the genes provide the means of converting life energy that exists only in a wave form, to a chemical form. Genes provide communication between life and matter so that living things can exist. Inherited DNA patterns distinguish one body from another but the shape they take, being that of human, mouse, or monkey, for example, is determined by the life-force in the body.

There is a life-force in living things no less real than the molecules and atoms that make up the body. It is the life-force that controls behavior of the cells. How ridiculous to say otherwise, unless there is a hidden agenda. To be recognized as an authority on cancer, and use this position of power and trust to misinform the public is a breach of public trust.

On the jacket of the book *One Renegade Cell,* we find this supportive reference by none other than Richard D. Klausner, M.D. Director, U. S. National Cancer Institute. Dr. Klausner says:

> This is an engaging, understandable and accessible narrative of one of the great scientific stories of our time — the struggle to understand cancer. It paints the gradual and impressive illumination of the mysteries of cancer, recognizing that we have a long way to go but that we seem to have found the roads upon which we must travel.

The concepts expressed by the author of One Renegade Cell are those of mainstream medicine and cancer specialists throughout the world. In Canada, we have *Everyone's Guide to Cancer Therapy*, to explain the genetic cause of cancer. We read (Page 3):

Understanding Cancer

> A cancer cell has an abnormal chromosome from genetic change or damage. **The altered gene starts sending the wrong message** or at least a message different from the one it should give. A cell begins to grow rapidly. It multiplies again and again until it forms a lump that's called a malignant tumor. Or cancer.

Here again we find that genes are given a third function. Altered genes send messages, all on their own. If they start "*sending the wrong message,*" they cause cancer. What is there about an altered gene that gives it more power and authority than a normal gene? Where is the proof? Why should we belief that statement?

This large seven hundred-page text has contributions from 127 cancer specialists and the cover reads, "Adapted by the Canadian Medical Association." This book is the authority in Canada by which cancer victims evaluate approved treatments for cancer and avoid unproven treatments. Included in the text, Chapter 13, is a large section warning cancer patients to stay away from unproven therapies such as metabolic therapy and oxygenation of cells. Misinformation on cancer goes far beyond errors of opinion on the function of genes. Misinformation is in direct conflict with medical teaching and reality. We will review this later in Chapter 22, *Ruthless ongoing suppression of effective cancer cures.*

If we look for a second opinion on the function of DNA, we find a significant statement in *Harper's Review of Biochemistry*, The biochemistry text concludes that the cause of DNA synthesis is not in the genes or cells, but may be an intrinsic property of the chromosome (Page 383):

> The nature of the signals that regulate DNA synthesis at these levels is unknown, but the regulation does **appear to be** an intrinsic property of each individual chromosome.

There are no references in biochemistry that trace the pathway showing how defects in genes or chromosomes cause cancer. "Appears to be" is not proof that they do. "Appears to be," also says they do not know. The theory that DNA, genes, or chromosomes control replication are only assumptions that are now promoted as dogma and fact. The theory has never been proven. That is why more research is needed to find the cause of cancer. In my opinion, the intrinsic property of the chromosome is the ionic hydrogen bond that responds to the presence of an ionic current of injury.

The complete hypocrisy of the defective gene theory becomes evident when you realize that the normal life function of tissue repair is initiated by an event outside of the genes. Cells multiply upon demand to repair the injury and replication stops when the injury is repaired. It happens every time we damage the skin of our hands or knees. This process leads to cancer if the repairs are not made and the rejected cells find a low-oxygen environment to mature as fermentative cells.

The current of injury is used every day in modern medicine. Mainstream medicine measures the severity of heart attacks using electrocardiograms that measure the strength of the current of injury. The strength of the current of injury is always proportional to the size of the injury. Since the heart is such a vital organ, the body seeks to repair damage as quickly as possible. There is a high current of injury associated with heart attacks.

In skin tissue damage, the same rule applies. The current of injury initiates replication and repair of cells in proportion to the injury, and therefore is the signal that causes genes to replicate.

When one realizes that cancer was produced in laboratory mice in 1913, by Nobel Prize winner Dr. Johannes Fibiger, using parasitic worms from horses, one must question any theory of cancer that totally ignores such significant research. The obvious neglect of this research in information on the possible cause of cancer supports a theory that a significant cover-up is in progress.

Do genes have a third function of sending messages and controlling cells in our body? Weigh this issue very carefully for it is the very foundation upon which is built the whole empire of the cancer industry including cancer research and gene therapy. Your donations for cancer research go to this end.

If genes have the third function, then the investment of billions of tax-revenue dollars and public donations into the genetic cause of cancer is meaningful. However, if the concept is false, the billions of dollars invested in cancer research are being wasted. More significant, millions of people will die of cancer because researchers are looking for the cause of cancer in the wrong place. They will never find it and there will never be a cure for cancer. Donating to cancer research creates false hope and defrauds the public of their money.

Let's take an in-depth look at DNA and genes to find out why defective genes do not cause cancer.

Do you visualize a gene as some vague vitalistic entity that gives rise to traits such as blue eyes or skin color? If your concept of a gene is vague, you will tend to believe anything anyone in authority tells you. You have no way to recognize nonsense and misinformation. It is important that you learn to recognize the molecular structure of genes to understand why defective genes cannot cause cancer.

The definition of genes in four parts

There are many variations to the definition and description of genes. The definition of a gene in the 1997 textbook *Human Genetics* (Page 383-384) ends by describing genes as "...*overlapping fuzzily defined regions on a sequence*". This definition illustrates how little is actually known about genes or it is used to help maintain confusion over the function of DNA.

Most textbooks define genes as follows:

A gene is a sequence of nucleotides

in DNA

that codes for

a functional product.

What does that mean? Let's take a close look at the four groups of words and phrases used in the definition.

Nucleotides are molecules in the *nucleus* of the cell. Nucleotides are combinations of nitrogen, hydrogen, oxygen, and carbon making up stable molecules formed in ring-shaped structures. These ring structures, once formed, are very stable. A very similar nucleotide called benzene is so stable that compounds of benzene form a special division in chemistry called aromatics. Dyes are benzene-based molecules and dyes hold their color because of the stability in the benzene molecule.

This equally stable structure of DNA nucleotides gives DNA the capacity to store and reproduce as templates for construction of functional products. The stability of nucleotides in genes accounts for the stability of living things and the continuity of life.

Giving genes an independent life function would eliminate the stability of life because all genes are essentially the same. There are only 64 possible bases, shared by all living things. If genes dictated their own replication, there could be only 64 life forms. If new combinations of genes created new life forms, why would there be such stability in living things and defective genes at the same time? America has over 10 million cancer patients. Shouldn't there be millions of new cancer-free species too. Giving genes control of the body simply doesn't make sense.

DNA is an abbreviation for deoxyribonucleic acid, the principle molecule carrying genetic information in almost all organisms. Any general reference to DNA includes reference to the related components transcribed or copied from DNA in the nucleus such as RNA, tRNA (transfer) and mRNA (messenger). RNA is formed in the nucleus and exits into the cytoplasm to direct assembly of functional proteins. DNA is also found in the mitochondria or energy-producing units within cells. Mitochondria reproduce independently of the replication cycle of the cell and carry their own genetic structure. If mitochondria are a separate life form with the cell, why don't mitochondria cause defective genes or mutated cell wall membranes? Answer: mitochondria produce cell wall components compatible with normal human cells and defective genes that cause cancer do not exist.

The DNA structure is a natural consequence of the atomic valences of atoms and the quantum theory. There are only four base molecules that fit the DNA crystal structure. These are Adenine, Thymine, Cytosine, and Guanine. You may recognize adenine in ATP (Adenine triphosphate.) A fifth molecule called Uracil takes the place of Adenine or Thymine to form RNA in combination with a change in the sugar base that ties the cells together. RNA assembles or translates atoms and molecules in the cytoplasm into functional enzymes with the same crystal form and resonant qualities as in the original DNA. That's how enzymes are formed.

The four DNA molecules join in only two pairs:

1. Adenine with Thymine (expresses as A-T or T-A) and

2. Cytosine with Guanine (expressed as C-G or G-C).

To help remember the combination sequence, look at how well the circular letters C and G combine (CG). Similarly, notice how well the stick letters AT and TA combine. Combinations of CG's and AT's are bases. Three bases work together as a set called a codon. The word codon is derived from the codes used to identify the set of bases. Codons are continuous triplets of RNA that specifies a particular amino acid.

For an in-depth but easy to follow understanding of the genetic code go to the Internet. There are hundreds of powerful demonstrations. Information is also available in many books such as the 1997 book by David E. Brody and Arnold R. Brody, Ph.D. called *The Science Class You Wish You Had.*

Understanding the genetic code is the first step in understanding the function of genes. The major concepts are easy to understand.

Codes for specifies the arrangement of bases in RNA and identifies the amino acid produced by the gene. By way of an analogy, during wartime, messages are sent by code. A wartime code can be anything, but in DNA code, the code consists of four letters, A, T, C, G. These letters, of course, designate the four nucleotides in DNA. In RNA the code consists of four letters A, C, G, and U. The letter U stands for Uracil, the unique nucleotide in RNA. In both DNA and RNA, all words have a precise length of three letters so that a three-letter code in DNA will always produce a three-letter code in RNA with the replacement of an A or a T (the stick letters) for a U. For example, the DNA code AAA becomes the RNA code UUU and codes for the amino acid phenylalanine. Similarly, the DNA code TAC becomes the RNA code AUG and codes for the amino acid methionine. There are only 64 three-letter codes possible, making up the Universal Genetic Code. Three of these codes (ATT, ATC, and ACT) are used to identify termination points in genes. These are transcribed into RNA as UAA, UAG, and UGA enabling genes to be identified as functional blocks, isolated, cut, harvested, spliced and replicated as such. This is how scientists harvest genes from one life form to splice into another life form. Other groups of letters identify functional parts.

The study of defective genes relates almost entirely to the genetic problems of cells producing or failing to produce essential amino acids and structural proteins, or of not producing enzymes to digest certain essential amino acids in metabolism. None of these defects cause cells to multiply out-of-control because that is not the function of genes. Genes store information and transfer information. End of functions. Genes do not take off and do their own thing, like dictating replication when they wish, or differentiate the cell to function anaerobically, or control the shape and behavior of the body.

None of the defects cause cells to stop the oxidative process and revert to fermentation.

If you believed defective genes cause cancer, or even may have caused cancer, do you see how you have been misled by misinformation? The theory has no scientific basis. It is simply not possible.

Defects in genes are related directly to what information is stored and how accurately it is transferred. Defects that may lead to cancer cause metabolic problems that may lead to structurally weak cell walls in arteries and veins, for example, or the incapacity to produce defensive enzymes, or the incapacity to break down proteins leading to allergies and fermentation. Defective genes do not cause replication nor do they send messages to replicate. Defective genes in cells of storage vessels and ducts cannot produce growth hormones. Human growth hormone is produced only in the pituitary gland. Tumors release growth hormone because parasites produce growth hormone that contaminates human cells. Defective genes are not involved.

All of the DNA bases in a cell make up the cell's genome. A base is a combinations of two crystal-like molecules (A-T or C-G) bonded together to form one larger crystal-like molecule. The bond holding the A crystal to the T crystal consists of two ionic hydrogen bonds. The bond holding the C crystal to the G crystal consists of three ionic hydrogen bonds. The relative *instability* of the ionic hydrogen bonds accounts for the capacity of DNA to divide without disturbing the nucleotides. The secret of DNA replication is in the bonding mechanism that is only about one-twentieth as strong as the chemical bonds forming DNA nucleotides.

The two major structures forming nucleotides or building blocks of DNA are called purines and pyrimidines.

1. *Purine* is a word made up by combining the Latin words *pure, uric and ine*. Purine thus refers to the uric acid group of organic compounds in the body. The group gets its name from urine, from which it was first isolated. Purines have a double-ring (side by side) structure. The DNA components Adenine and Guanine are purines because they have a double-ring structure.

2. *Pyrimidines* have a single-ring structure. The DNA components Cytosine and Thymine have a single ring structure and are thus referred to as pyrimidines.

The nucleotides consist of one nitrogenous molecule, one deoxyribose molecule, and one phosphate molecule. These are attached to form strings or groups called genes and chromosomes. The phosphate molecules carry the life-force along the genetic structure much like a nerve carries electric energy.

These are the same phosphate molecules found in membrane cells. They are also the same phosphate molecules built by plants using minerals from the earth and energy from the sun. In plants, they are called glucose-1-phosphate with a six-sided structure. In DNA the stability of these phosphate molecules comes from their combination with stable five-sided sugar molecules called pentose phosphate. Pentose phosphate is produced by fermentation, but not by oxidation, which explains why cells that replicate first switch from oxidation to fermentation of glucose. This will be discussed later.

Genes are specified by the terminal codons described above. There are 46 chromosomes in the human cell, with millions of genes. The average chromosome contains a DNA molecule approximately five centimeters long. If all the DNA molecules were combined, they would be about two meters or seven feet long. The process of assembling chains of nucleotides to form genes is referred to as polymerization. This gives rise to the name of an enzyme that builds these structures as *DNA polymerase*. This enzyme controls DNA replication because it guides the formation of new strings. Nothing else will do so. Without this enzyme and coenzymes, replication cannot take place. Coenzymes are part of an enzyme, not a cooperative or secondary enzyme. Coenzymes perform secondary functions that follow other functions, much like a chain of dominoes falls one after another in a flowing motion. The 191 amino acids in growth hormone make up a long chain of coenzymes called growth factors.

Chromosomes get their name from how they were first discovered. According to Isaac Asimov, the protein molecules in the nucleus were first discovered by staining. Around 1882 the German biologist Walther Flemming discovered small thread-like granules in the cell nucleus and called them *chromatin* for the Greek word for color. By 1888, the threads became known as *chromosomes*. Later, when he observed how these threads divided, he described the process as *mitosis* from the Greek word for thread.

In the process of *mitosis*, the number of chromosomes is doubled so that each daughter cell has a complete complement of the genetic structure of both parents. In the process of egg fertilization and division, called *meiosis*, the number of chromosomes is halved so that the newly fertilized egg cell has a complete set of genes with half from each parent.

For an educated person to assume that all this happens through some chemical-mechanical force is beyond my comprehension. It would be far easier to put the pieces of a clock in a box, shake the box a few times, and expect to find a fully functioning clock inside.

DNA nucleotides are very stable molecules. Our body in the process of acquiring DNA nucleotides from food secretes intestinal digestive juices or enzymes that isolate and release the nucleotides intact. These are later used to build protein structures and DNA molecules. The more natural our food the healthier we will be because the assembly process goes faster. The body is designed to process living food first, modified living food second and chemicals not at all. These nucleotide structures can also be cut intact from the mycelia of fungi and are called "Yeast Artificial Chromosome." Fermentation of trapped blood sugars (a fungal process) produces a ready supply of DNA nucleotides for cancer growth in adjacent cells. That is why cancer can grow so rapidly. When one recognizes that every cell has billions of DNA bases, one realizes that cancer cells speed assembly by bringing in sub-assemblies produced in fungal mycelia. Considering the time required for mitosis, the capacity of childhood tumors to form from a single defective cell is mathematically impossible. Childhood cancer can only be explained by the microbial cause of cancer.

Genes can be pictured as a twisted ladder, circular staircase, or a double threaded screw made up of DNA bases. If you imagine cutting a ladder in half, lengthwise through the rungs, each half would be like a *strand* of DNA. The outside railings would be like the deoxyribose sugar chain of molecules holding the rungs in place. Ribose sugar is also a stable molecule consisting of a five-sided pentose structure. These DNA strands serve as templates to form strands of RNA. The pattern in DNA is transcribed into the pattern in RNA based on the molecular attraction of atoms and molecules. RNA is always a single strand because it is a copy of a single strand of DNA.

DNA has the sugar *D*eoxyribose whereas RNA has the sugar *R*ibose holding the bases together. Deoxy means an atom of oxygen has been removed from the ribose molecule. By removing one atom of oxygen from the molecule, the ionic hydrogen bond in RNA is less stable and easily transported by the cell to function in the cytoplasm. Hence, we have DNA and mRNA. In mRNA the nucleotide Thymine is replaced by the nucleotide Uracil so that a molecular difference is established between RNA and DNA. RNA does not become DNA during the replication process. The two molecules or crystals are uniquely different and RNA does not fit into DNA nucleotides with equal stability.

A functional product is an enzyme or protein that will perform a specific function for the cell or a protein that will serve a structural function. There are roughly 50,000 functional products already identified. Enzymes are functional products different from proteins although enzymes contain nucleotides similar to proteins. The words *enzymes* and *proteins* are often used interchangeably in older texts because the dual function had not been identified.

Enzymes have a functional end and a non-functional end. The non-functional protein end contains the address for delivery within a cell's structure, and the functional end contains magnetic, paramagnetic, or diamagnetic molecules that modify chemical actions. Paramagnetic molecules are attracted to magnetic molecules, and diamagnetic molecules are repelled by magnetic molecules. I theorize that the life-force is able to polarize magnetic fields causing enzymes to twist and turn so that chemical actions can be modified by both pushing and pulling. At present, how enzymes and catalysts function is still a mystery, but adding the capacity to repel objects adds a whole new dimension. A catalyst modifies a chemical action without entering it by way of diamagnetic forces.

In permanent magnets, the magnetic moments of atoms in the material can be permanently aligned to form magnetic fields. In enzymes, the addition of iron, and cobalt (Vitamin B12) produce permanent magnets. In paramagnetism, the atoms or molecules of the substance have ionic bonds that are capable of being aligned in the direction of the applied magnetic field. As such, they are attracted to the magnet, but lose the magnetic field as soon as the parent magnet is removed. DNA molecules have ionic hydrogen bonds that can be polarized by an ionic field. Water molecules are slightly diamagnetic at all times. The combination of organic compounds with oxides of minerals give all cell components a paramagnetic and diamagnetic capacity.

The diamagnetic force is the weakest, the paramagnetic force can mask out the diamagnetic force, and molecules with built in permanent magnets can modify the paramagnetic forces. The selective application of these opposing magnetic fields by the life-force enable living things to control biochemical actions and growth.

The significance of minerals in the diet becomes apparent when we realize that minerals provide the only permanent magnets in the body. According to P. W. Atkins in his text *Molecules*, hydrogen bonds occur only between molecules that can strongly attract electrons. The three important elements capable of forming weak hydrogen bonds are oxygen, nitrogen and fluorine.

We don't hear much about the function of fluorine in the body other than to fight bacterial tooth decay. However, it does appear essential for growth and could play an important part in replication of DNA and control of bacterial infections such as cholera and diphtheria. Since cancers start with infections, a lack of fluorine could be a major cause of cancer. Fluorine may have an essential role in production of antigens to support the immune system.

In the book, Paramagnetism, Philip Callahan writes (Page 8):

...late investigations that fluorine is regularly found even in white and yellow birds' eggs, we must acknowledge it is something essential to the organism. Chickens get this fluorine and other earthly constituents when they have a chance to pick up little slivers of granite. Where this is denied them, as in a wooden hen house, they succumb to chicken cholera and chicken diphtheria.

For a complete explanations of paramagnetism see Philip Callahan's book, *Paramagnetism, Rediscovering Nature's Secret Force of Growth.*

The DNA nucleotide base is fascinating, but it is still only a collection of molecules without the attributes necessary to dictate when cells should multiply. DNA is as dead as any other combination of atoms. The big difference between DNA and other large molecules is the ionic hydrogen bonds between the nucleotides.

DNA taken from previous living things will replicate in the DNA polymerase chain reaction, but DNA does not replicate on its own. A life-force or energy field is necessary to initiate DNA replication.

Amino acids or proteins are functional products similarly transcribed from DNA in expressed genes. A strand of DNA is used as a template to form a strand of RNA. The only molecules in RNA are A, C, G, and U. *(Thymine having been replaced by Uracil.)* An amino acid is transcribed from sets of three such bases starting alphabetically as AAA, and ending alphabetically as UUU.

Although there are 64 possible combinations, there are only 22 amino acids because some amino acids can be formed by two or more triplets. Arginine, for example, can be formed by six different triplets. None of these 64 triplets can cause cancer and no other groups are possible.

By combining long chains of these groups, millions of different proteins can be formed. Defective proteins and cells come from errors in arranging these groups, not in the basic purine to pyrimidine structure (except in some very limited cases).

Cancer occurs only when metabolism switches from oxidative metabolism and production of abundant energy in the form of ATP to a form of metabolism with reduced ATP production through fermentation. Cancer cells are normal human cells with changes in the cell wall and genes expressed for metabolism. Reduced respiration can occur from lack of sufficient oxygen or lack of necessary enzymes. Genetic defects and mutations cannot force a change in metabolism. Toxins and pollutants destroy metabolic enzymes causing a switch in metabolism. Contaminants from fermentation of glucose in scabs and blood clots can cause a switch in gene expression during replication of adjacent cells. Defective genes and cells are a result of cancer-causing conditions produced by factors outside of the cells.

Let's summarize and review by putting the components of the nucleus into order by size, shape, or function.

DNA

1. Atoms of hydrogen, oxygen, carbon, and nitrogen form stable ring-shaped molecules called Adenine, Cytosine, Guanine, Thymine, and Uracil for RNA.

2. The molecules of Cytosine, Thymine, and Uracil are single ring structures called pyrimidines.

3. The molecules of Adenine and Guanine are double-ring structures called purines. In DNA, a purine molecule joins to a pyrimidine molecule to form a DNA base. These bases are crystals connected to a phosphate crystal that energizes the gene giving it a vibrational frequency. Genes have thousands of bases made up of combinations of A-T's and C-G's. Only about 2% to 3% of these bases are used for production of functional products. The balance is called junk genes. (I theorize that these so-called junk genes probably function on a spiritual level and don't have to be expressed because they do not produce functional products. These genes are probably the most valuable, otherwise the life-force would not maintain them.)

Genes

4. Three bases of DNA function together to form a codon. Groups of codons string together to form genes. Enzymes are transcribed from groups of codons in DNA to their equivalent in RNA.

5. In RNA, Adenine and Thymine is replaced by Uracil. RNA is transcribed from DNA to form a template. The template exits the nucleus to guide assembly of enzymes in the cytoplasm of the cell or in a structure called ribosomes.

Chromosomes

6. All of the genes in our cells are referred to as the genome. Genes also string together to form chromosomes with separation points made by terminator genes. There are 46 chromosomes in normal cells; 47 chromosomes in mongoloids. The extra chromosome causes defective human parts but does not cause cancer.

7. Chromosomes are packaged tightly wound in the nucleus of the cell. Each chromosome consists of two strands (one from the male and one from the female) that are twisted around each other in the form of a double helix. There are 23 pairs or 46 chromosomes in a normal cell. These chromosomes are safely packaged inside a membrane forming a nucleus so that random defects do not occur. The chromosomes and genes are bonded only by ionic hydrogen bonds which respond to the current of injury or normal growth to initiate replication of DNA.

Nucleus

8. All of the material within the nucleus is called nucleic acid. All of the nucleic acid within the trillions of cells in our body taken together would fit into a teaspoon. Genes are therefore extremely small and powerless on their own. The active 2% to 3% of genetic structure is an extremely small portion of the human body.

A single defective gene or renegade cell is simply not capable of overtaking the human body and causing all the changes necessary to cause cancer. The cancer cell can only exist in a low-oxygen reduced respiration environment. These environmental changes are caused by microbial infection. The theory of one renegade cell causing cancer is ridiculous.

Genes serve as templates to produce functional products. Genes are important in research on the cause of cancer because genes produce functional products such as proteins and enzymes that control metabolism and respiration. Smoking and other toxins destroy these enzymes resulting in reduced metabolism and increased fermentation.

Microbes have similar genes that produce similar enzymes that destroy or take over functional products produced by human genes. That's how fungi and bacteria cause diseases such as cancer. That's how viruses cause viral diseases. Viruses cannot make large human cells replicate.

In addition, defective genes and chromosomes cause defective human parts and conditions such as Down syndrome. By reviewing these genetic faults, we can see that cancer cannot be caused by any known or possible genetic fault. Cancer growth relies on healthy genes to produce enzymes for growth and replication in a complex anaerobic process with the breakdown of large carbohydrate and protein molecules, rapid assembly of new molecules, respiration, and removal of wastes. There is nothing defective about cancer cell metabolism.

The following quotation from Harper's *Review of Biochemistry* helps describe the structure of DNA and the influence of heat and salt concentration to separate the two strands of DNA. (Page 362. My emphasis on hydrogen bonding added):

> The B form, the overwhelmingly dominant form of DNA under physiologic conditions, has a pitch of 3.4 nm per turn. Within a single turn, 10 base pairs exist, each planer base being stacked to resemble 2 winding stacks of coins side by side. The 2 stacks are held together by *hydrogen bonding* at each level between the 2 coins on opposite stacks and by 2 ribbons wound in a tight right hand turn about the 2 stacks and representing the phosphodiester backbone.

> The double stranded structure in solution can be melted by increasing temperature or *decreasing* salt concentration. Not only do the 2 stacks pull apart but also the bases themselves unstack while still connected in the polymer by the phosphodiester backbone.

Harper's Review of *Biochemistry* connects DNA separation to the decreased salt levels in the cell. In the *textbook The Organization of Cells and other Organs* by Laurence Picken, there is an interesting theory that ties the current of injury to the *decreased* potassium level in the cells as well. We read (Page 325):

> It was Bernstein who put forth the hypotheses that the plasma membrane of muscle is permeable to ions present in high concentration in the interior of the fiber; that a potential difference exists across the surface of the uninjured fiber due to the formation of a Helmholz double –layer (sic?) by the limited outward diffusion of potassium ions; and that an injury current arises whenever the plasma membrane is damaged so that its permeability increases. The injured region then behaves as the negative pole to the positive pole of the intact surface; potassium ions leave through the injured area and sodium ions enter.

Based on this theory, it is not the salt level that dissolves the DNA ionic hydrogen bonds, but the increased electrolytes. In the DNA chain reaction for production of DNA profiles, we are told the process includes cycles of heating and cooling. I suspect there is more to it than that. A change in electrolytic capacity probably accounts for the reason why DNA separates because the DNA bonds are weak ionic hydrogen bonds. There is nothing all that mysterious about initiating replication of DNA because scientists do it for the DNA polymerase chain reaction.

Following DNA separation, high-energy molecules are required to separate genes one from another at terminator points, allowing for their replication in genetic groups. I theorize that this is where high-energy pentose-phosphate molecules come into the scene. Pentose molecules are produced through the progressive breakdown of glucose in fermentation, but not in oxidation. That is why fermentation of glucose leads to cancer and oxidation of glucose stops cancer. ATP and enzymes are also needed to pull chromosomes apart and assemble new nucleotides.

Viruses cannot possibly mutate DNA to cause cancer

In the text, Human Genetics, we read (Page 197):

Viruses are, in a sense, jumping genes. A virus's nucleic acid—DNA, or RNA converted to DNA using reverse transcriptase—inserts into a host chromosome, sometime impairing the function of a residual gene.

What is a virus? Its easy to imagine a gene jumping from one chromosome to another during mitosis, (*jumping genes are called transposons*), but how does a virus get into the genetic structure. A virus must be composed only of nucleotides found in DNA? What is the difference between a segment of a gene and a virus? If a virus invades a gene, such as the so called RNA virus that causes AIDS, how does it do so? Genes are crystals composed of only four nucleotides joined in pairs. A virus must be very similar to a gene in order for a virus to invade a gene.

The physical limitation in a DNA base combinations of A to T and C to G explains why viruses, chemicals, oxygen atoms and other molecules cannot enter the DNA structure to cause defects or mutations leading to cancer. (*However, these carcinogens can mutate the cell-wall membrane.*) The only combinations are nucleotides A to T and C to G. You cannot have A to virus or A to retrovirus, or A to anything else other than T. That's why viruses do not cause defective genes that become oncogenes. If the DNA structure is interrupted or damaged, it loses its DNA stability and resonance. It can no longer transcribe functional products or enzymes. Chemicals and energy forces such as x-rays can destroy DNA but these cannot mutate DNA into a functional product or produce a renegade cell.

Adenine, Thymine, Cytosine, and Guanine have the molecular ring-structure to form stable DNA bases. Viruses are not bodies formed in nucleotides of purine or pyrimidine although they have some DNA bases in their structure.

Lloyd Motz describes a virus as a series of nucleotides within an outer coat or shell. A virus is not physically similar to a pyrimidine or a purine molecule and therefore does not fit into the genetic structure of DNA. Similarly, the virus structure does not fit into the structure of RNA. Sections of the virus may fit in as a combination of bases, or part of a strand, but such variations do not function as DNA or RNA to produce functional enzymes or existing normal genes that do.

Who is Lloyd Motz?

After researching defective genes as the cause of cancer, and finding it did not make sense, I looked for more information on genes from non-medical sources. It was a long and arduous search. I finally found two valuable chapters in a 1975 edition of a cosmology text called *The Universe, Its Beginning and End*, by Lloyd Motz. Not only does the defective gene theory not make sense, the viral cause of cancer is even more senseless.

Back in the 1970's, Lloyd Motz was Professor of Astronomy at Columbia University in New York. While writing articles for a scientific journal called *Chemical Engineering*, he was recognized for having the capacity to express complex ideas in simple language. In 1973, he was commissioned by publisher Charles Scribner's Sons to write a cosmology book in nontechnical language for the public. Not only is his writing easy to follow, he writes from a purely scientific view. His description of DNA is unlike any description found in modern medicine textbooks.

In his book, after describing how the earth and atmosphere were formed, he wrote about *"The Structure of Atoms and Molecules,"* followed by a chapter *"The Origin and Nature of Life."* In this text, the quantum theory is used to explain the structure of viruses as well as the scientific basis for the DNA structure and the uniqueness of living things.

Lloyd Motz describes the DNA structure and how molecules form as a consequence of the atomic theory. None of the medical texts presented or described this very vital issue. He wrote (Page 251):

It should be noted that there is nothing in the mechanism of the formation for DNA from atoms of hydrogen, carbon, nitrogen, and oxygen and their own molecular combinations that cannot be accounted for by the atomic valences and molecular bonds, all consequences of the quantum theory and the electromagnetic force.

The above information is significant in regards to the defective or mutated gene theory because it erodes belief in the power of DNA to control replication of itself. The "spontaneous arrangement of atoms and molecules into the basic building blocks of life is a direct consequence of the physical laws that govern atoms and molecules." There is nothing inherent in a gene that is not also inherent in other molecules found in nature. Genes do not have the capacity to issue orders any more than other molecules have this capacity. There is nothing in the quantum theory and electromagnetic forces in assembling DNA that gives DNA the power to dictate and control cell division.

Replication is not a conscious effort from within DNA to replicate, nor is it a conscious effort from segments of DNA called genes or packages of DNA called chromosomes. DNA is a stable molecule used by living things to store information. Therefore, DNA does not cause itself to replicate. We must look elsewhere for the cause of DNA replication and cancer.

In order to defend the defective gene theory of cancer a long chain of misinformation is required. That first error or lie gives rise to numerous other errors. There must be a master gene or oncogene, there must be suppressor genes, there must be a cell cycle and therefore there must be a cell-clock. In order for cancer to start there must be mutations to the genes and suppressor genes and so on. Millions more dollars are needed now to figure it out!

If genes do not act on their own to initiate replication, none of the secondary conclusions are valid. The defective gene theory of cancer is therefore false. It all comes down to one question: "how is information transferred?" Are genes dead or alive?

In the book, *The Body Electric, Electromagnetism and the Foundation for Life*, authors Robert Becker, M.D. and Gary Selden write about the mindset held by the majority of medical scientists (Page 91):

> I was approaching the body's system of information transfer from the periphery, asking "What makes wounds heal?" They'd started from the center asking, "How does the brain work?" We were working on the same problem from opposite ends. As I contemplated their findings and all of biology's unsolved problems, I grew convinced that life was more complex than we suspected. I felt that those who reduced life to a mechanical interaction of molecules were living in a cold, gray, dead world, which, despite its drabness, was a fantasy.

The defective gene theory of cancer is a fantasy based on an unrealistic supposition that genes are the first or primary cause of human activity and DNA replication based on some form of mechanical interaction of molecules. The stability of DNA and life does not allow for mechanical interactions guided by mechanical structures. The principle of life is needed to explain DNA function of assembling nucleotides into functional products and body form.

Essential difference between living and non-living things

If we are to assign genes with the capacity to give orders and direct life functions, we must assume they are alive. They must have intelligence in order to make decisions. They must have some freedom in order to make the wrong decisions and give the wrong orders. If they give the wrong orders unwillingly, they must then be guided or forced by another mysterious life-force. There is no logic in such reasoning because it does not correspond to the real world.

Why not look for the cause of cancer in the life-force giving human traits to new cells in the body by expressing dormant genes, or parasites living in the body and giving non-human traits to new cells as they develop? Both of these possibilities are based on known research.

Lloyd Motz compares living things to non-living things by comparing salt crystals, DNA molecules and viruses. All of these things have the capacity to reproduce. Are they all alive, dead, or somewhere in between? The basic question is what constitutes life. Capacity to reproduce is not the sole criterion because salt crystals reproduce. Salt is a molecule of sodium and chlorine, not a living thing.

Lloyd Motz provides this valuable insight into the difference between living and non-living things, (Page 244):

> The most striking thing about any single living organism is that it is a unique group of atoms and complex molecules that— contrary to the natural tendency of all inanimate systems to evolve to states of complete disorder and equilibrium—produces orderly events and higher states of order by assimilating matter and producing from it exact replicas of its own basic entities—in cells.

Lloyd Motz contrasts living things to crystals because both reproduce themselves. Crystals are not alive. Place crystals of salt in water and the salt goes into solution. Remove the water and salt crystals form naturally. The crystals reproduce only through the atomic forces within the atoms causing salt, for example, to reform in a periodic crystal structure. In contrast, the living cell reproduces itself from organic and inorganic atoms and molecules that are different from itself, whereas crystals only reproduce with atoms that are the same as itself.

If the dividing line between living and non-living things is based on how replication occurs, DNA nucleotides are clearly in the same category as crystals and other lifeless matter.

The most significant difference between a crystal of salt and a crystal of DNA is that many more atoms and a greater variety are involved in DNA.

From the pool of atoms and nucleotides within the cytoplasm of a cell, the atomic forces within atoms cause the molecules to form purines and pyrimidine structures. When these molecules are formed, because they have such a high threshold of stability, the purine nucleotides connect with the pyridine nucleotides without either being destroyed or changed. This is accomplished through the ionic hydrogen bond. One structure is built upon the other.

When these crystal-like molecules are attached to pentose phosphate molecules, they become energized and more life-like. They build one upon another due to their stability. They form crystals of chemically bonded molecules held together by much weaker ionic hydrogen bonds. These ionic hydrogen bonds will be discussed later.

The same atomic forces draw millions of molecules into long chains or polymers that form strands of DNA. There is nothing in the basic DNA structure that is not a direct consequence of the quantum theory and atomic valances. The DNA molecule is not alive. DNA molecules combine with the same periodic repetition as salt crystals, C to G and A to T. Combinations of non-living molecules do not impart life. DNA cannot give orders, make decisions, or direct life processes. Only living things can do that.

Living things have the unique capacity to organize the DNA bases resulting in a modified enzyme or functional products to adapt to their environment. Living things are a form of wave energy, and the ionic hydrogen bond is a form of wave energy. Electrons are not involved. Living things, thoughts, and emotions can express genes to produce functional products. The ionic hydrogen bonds in DNA account for the variety of living things as well as evolution. DNA has not evolved for billions of years because DNA is only a collection of atoms dependent on the valences of chemicals in the molecule. The life form changes but DNA remains changeless.

Radiation and toxic chemicals (a mutagen) can destroy existing DNA combinations causing genetic defects. This process is the opposite to living things which assemble new combinations in a higher order. Genes destroyed by radiation or toxins do not become functional genes. Such genes do not become templates that serve a functional purpose. Chaotic destruction by non-intelligent forces does not equal organized construction guided by an intelligent being.

The inherent stability of the pyrimidine-purine molecular structure accounts for the stability of life. If genes were alive and free to decide the behavior of the cell, there would be no explanation for the stability of life as we know it. Nucleotides of DNA are simply organic crystals in stable molecules energized by pentose phosphate crystals.

When organic crystals are immersed into water to form a solution, they are referred to as crystalloid. Crystalloid solutions carry an electric current efficiently and are known as electrolytes. Crystalloid molecules in solution will pass through cell-wall membranes enabling cells to function like batteries to produce and use energy. Crystalloids are the spark of life but they are not living things. A crystalloid is a crystal in solution, like the liquid crystals in modern digital watches. Crystalloids are capable or resonating with magnetic pulses of living things, magnets, and electrical fields as well as capable of modulating existing ionic fields by polarization. Crystalloids are the spark plug of living cells.

One cannot deny a connection between the earth's magnetic field, crystals, and living things. Birds have the capacity to migrate for thousands of miles and return to their nest due to a magnetic crystal in their brain. Monarch butterflies can fly from Mexico to Canada, pass through several life stages, and have the last generation return to a specific tree in Mexico to spend the winter. The capacity to convert electromagnetic stimuli through resonance of the earth's magnetism is accomplished by magnetically sensitive nucleotides in their bodies. How this functions is a mystery, but we know it does function.

Let's look now at the function of viruses and research the viral cause of cancer.

The smallest living things, according to mainstream medicine, are viruses, although several researchers have identified even smaller things through darkfield microscopes and systems that magnify an image electronically. Since viruses are considered a possible cause of cancer, I will focus on virus-sized life forms only.

David M. Locke has written extensively about the nature of viruses. In the 1970's, he was a professor at the Illinois Institute of Technology as well as an associate in biochemistry at Rockerfeller University. In his book *Viruses, The Smallest Enemy* there is a description of viruses that reads as follows (Page 3):

The Nature of Viruses

What some chemists have found can be summed up quickly: a typical virus is composed of several kinds of rather large molecules—the proteins and nucleic acids mentioned above—held together in a definite pattern....The natural packing of the individual protein and nucleic acid molecules into the virus particles has also been studied and found to follow purely physical laws, like those that regulate the formation of crystals. With several viruses, it has even proven possible to take the particles apart, purify the individual molecular components, and then put them back together again in such a way that they form intact, fully infective viruses.

Usually, virus particles have quite simple structures. Two patterns predominate: rods and spheres. The principle structure components are protein molecules—hundreds of identical proteins subunits packed in an orderly manner, rather like bricks in a chimney. The rod-shaped structures are, to be more precise, helical—which means subunits are arranged in a continuous spiral, like the lighthouse staircase. And the spheres are really polyhedra, solid forms with a great many polygonal faces very much like globes covered with tiny mirrors that rotated in dance halls of another era.

In *Life the Unfinished Experiment* by S. E. Luria we can find additional scientific description of the rods and spheres that help explain why viruses do not fit the genetic structure (Page 92):

> In one of the simplest viruses, called tobacco mosaic virus from the disease it produces in the tobacco plant, there are 2130 identical protein molecules, forming a hollow tube within which the nucleic acid molecule rests. In one of the largest viruses, the cold-producing adenovirus, the shell consists of many thousand-protein molecules organized in a perfect geometric crystal-like form, with twelve vertices and twenty faces—the polyhedran called an icosahadren. At the tip of each of the vertices there is a spike made of different proteins.

Notice that descriptions of viruses by non-medical writers tend to paint a totally different picture than those of modern medical writers. Medical writers describe viruses as the cause of defective genes and gloss over inconsistencies in shape and size. They also gloss over the fact that viruses exist in rods and spheres. Instead, they present virus as bits of free-floating DNA or RNA. The medical description is misinformation to support research on viruses as the cause of cancer. The possibility that viruses cause a functional change in DNA structure causing cancer is zero. The possibility that a viral cell-wall membrane can mutate a human cell-wall membrane is also zero because the components are too different to be interchanged. The limited amount of DNA in a virus, not capable of replicating on its own, cannot control how much larger cells replicate. Cancer is only caused by life forms with the same ancestry so that parts produced by one can be switched to the other. Viruses do not metabolize food nutrients and therefore virus cannot cause a change in metabolism as found in cancer cells.

From the above description, there is little or no possibility that a virus can combine with DNA to mutate genes and take control of cell functions. The vast physical differences do not justify such speculation. DNA molecules are limited to A-T and C-G combinations. Viruses are not similar to segments of DNA or RNA. Viruses are more like a pig in a poke than functional DNA nucleotides. Viruses influence health by contaminating the cytoplasm of the cell and disrupting cell functions. We speak of viral infections for this very reason.

We learn that viruses come in two main patterns, rods and spheres, in much the same way as bacteria. Viruses could be an early life-form of bacteria or fungi which also come in rods and spheres. Numerous researchers now claim they all microbes are pleomorphic and exist in many forms. This possibility is not promoted in medicine because it goes against the basic germ theory of disease and treatment for disease. If virus develop into larger life forms by assembly of more nucleotides, what do they become? Viruses, fungi, and bacteria come in rod and round forms but there are no viruses as large as bacteria. What force limits the size of a virus? If DNA in humans can replicate on its own to form a massive cancer tumor, and if a virus is DNA, why can't a virus replicate as a cancer tumor and become a large virus?

Locke describes rod shaped viruses as helical or shaped like a lighthouse staircase—practically the same description as rod shaped bacteria. Spherical viruses appear to be a ball-shaped structure made up not as a perfect circle but as a group of hexagonal faces—the same description as used for coccoid bacteria. As D. M. Locke states: "the natural packing of the individual protein and nucleic acid molecules into the virus particles has also been studied and found to follow purely physical laws, like those that regulate the formation of crystals." These creatures take on the same shape because of the physical forces within atoms and molecules.

The principle of life is not within a physical structure but outside of it. Living things guide the purely physical function of DNA formation. DNA does not dictate to living things and defective DNA does not cause spontaneous replication and functional proteins.

Since DNA bases combine only as C to G and A to T, and all combinations are a consequence of atomic forces, DNA is not a living thing. Genes are not independent living things, and chromosomes are not independent living things. Non-living things do not spring to life and decide to multiply. Therefore, genes do not cause out-of-control replication and cancer. Genes require a life-force to generate replication. A virus can only multiply inside a living cell because it needs the electromagnetic stimulation of a living cell to initiate replication. Human genes have vibrant energy, because they contain phosphate molecules.

Lloyd Motz describes the function of genes to act as templates for the life-force. After describing the quality of living things to perform the complex physical, chemical and biological operations called life, he writes (Page 245):

> Thus, although the living organism is a highly ordered structure, its orderliness is not the simple periodic order of the crystal: it is a combination of diverse periodicities subtly woven together, and the genes themselves, which guide the entire structure, are complex patterns of periodicities that act as templates for the orderly processes in, and the precise reproduction of, each cell.

Genes act as templates to guide the processes of life in cells and the precise reproduction of cells. By way of comparison, templates guide your pencil as you make precise drawings, but the template does not control the pencil. You do. The template controls how the line is drawn but you control whether or not the line is drawn. Genes control how replication takes place, but a living thing or outside forces decides if replication takes place.

Let's look now at genetic mutations to see if they can cause cancer. Can viruses cause a mutation in DNA molecules that will lead to cancer? Can a virus give life to a gene? The answer is no.

A virus cannot combine with or take the place of other DNA nucleotides. The outer protein shell of the virus eliminates that possibility and the viral nucleotide structure does not fit. The DNA structure is complete or saturated in a tight spiral and more nucleotides cannot combine with existing DNA except during replication.

Viruses with DNA influence health by entering the cytoplasm of the cell, not the DNA nucleotide structure protected inside a membrane. Lloyd Motz explains scientifically how viruses insert themselves into the cytoplasm of cells; and similar explanations are available on the Internet or other biology books. In his book, *The Universe, Its Beginning and End*, (Page 257), we read:

> Apparently a virus is a bagful of pure genetic material that comes to life only when it is in contact with a living cell; otherwise, these minute creatures collect themselves into inert, lifeless crystals.

The process by which viruses attack living cells is now understood; a single virus attaches itself to the wall of a cell, in accordance with the genetic instructions imprinted on its DNA, and then, via some kind of appendage of its own skin (which is all protein, like the stinger of a wasp) pierces the cell wall and injects all of its DNA into the cell, leaving behind its empty protein coat.

At this point the intruding DNA of the virus is attacked by the natural immunological defenses of the cell, which in most cases destroy the foreign DNA. But if these cell defenses are not strong enough to devour the injected DNA molecules, these molecules, using their own genetic code, induce the cell to manufacture new viruses from its own nucleotides and amino acids, and within 10 minutes of the intrusion, new empty protein virus coats are formed inside the cell.

Viruses appear to lack the capacity to generate energy and must receive energy from much larger cells capable of producing a significant quantum of energy to cause viral DNA to replicate. It appears that a virus inserts its stinger into a cell-wall by piercing the membrane, creates an immediate current of injury in the host cell, and utilizes this current of injury to replicate its own DNA.

Note that viruses outside of a cell are inert lifeless crystals. The important point about viral infection is that the virus appears to come to life only after it absorbs an electromagnetic stimulus from the cell-wall membrane while the virus is still outside of the cell wall. This is the ionic energy field that becomes the current of injury when a cell-wall membrane is injured. A virus is able to tap into a meridian of energy on the cell wall with its protein stinger. It is then capable of injecting its own DNA into the cytoplasm of the cell and using the ionic energy of the cell to replicate existing DNA and assemble new ones, based on random combinations due to the population differences of nucleotides in the cytoplasm. Energy from the cell enables the virus to replicate DNA and manufacture more viruses from nucleotides in the cytoplasm. One could assume that if several viruses are multiplying simultaneously, mutations would occur, due to random selection of component parts. Viral mutations could occur through random infection of one cell by more than one virus. For example, if both red and green viruses invade a single cells, and red viruses produce red components adjacent to green viruses producing green components, we could end up with red-green viruses.

The first function of the virus is to build new coats. A virus does not inject its nucleotides into saturated molecules of DNA nor does it multiply and reside as free-floating DNA or RNA nucleotides. According to Lloyd Motz, "within 10 minutes of the intrusion, new empty protein virus coats are formed inside the cell."

In the National Cancer Institute's publication *Science and Cancer* the description of viruses is more supportive of the capacity to cause genetic changes and mutations because 'structurally they are either DNA or RNA nucleotides'. This medically orientated description of viruses illustrates misinformation to confuse the public. We read (Page 54):

> The world of viruses is a large one, and includes entities that are quite different in size and in chemical structure. Basically, viruses are giant molecules of the same chemical structure as the components of animal and plant cells. Viruses are cell parasites in that they can replicate only within animal or plant cells. They are structurally either deoxyribonucleic acids (DNA) or ribonucleic acids (RNA), a series of nucleic acid components (purines and pyrimidines) attached along backbones of sugarphoshoric acid building blocks. The nucleic acids during the extrascellular phase of virus existence are contained in a protein coat, which is shed when the virus enters a cell.

How can one read the description of a virus from The National Cancer Institute without believing that viruses could easily cause defective genes? Allow me to repeat these two references for sake of comparison. We are told by the national Cancer Institute:

> *They (viruses) are structurally either deoxyribonucleic acids (DNA) or ribonucleic acids (RNA), a series of nucleic acid components (purines and pyrimidines) attached along backbones of sugarphoshoric acid building blocks.*

Compare the above description to the following one by S. E. Luria:

> *In one of the simplest viruses, called tobacco mosaic virus from the disease it produces in the tobacco plant, there are 2130 identical protein molecules, forming a hollow tube within which the nucleic acid molecule rests. In one of the largest viruses, the cold-producing adenovirus, the shell consists of many thousand-protein molecules organized in a perfect geometric crystal-like form, with twelve vertices and twenty faces—the polyhedran called an icosahadren. At the tip of each of the vertices there is a spike made of different proteins.*

By way of comment, both authors state that a virus sheds its coat when it enters a cell. In Motz's description, viruses build new coats before they replicate inside the cell. In NCI's description, the old viral coat is shed outside the cell and no mention is made of the new viral coat being the first step in replication. Similarly, in the more scientific description of genes by David Locke, we read (Page 3): "some viruses may dispense with their protein (coat) altogether and exist only as nucleic acid, but this is the exception, hardly the rule."

In the NCI description of viruses, we read "they are structurally either deoxyribonucleic acids (DNA) or ribonucleic acids (RNA). In the more scientific descriptions, such as that by David Locke, the similarity of viruses to DNA and RNA is totally unfounded. Lock describes viruses by saying: "Usually, virus particles have quite simple structures. Two patterns predominate: rods and spheres. The principle structure components are protein molecules—hundreds of identical proteins subunits packed in an orderly manner, rather like bricks in a chimney."

I believe this point is very significant. Inside cells, a virus is a life-form with a body formed by a protein coat. Inside cells, viruses do not exist as free-floating globs of DNA or RNA forcing defects and mutations on human DNA and causing controller-genes to go haywire. The capacity for virus to mutate existing DNA structures is very limited if viruses are contained within a protective protein coat on one hand and genes are saturated molecules inside a deoxyribose (sugar) coat on the other hand.

In DNA, nucleotides join together due to immutable laws of nature in a crystal-like pattern of either Cytosine to Guanine or Tyrosine to Adenine. Viruses do not attach themselves as lengths of human DNA or even DNA nucleotides because the atomic forces don't cause or allow them to do so.

Based on descriptions of genes and viruses, the theory that virus cause genetic mutations leading to cancer is without scientific merit. While some genetic changes do occur, such changes are not frequent. An estimated ten million people are now being treated for cancer—far more than can be explained by mutated genes and viral oncogenes.

The following quotation from *Harper's Review of Biochemistry* (Page 404), helps confirm this vital issue about genetic mutations.

Mutations

A mutation is a change in the nucleotide sequence of a gene. Although the initial change may not occur in the template strand of the double-stranded DNA molecule for the gene, after replication, daughter DNA molecules with mutations in the template strand will segregate and appear in the population of organisms. Single base changes may be **transitions** or **transversions**. In the former, a given pyrimidine is changed to the other pyrimidine or a given purine is changed to the other purine. Transversions are changes from a purine to either of the 2 pyrimidines or the change of a pyrimidine into either of the 2 purines.

Since the four nucleotides are similar, they can combine as molecules, but they lose their DNA stability and function if they change. They will not replicate precisely due to lack of stability. They do not have the capacity to store knowledge and repeat it without error. Life cannot be built upon these unstable molecules.

Based on the atomic theory and observed mutations in biochemistry, there are no scientific reasons to theorize viruses being capable of creating oncogenes that cause cancer. It is also illogical to say defective genes initiate the replication processes of a much larger chromosome. The theory is too far from reality to be of scientific value.

When one reviews the misinformation promoted by the U.S. National Cancer Institute, regarding the form of viruses, and realize that this false information is medical dogma costing people billions in search of the cause of cancer, one must question all of their other statements. I believe cancer specialists know the cause of cancer simply because they are so careful to avoid any mention of the true facts such as the current of injury and microbial growth hormones and fungal cell-wall chitin. Cancer information for public knowledge is carefully structured, censured, and controlled.

Retroviruses or mutant enzymes do not cause cancer

If virus and mutant genes cannot cause cancer, do retrovirus or mutant enzymes or lack of enzymes cause cancer? Specifically, does the lack of a suppressor gene cause cancer? The answer is no.

Harper's Review of Biochemistry text explains how enzymes are transcribed from expressed genes and how mutations occur (Page 86):

The primary structure of an enzyme, like that of all proteins, is dictated by the trinucleotide (triplet) code of its messenger RNA (mRNA). The sequence of nucleotide bases of the mRNA is in turn dictated by a complementary base sequence in a DNA template or gene. Information for protein synthesis, stored in DNA, thus determines a cell's ability to synthesize a particular enzyme.

Mutations alter the nucleotide sequence of DNA and result in synthesis of proteins with modified primary structures. This may alter structure at higher levels of organization if the new amino acid is significantly different from the old. Mutations may cause partial or complete loss of catalytic activity or, rarely, enhanced catalytic activity. Since mutations are of various genetic loci can produce enzyme with impaired activity, a large number of molecular diseases can result.

The closest we get to information that defective genes cause cancer is that *"a large number of molecular diseases can result"*. Cancer is not specifically mentioned. Since these genes are in cells operating in the oxidative mode, only oxidative enzymes will be transcribed. Out-of-control replication occurs only when the cell operates with reduced oxygen allowing microbial enzymes to take control of replication cycles, stop the oxidative process and maintain rapid fermentation.

Biology texts have references to defective genes from retroviruses. Defects occur by wholesale insertion of a virus between segments of the genetic structure or segments of a strand. In *Harper's Review of Biochemistry* we read (Page 366):

> The genetic material for some animal and plant viruses is RNA rather than DNA. Although some RNA viruses do not ever have their information transcribed into a DNA molecule, many animal RNA viruses, specifically the retroviruses, are transcribed by an RNA dependent DNA polymerase to produce a double-stranded copy of their RNA genome. In many cases the resulting double stranded DNA transcript is integrated into the host genome and subsequently serves as a template for gene expression and from which new viral RNA genomes can be transcribed. *(Note: the total gene package is called the genome.)*

At first glance, it sounds as though RNA viruses and retroviruses can invade DNA to cause genetic defects that could cause disease. But look more closely and we find that the only possible product transcribed from such insertions is another copy of itself. RNA inserted into DNA can replicate itself, but it cannot transcribe other functional proteins or enzymes that control replication cycles or metabolism. Allow me to repeat that vital statement from the above quote: **"In many cases the resulting double stranded DNA transcript is integrated into the host genome and** *subsequently serves as a template for gene expression and from which new viral RNA genomes can be transcribed."*

RNA cannot become DNA even if it enters the host's genome. RNA has the nucleotide Uracil replacing Thymine and the sugar ribose replacing deoxyribose. Since ribose in RNA is different from deoxyribose in DNA, the total complement of atoms does not fit the atomic structure to produce a stable molecule. RNA viruses cannot function as DNA to produce enzymes that would cause a cell to switch to anaerobic metabolism. RNA viruses cannot make phospho-lipid cell-wall components. RNA virus in DNA can replicate only more copies—like looking into a mirror. The theory or concept that a retrovirus is capable of producing enzymes that would take over cellular function is ridiculous. What is stopping the billions of normal cells and immune defenses from functioning normally and taking control of the viral oncogenes?

Similarly, viruses containing DNA (rather than retroviruses) infect and multiply in the cytoplasm of the cell, not the nucleus or DNA. DNA molecules are saturated and cannot accept more nucleotides.

The fact that viruses live only in the cytoplasm of the cell explains why virus can be killed by electrical energies and magnetic impulses the same as any other parasite. Since viruses thrive in the cytoplasm, they cannot avoid electro-magnetic frequencies in the lymphatic system.

Mutations in proteins result in diseases with defective human parts. None result in cancer, not even those found as birth defects. If cancer were a defective gene disease, we should experience a high frequency of birth defects combined with cancer.

If errors occur during the assembly process of the amino acid sequence, mainstream medicine recognizes this error as a defective gene. The gene is wrongly classified as being defective for the simple reason the assembled protein is defective. That's like saying your fax machine is defective every time you have a transmission error. Did you ever receive a fax with transmission errors that gave you a coherent but wrong message? Garbled transmissions in DNA produce garbage, not functional enzymes that take over metabolic processes.

Assembly errors from components of human RNA cannot cause cancer. A human cell with expressed genes for transcribing tRNA (*short for transfer RNA*) for enzymes that support the oxidative cycle cannot accidentally assemble enzymes that will support the fermentation process. It follows without question that the search for the genetic cause of cancer is a waste of cancer research resources and leads to the needless death of millions of people every year.

In summary, mainstream medicine argues that defective genes cause cancer by producing the wrong functional products that supposedly control replication and growth. It also supports the concept that cancer is a result of suppressor genes failing to produce functional products that normally stop excessive growth. It also claims that cancer cells have lost the function of contact inhibition, meaning cells stop multiplying as soon as they contact another cell. Nothing can be further from the truth concerning cancer.

The current of injury associated with damaged tissue produces the signal for replication. Parasites and ammonia can damage tissue to turn on the field of injury. Fungi and bacteria produce the DNA polymerase and co-enzymes that control replication leading to mutated cells. Lack of normal repair to the damaged cells keeps the new cells from knitting over the injury, the current of injury stays on full time resulting in out-of-control replication of cells. Cells do not have a contact inhibition faculty. The current of injury forces continual multiplication

Additional damage to epithelial cells by parasites, surgery, a biopsy, or ammonia, results in new cancer springing up in other places such as the lungs.

There is no possibility that human genes can suppress parasites from damaging tissue and microbes from producing DNA polymerase enzymes and coenzymes that differentiate replicating cells into more embryonic cancer cells.

However, you can control production of microbial enzymes in your body by eliminating parasites. You can suppress microbes from producing DNA polymerase in your cells. You can kill parasites and eliminate them with herbs, oxygen therapies, colonics, magnets, ozone therapies, and electronically functioning devices. You can eliminate the source of enzymes for a permanent cure, not just a temporary remission. All you need to do is selectively destroy the capacity of microbial enzymes to function. Magnetic pulses and modified electrical impulses can destroy enzymes and microbes without damage to human cells and enzymes because human cells and enzymes operate at a much higher frequency. Cancer can be cured in many ways that are better than surgery, radiation and chemotherapy.

Genetic liabilities do not cause cancer or any disease.

The concept that genetic liabilities cause disease needs to be reviewed. Genetic liabilities are presented as an explanation to separate victims of disease from people who stay healthy. If you experience cancer, it is not your fault and there is nothing you can do about it. Your genetic defects are liabilities leading to cancer and disease. Not so.

The McGraw-Hill Encyclopedia entry under "Human Genetics" tells us in broad terms that any change in DNA is a mutation whether it applies to the structure of the gene or to a change in DNA that alters the genetic code and leads to synthesis of an altered protein. It then goes on to tell us that everyone carries many mutations with possibly as many as 20% of our genes mutant in some form or other.

In order to rationalize how people can have both normal health and thousands of defective genes, the significance of defective genes is now reduced by saying we have *"genetic liabilities."* Liabilities may cause disease due to an environmental stress factor. Hereditary cancer starts with having a genetic liability. Presumably, if you didn't have the liability you couldn't get cancer. Therefore, genetic liabilities cause cancer. The reason why some people experience cancer and others don't and why cancer is hereditary, rises from these genetic liabilities.

Does that make any sense to you? I hope not. Isn't it obvious that the environmental stress factor causes the disease? Without the more significant environmental factor that activates the liability, disease would not occur. For example, a match has the capacity to start a fire, but fires do not start unless someone lights the match. After the fire is started, we don't blame the match. The gene, defective or not, is a mechanism. The stress factor is the cause.

The deceptive statement that everyone has numerous "genetic liabilities" leads to the conclusion that all diseases are "possibly gene related." When we hear "possibly gene related" we are led to assume defective genes are the cause of all diseases.

The simple truth is that every disease is positively gene related, because enzymes control all cellular activities and all enzymes are copied from genes That does not mean the genes are defective nor should we assume that nothing can be done to eliminate the disease. Nor does it mean that we have genes for laziness or genes for committing suicide. These are acts of a free will or a disturbed mind. These are not diseases.

Even starvation is a gene-related condition because the body cannot assemble proteins for body function. How can you have a disease that is not somehow gene related? The lack of effective human enzymes or the influence of microbial enzymes and mycotoxins cause all human diseases. Therefore, all diseases are gene related.

Genes defined as a response mechanism

The fatal flaw in the defective gene theory lies in the definition, which fails to recognize genes as response mechanisms or templates. The definition also ignores the function of 97% of the bases that make up the chromosomes. I suspect the two issues go hand in hand. If genes were seen as a response mechanism, there would be no logic in researching genes as the cause of cancer. The cause would be in whatever it is the genes respond to.

Ricki Lewis' textbook *Human Genetics* (Page 384), reports that only "one encoding gene occurs in about every 40,000 to 50,000 bases." That's incredible! An encoding gene takes only three bases to form an amino acid template and most genes are only a few thousand bases long. The majority of bases in genes do not even produce functional products. The definition of a gene is incomplete if it does not include the great majority of DNA bases. Defining genes as nucleotides in DNA that codes for production of functional enzymes leaves out the function of regulatory genes that sense the emotional and spiritual and chemical environment of the cell. It also ignores the possibility that 97% of the genes are used for producing life energy used by the cell for autonomic control of bodily functions.

In the text, *The Secret of Life*, (Page. 18), by Levine and Suzuki, we learn more about the function of these bases.

DNA's four-element code also needs long strings of A's, G's, C's and T's to encode information; scientists estimate that *each of our cells contains roughly 6 billion of them.* Even a typical small gene consists of a least 3,000 base pairs, and many genes are much longer.

Each of our cells contains six billion bases not used for enzyme production, but their function is not included in the definition of genes. Genes respond to our emotions and thoughts as well as to the cellular environment. The definition of genes should include the fact that genes respond to stimuli from within cells as well as from stimuli from the body. A better definition of genes should include references to all genes and so called 'junk' genes.

A gene is a sequence of nucleotides that CODES in DNA, *capable of receiving stimulants from the vibrational frequencies of sunlight and sound as well as intellectual, emotional, lymphatic and cellular signals* **and is capable of responding, in time, with functional products to serve the needs of the cell or body.**

Perhaps another clause should be added that says genes are liquid crystals, resonating with the earth's energies, and producing wave energy used by living things to sustain the life-force.

The added response-clause gives functional value to the 97% of nucleotide bases that do not produce functional products or support replication. The above definition would help researchers sharpen their focus. It would take research for the cause of disease away from defective genes and focus research on the cellular conditions and stimuli that cause the genes to produce the functional products. It would take research, for example, into the current of injury as the cause of replication.

DNA responds to the cellular environment and the contents of the cytoplasm of the cell. If the cellular environment is polluted by a death wish or emotions, this problem must be taken care of first. A wild animal caught in a trap can die from stress within a few hours without being physically harmed. If the person harbors resentment, envy, hate, fear, and other emotions that upset metabolism, he or she must also eliminate these stresses.

Books are now available suggesting that we can consciously repress genes we do not want expressed, or express genes we want expressed. If true, this would help explain some of the mysteries of life that are beyond scientific understanding or deemed to be miraculous. This vast topic is not significant to the main purpose of this book and need not be discussed any further. If you want to research this topic further, please look up Theresa Dale's book, *Transform Your Emotional DNA*, ISBN 9-9652947-6-5. The text is based on the assumption that DNA is controlled by our thoughts and emotions as well as the life-force or spirit within our bodies.

In the book *Light, Radiation and You* by John N. Ott, we read about the influence light has on growth and development of plants and animals. In addition, there are several references to curing physical diseases by using mental imaging. On pages 107 to 110 we read about 4 ½ year old Sara who had tumors behind the left eye. Surgery of the eyeball was recommended, but would probably be of little value as the growth was not in the eyeball itself. Amazingly, the problem was cured by mental imaging. Ott writes as follows:

> To explain medically and scientifically, the value of the 'visual imagery' that we used, we know that as a wholistic modality, 'visualization and expectancy' are attached to one's own volitional effort, the skill is developed and embodies genuine self-regulation of the autonomic nervous system. This, in turn, can affect organic and functional changes in one's body. This has been proven time and time again with biofeedback instrumentation, as demonstrated by Drs. Elmer and Alyce Green at the Menninger Clinic, Carl O. Simonton, M.D., oncologist, as well as in hospitals, medical schools, etc. throughout the world.

The concept that mental imaging affects one's *autonomic nervous system* followed with measurable organic and functional changes in one's body supports the concept that genes are expressed according to the thoughts and desires of the individual. Mental imaging helps cure disease and supports evolution. We become what we think about.

For people who believe in reincarnation, the existence of millions of genetic bases not involved in producing functional products for life on earth suggests that different groups of these dormant genes could be expressed in another life form. The characteristic of people we call "personality" and hereditary features may have resulted from expressed genes during our youth. Just because 97% of the genes are repressed today does not mean they have always been repressed in our lifetime.

Medical texts and books by alternative health specialists discuss how mental imaging can play a large part in health and restoration of health. This point brings us to consider the opposite effect. Can biofeedback or stress cause cancer?

Cancer not caused by trauma, stress, emotions or worry

Can cancer be caused by negative human thoughts and emotions causing defective genes or out-of-control replication?

Numerous authors believe that many diseases, including cancer, follow from emotional problems and stress. The concept is important to an understanding of cancer because emotional problems—loss of a loved one, accidents, trauma, stress, and shock, appear to be related to cancer. What is the relationship? Specifically, what causes cells to multiply out of control following a shock?

It seems to me that we can identify a direct relationship between stress and metabolism. Stress destroys enzymes and depletes our body of functional products. Stress leads to lack of enzymes for oxidative metabolism and increases fermentation of nutrients, which in turn leads to replication of cells. Stress disturbs nutritional habits and hormonal balance, depletes the immune system, allows parasitic and fungal growth that in turn leads to cancer. In most cases where stress or shock appears to initiate cancer, it takes months or years for cancer to develop. We can be sure that stress does not cause cells to multiply directly, or to mutate DNA and cause cancer.

The incredible precision of replication in DNA nucleotides is based on the electromagnetic forces in the atoms and molecules of DNA. That is why the DNA profile stands up in court as evidence that cannot be dismissed. Replication of target genes and production of identical profiles can be repeated over and over if required. It is a simple mechanical process totally controlled by a thinking person following the pattern of normal growth and replication.

DNA is capable of storing information, and DNA crystals are capable of being duplicated in living creatures but not so in dead creatures. DNA is dependent on life to give it the power to replicate.

DNA is a template. DNA responds DNA cannot cause anything except errors in duplication. Errors cause defective parts, not cancer.

7. Defective genes produce defective human parts, not cancer

Now that we know that genes are templates for production of functional products, we can see that defects occur outside of the basic molecular structure of purine and pyrimidine molecules. Understanding how genes are coded within the Universal Genetic Code is also necessary to understand description of genetic faults.

When genes go awry during replication, we get deformities such as extra fingers or toes. In lesser creatures, we may find two heads or four wings where there should be only one head or two wings, and so on.

Children from Chernobyl and Hiroshima, and children born of women, who suffered thalidomide drug poisoning, were born with defective parts, not cancer. Some may have died later from cancer, but that does not say they died from birth defects causing cancer. If defective genes caused cancer, we should experience infants with cancer on a large scale. Children are not born with cancer because the current of injury is not turned on to make infected cells multiply.

Researchers now claim they have discovered 9000 defective genes, but none of these cause cancer. Doesn't that tell them something? Why are they still looking?

No common genetic disorders are directly related to cancer

Defective genes are possible and common if we mean the proteins produced by them or if the arrangement of codons is defective. (*Codons are continuous triplets of RNA that specifies a particular amino acid.*) The components of the codon are structurally perfect, but the combinations are imperfect. Let's review several known defective-gene conditions to prove that defective genes cause defective human parts, not cancer.

Normal genes provide templates for development of normal cells. If a cancer cell can be identified as a specific tissue or epithelial cell, cancer occurred after replication. If the DNA does not show any defective genes, the defect must be in the cytoplasm or the cell-wall membrane. In cases where the cell is not recognizable, one still must identify the source of the Epidermal Growth Factor or coenzymes that caused the cell to differentiate (*develop special cell traits*) into whatever it is. If the growth factors are not from a human cell, they must be from a microbial or parasitic cell because growth factors come only from living things.

Let's review some common genetic diseases.

Myotonic dystrophy is a trinucleotide repeat

(Inability of muscles to relax after the need for contraction has passed.)

In *Human Genetics*, (Page 196), we read:

> With the ability to sequence genes, researchers found startling evidence that myotonic dystrophy was worsening with each generation because the gene was expanding! The gene for the disorder, on chromosome 19, has an area rich in the DNA trinucleotide CTG, which is repeated over and over, like a molecular stutter.

> A person who does not have myotonic dystrophy has from 5 to 37 copies of the repeat, whereas a person with the disorder had from 50 to thousands of copies. The higher the number of repeats, the more severe the disorder, or the sooner it appears.

Down syndrome is a chromosomal repetition

In the text *Human Genetics* (Page 193), we read:

> In Down syndrome, for example, the defect is chromosomal. Chromosome 21 is replicated three times instead of the normal twice, leaving the person with 47 chromosomes rather than the normal 46.

Here again, the mutation occurs in the arrangement and quantity of chromosomes rather than in the individual genetic base structures.

Sickle Cell disease is a nucleotide substitution

The first genetic disease to be understood at the molecular level is Sickle Cell Disease. According to *Human Genetics* (Page 186), the genetic changes are as follows:

> Using protein-sequencing techniques that had recently been invented, Ingram identified the miniscule mutation responsible for sickle cell disease. It was a substitution of the amino acid valine for the gutamic acid that normally is the sixth amino acid in the betaglobin polypeptide chain. At the DNA level, the change was even smaller—a CTC to a CAC, corresponding to RNA codons GAG to GUG. Eventually, scientists found that this mutation causes hemoglobin to crystallize in low-oxygen conditions, bending red blood cells into sickle shapes that cause anemia, joint pain, and organ damage.

A brief look at the Universal Genetic code tells us that CTC results in the production of glutamic acid and CAC results in production of valine. Excess valine created the problem.

Huntington's Chorea disease is a trinucleotide repeat

Huntington's disease results in the degeneration of nerves in the brain. While searching the Internet under Huntington's, for more details, I found the following statement concerning this genetic fault.

> **No genes involved in cancer have been found to be associated with trinucleotide repeat mutations although there are at least eight genetic disorders of this type.**

"No genes involved in cancer have been found..." sums up the basic truth about all defective genetic errors. None are related to cancer because cancer is not a genetic fault disease. Cancer is a cell-wall membrane disease following from mitosis of infected cells.

In the textbook *Genes and the Biology of Cancer* (Page 93), Dr. Varmus describes in detail the three-dimensional structure of a protein determined by x-ray crystallography. He writes as follows:

> By diffracting x-rays through ordered crystals composed of a single protein, the position of virtually every atom in the protein can be determined.

How can genetic researchers miss a genetic defect if they can identify and study every atom in a protein? We must look elsewhere for the cause of cancer.

Let's make a mental note of the fact that x-ray diffraction has identified proteins to be ordered crystals. Crystals have the capacity to resonate from a vibrational frequency. Enzymes are proteins with a resonant frequency that enables them to moderate chemical actions without sharing electrons or developing other chemical bonds. The mystery of how enzymes function will be discussed later following a description of paramagnetism.

8. The current of injury initiates replication of DNA

In this chapter, we will study the current of injury that results in the normal process of DNA replication, and review how cells are mutated during the assembly process to become cancer cells.

Heart attacks and injury to membrane tissue produces a zone of increased electrical activity called a current of injury. The zone of the current of injury is directly proportional to the size of the injury as well as to the vitality of the body. A strong, healthy and energized body produces a stronger current of injury than is produced by a devitalized body. The current of injury results in healing of injured body parts and the rate of healing is directly related to the health of the individual. That is why young bodies heal faster and why the incidence of cancer does not occur frequently among healthy and active teenagers.

The current of injury explained

In Arthur Guyton's, *Textbook of Medical Physiology* current of injury is discussed in conjunction with heart attacks and cardiac abnormalities. He writes (Page 192):

The Current of Injury

Many different cardiac abnormalities, especially those that damage the heart muscle itself, often cause part of the heart to remain partially or totally depolarized all the time. When this occurs, current flows between the pathologically depolarized and the normally polarized areas. This is called the current of injury. Note especially that the injured part of the heart is negative, because it is this part that is depolarized while the remainder is positive.

The current of injury results when "current flows between the pathologically depolarized and the normally polarized areas" of muscle tissue. The current of injury is a polarizing force. The heart beat normally functions according to a rhythmic polarization and depolarization of the heart muscles.

When some muscles remain depolarized, the heartbeat stops or fails to beat properly.

Guyton goes on to teach:

"... many stray currents exist in the body, such as currents resulting from "skin potentials" and from differences in ionic concentrations in different parts of the body. . . Often the heart muscle does not die because the blood flow is sufficient to maintain life even though it is not sufficient to cause a repolarization of the *membranes. As long as this state exists, a current of injury continues to flow during diastole.*"

Diastole is the period of dilation of the heart muscle that alternates with contraction to pump blood. In the process of a heartbeat, polarizing and depolarizing cause contraction and relaxation of muscles. Following a heart attack, the current polarizes the injured area and the current stays on as long as the polarized conditions exist in the muscle tissues. The heart muscles cannot be polarized and depolarized in a rhythmic manner.

In the above reference, Dr. Guyton indicates that the current of injury is used to polarize the depolarized tissue. The injured part is negative. The current of injury flows from the healthy or "polarized" to the injured or negative or depolarized area. The current of injury is an increased region of high ionic activity that exists over the injury, but does not flow elsewhere. The current of injury stays on until the injury is repaired.

Dr. Guyton teaches that there are three possible causes for the injury to heart muscles. He writes (Page 192):

Some of the abnormalities that can cause current of injury are:

(1) mechanical trauma, which makes the membrane remain so permeable that full repolarization cannot take place,

(2) infectious processes that damage the muscle membranes, and

(3) ischemia of local areas of muscle caused by coronary occlusion.

A coronary thrombosis is a heart attack. Ischemia refers to localized reduced blood flow and coronary occulsion refers to blocking of an artery to stop blood flow within the heart muscles.

The important point within the above reference is item (2): the current of injury may be caused by an infectious process that damages the muscle *membrane.* Veterinarians regularly treat pets for heartworm parasites.

Infection can damage membrane tissue that forms around heart muscle and valves. In other words, parasites can cause heart attacks and turn on the current of injury by damaging heart tissue membranes. In the same way, outside of heart tissue, the damage of epithelial tissue in organs and ducts by parasites causes a current of injury to begin replication in order to repair the damage. Replication of cells begins with the current of injury. Parasites and infection are often the cause of cancer. Physical injury, nutritional deficiencies, a biopsy, mammogram, drugs, pollutants, excess hormones, etc. are others.

The current of injury is all that is needed to explain why some cells multiply out of control to cause cancer. Controller genes or defective genes sending the wrong message or defective genes failing to stop replication are not required to explain the cause of DNA replication. Parasites can cause the current of injury that leads to cancer. Unfortunately, there does not appear to be any references available in my copies of medical textbooks to the current of injury causing DNA replication and cancer.

In the book, *Cross Currents*, Robert O. Becker, M.D., describes how he discovered that the nervous system of animals operates on both direct current and alternating current. The more primitive system is the direct current type, and was used for sensing injury and accomplishing repair. Although nerves are not involved, the system encompasses all cells in the body and is still used today. This is the energy that causes replication of DNA to repair an injury.

In the book, *The Body Electric with the subtitle, Electromagnetism and the Foundation of Life*, by Robert O. Becker and Gary Seldon, the current of injury is discussed for more than one hundred pages. Substantial proof is given that the current of injury causes replication of broken bones and epithelial tissue. The connection to cancer is not mentioned but becomes obvious when you read that cancers start with an abnormal growth or cyst or an injury that does not heal. The text also eliminates other possibilities that one might consider as the cause of DNA replication.

On page 87, we find reference to research showing that normal body energy levels are not related to replication and growth.

> Another problem is the fact that, although nerves are essential for regeneration, the action potentials are silent during the process. No impulses have ever been found to be related to regrowth, and neurotransmitters such as acetylcholine have been ruled out as growth stimulators.

Growth is not controlled from the brain center by measurable electrical impulses along nerves. On page 92, we find reference to research showing that ionic currents in solutions do not cause replication either.

> Ionic current is conducted in solutions by the movement of ions—atoms and molecules charged by having more or fewer than the number of electrons needed to balance their proton's positive charges. Since ions are much bigger than electrons they move much more laboriously though the conducting medium, and ionic currents die out after short distances.

The above references support the concept that a current of injury is really not a current at all, but a field of ionic energy that surrounds the injury for the purpose of polarizing the nucleotides and initiating replication. I theorize that the ionic field disturbs or polarizes the ionic hydrogen bonds in DNA to initiate replication. This step needs further research. I have not found an explanation that describes exactly how the current of injury causes DNA to replicate, but I believe the process is based on the type of bonding in molecules. Let's review some basic chemistry.

Bonds between atoms are formed by the attraction between electrons of one atom for the positive nucleus of the other atom. This type of bond also contains repulsive or disruptive forces that keep the atoms from collapsing into one unit. Repulsion between positive nuclei and repulsion between orbiting electrons set up a dynamic equilibrium that holds the molecule together but also opens the door for further bonding and chemical action. The unique vibrational frequency of each molecular combination establishes unique chemical and physical properties as well as a unique vibrational field.

Different atoms pull on bonding electrons to differing degrees and this difference determines whether a bond is considered molecular or ionic. When atoms have an equal or nearly equal pull on the bonding electrons, a more equitable relationship exists and a covalent compound is formed. When one atom has a much higher pull on bonding electrons than the other atoms, electron transfer occurs and an ionic bond is formed. A third type of bond exists in which electrons are not exchanged or shared at all and this is referred to as the ionic hydrogen bond. As we shall see later, DNA bases are formed by ionic hydrogen bonding.

Direct current battery starts limb regeneration in rats

In *The Body Electric*, Chapter Seven, *Good News for Mammals*, Dr. Becker illustrates how an artificial current of injury produced by a miniature battery implanted in the stump of a rat's leg caused the leg to grow back. Growth of new legs in mammals such as rats is not a normal phenomenon.

On page 153, there is a diagram of a rat's front shoulder with the leg cut off. Connected to the shoulder bone stub there is a miniature battery. Following this diagram are several smaller diagrams showing the progressive growth of new cells as the leg starts to regrow because of the artificial current of injury.

Following the diagram, Dr. Becker writes:

> I shall never forget looking at the first batch of specimens. The rat had regrown a shaft of bone extending from the severed humerus. At the proper length to complete the original bone there was a typical transverse growth plate of cartilage, its complex anatomical structure perfectly regular. Beyond that was a fine-looking epiphysis, the articulated muscles, blood vessels, and nerves. At least ten different kinds of cells had differentiated out from the bastema, and we'd succeeded in getting regeneration from a mammal to the same extent as Rose, Polezhaev, Singe, and Smith had done in frogs.
>
> ...Since the blastema always formed around the electrodes and since redifferentiation proceeded into organized tissue, we knew the current had stimulated true regeneration, not some abnormal growth. Mammals still had the means for orderly reading out of genetic instructions to replace lost parts.
>
> ...More important, we warned that if such a tiny force could so easily switch on growth, it must be very powerful, and we'd best know it thoroughly before using it routinely on humans, lest we give them unwelcome growths—tumors.
>
> ...So, to be exact, our electrodes had temporarily but drastically boosted the efficiency of the process as it normally waned with age in the rodent. Still, it was the first time that had ever been done in a mammal.

As I read this amazing report, I saw the complete cancer process for the first time. All of the mysteries about why cells multiply to cause cancer can be answered by reference to conditions that cause damage to epithelial tissue, a current of injury, internal bleeding, and fermentation of the blood clot.

An artificial current of injury cause a tumor in the rat's leg? The current of injury will not cause tumors. It just causes DNA to replicate. Microbial infection of cells causes membrane mutation during mitosis. Rejection of cells causes tumors. Fermentation of a blood clot infects adjacent cells and modifies the cellular environment and oxygen levels of them. The next cells to multiply are infected, mutated and rejected. The entire cancer process can be observed through injury to a membrane or bone fracture and microbial infection of adjacent cells.

There is no need for an oncogene that causes cells to multiply, nor is there any need to suppose the existence of a suppressor gene to stop replication. Turning on the current of injury starts the repair process, and shutting down the current of injury stops the replication process. Cancer occurs when the microbial DNA polymerase and coenzymes do not allow the new cells to develop normal membrane cells, heal, and close the gap properly so that the current of injury returns to normal. The difference in cell-wall membranes mutated by microbial proteins and chitin is all that is needed to understand why the current of injury is not turned off. Out-of-control replication of cells is a natural result of microbial DNA in infected cells replicating simultaneously with human DNA.

In *The Body Electric*, we read how fabricated energy fields reactivated dormant genes in red blood cells of humans. As a result, the current of injury applied to human red blood corpuscles, recreated red blood cells with DNA. (Page 140):

> In our series of slides the red cells went through all their developmental stages in reverse. First they lost their characteristic flattened elliptical shape and became round. Their membranes acquired a scalloped outline. By the third day the cells had become amoeboid and moved by means of pseudopods. Concurrently, their nuclei swelled up and, judging by changes in their reactions to staining and light, the DNA became reactivated. We began using an electron microscope to get a clearer view of these changes. At the end of the first week, the former erythrocytes had acquired a full complement of mitochondria and also ribosomes (the organelles where proteins are assembled) and they'd gotten rid of all of their hemoglobin. By the third week they'd turned into cartilage-forming cells, which soon developed further into bone-forming cells.

The current of injury process that causes DNA to replicate and form new tissue is not limited to amphibians. Children younger than eleven years of age are capable of growing new fingertips lost by accident. Human liver tissue is capable of new growth after surgery. In addition, the system for bone repair is the same in all vertebrates, including humans. On pages 147-148 we read:

> Except for the identity of the target cells, bone repair seemed to be basically the same in all vertebrates, proceeding through the stages of blood clot, blastema, callus, and ossification. In fish,

amphibians, reptiles, and birds, the red cells in the clot dedifferentiated in response to the electric field, especially the positive potentials at the broken ends of the bone. They redifferentiated as cartilage cells and continued on to become bone cells.

... By this time we'd become pretty sure that the marrow component of bone healing in humans involved the dedifferentiation of at least the immature erythrocytes, which still contained a nucleus, and possibly other cell types.

...The electrical forces turned the key that unlocked the repressed genes. The exact nature of the key was the one part still missing from the process. The current couldn't act directly on the nucleus, which was insulated by the cell's membrane and cytoplasm. We knew that the current's primary effect had to be on the membrane.

In is well known in modern medicine that fractured bones can be made to heal faster with an electromagnetic stimulus. The first such experience is recorded as follows:

...Fracture healing was ended by a straightforward negative-feedback system. As the gap filled in with new matrix, the bone gradually redistributed its material to balance the stresses on it from the action of the surrounding muscles during cautious use, in accordance with Wolff's law. Repair of surrounding tissues lessened and then stopped the periosteal injury current. As a result the electrical field returned to normal, shutting off the cellular activities of healing.

Wolff's law refers to the way a bioelectric field creates a magnetic field in much the same way as an electric current creates a magnetic field. *Periosteal* is a type of leg bone in frogs used for experimental purposes, and *periosteal injury current* refers to the current of injury around the damaged periosteal bone.

The important point in the above reference is that the current of injury is shut down by the repair. He writes: *"repair of surrounding tissue lessened and then stopped the injury current."* If this is true, and I have no reason to doubt it, we do not need suppressor genes to stop replication of cells. We cannot blame cancer on the lack of suppressor genes to stop the process. Cancer has nothing to do with defective genes that initiate replication or the lack of suppressor genes to stop replication. Injury disrupts the ionic field of cell-wall membranes, turns on the current of injury, and repair of injury turns it off unless an infection disrupts the healing process.

Another important point in the above reference is that "bone repair seemed to be basically the same in all vertebrates, proceeding through the stages of blood clot, blastema, callus, and ossification." All types of cells are equally stimulated by a field of injury. The blood clot and trapped blood proteins serve as an essential part of the healing process, probably because red blood cells in a blood clot can become new cells. Also, red blood cells conduct ionic energy and increases polarization of the adjacent cells. The blood clot conducts the current of injury across the gap. The connection between cancer and storage vessels and follows from infection of the blood clot. From this, we can conclude that anything that contributes to internal bleeding can lead to cancer. Nutritional deficiencies, chemical contaminants, and parasites that damage cell walls and organ membranes are good examples of carcinogens.

The current of injury explains why some cancer tumors grow rapidly and others grow more slowly. The paradox of a slow growing cancer tumor is answered by size of the current of injury and amount of blood in the blood clot. Research shows that the current of injury is in proportion to the injury, and it follows that the normal repair process is in proportion to the current of injury, and the rate of tumor growth is proportional to the current of injury. If parasites, cysts, polyps, or ulcers cause a large injury or a large number of small injuries, the rate of tumor growth is increased proportionately.

Some cancer specialists believe that doing a biopsy of a tumor results in increased rate of growth for the tumor and that doing a mammogram of breast cancer will increase the rate of growth. Obviously, if you put an incision into a tumor, burst some blood vessels, or injure adjacent flesh to reach the growth, you will have increased the size of the injury as well as the current of injury. You may recall that a Canadian study of more than 50,000 women showed that women of ages 40 to 49 who were given annual mammograms showed a 32% increased breast cancer mortality compared to those given physical examinations only. A similar study from Sweden showed a 29% higher mortality rate. These results can be explained through an increase in the current of injury.

All cells that protect the body, such as the outer skin, multiply often because they are more prone to environmental factors. Injury to the cell-wall membrane due to the environment could cause normal cellular replication. Ultraviolet rays from sunlight cause injury to skin cells, and some cancers are caused by sunlight. Perhaps lack of function, such as production of energy in the form of Adenosine triphosphate (ATP), switches on the current of injury to cause cells to multiply before they die. Consequently the cell components are renewed in a new cell-wall membrane, and the cell-function is renewed. In physical injury, cells are totally destroyed and lost, the current of injury causes adjacent cells to multiply and replace the lost cells. It is interesting that growth and repair of cells results from the death of cells. Cancer results from microbial infection of cells, injury to tissue, a blood clot, and initiation of the normal repair process by an ionic field. The secret lies in the type of bonds that hold DNA together.

The ionic hydrogen bond forms DNA and genes

The following information is taken from the Scientific American publication *Molecules*, by P. W. Atkins (Pages 10-11). Atkins states that the most common chemical bond is the *molecular bond* which occurs when two atoms share one, two, or three electrons. The second type is called *ionic*, and is a *magnetic bond* formed by the electrostatic charge between two unequally charged molecules or particles. The stable molecular and ionic bond that forms the six-sided pyridine and purine molecules gives DNA its stability.

The third type of bond is called the *hydrogen bond* that is formed by two molecules with a hydrogen atom or ion between them.

Weak ionic bonds of DNA nucleotides give DNA its flexibility to wind into a tight spiral or be expressed as active genes. In DNA, Adenine and Tyrosine are coupled by two ionic hydrogen bonds, and Cytosine and Guanine are coupled by three ionic hydrogen bonds. In RNA, the additional oxygen atom in ribose sugar probably allows for the RNA molecule to be more stable than the protein translated from it, but I could not find any references to ionic bonds in RNA.

On the Internet at the web sight http://www.science. utah.edu/beebe.html we learn about the work of three scientists at the University of Utah, College of Science, who measure the bonding force of different types of bonds. The Internet report contains these following statements relating to DNA bonding.

1. A hydrogen bond is the kind of weak bond that holds water molecules together, making water boil at a higher temperature than it would otherwise. A hydrogen bond is formed when negatively charged electrons in each molecule are attracted slightly to positively charged nuclei of adjacent molecules.

2. Such bonds are much weaker than covalent, ionic or metallic bonds, which hold atoms together within a molecule or crystal.

3. Hydrogen bonds hold together two strands of chemicals that give a double-helix shape to DNA. When a cell reproduces and its DNA is copied, an enzyme breaks apart the two strands.

Regarding the boiling point of water, Isaac Asimov, in a book called *The Left Hand of the Electron*, writes (Page 107):

> The hydrogen bond is about one twentieth as strong as an ordinary chemical bond, but that is enough to add up to 170 degrees to the temperature required to tear the molecules apart and set the liquid to boiling.

The hydrogen bond may be relatively weak, but it still has tremendous influence in living things, and has potential as a source of energy in place of magnetic fields. The bond is weak enough to be harnessed for energy.

Although the Internet report states an *enzyme breaks apart the two strands*, this need not be the case. Genes are maintained as units during replication, and genes are large molecules, far larger in length than the capacity of an enzyme to influence all of the bonds simultaneously. Enzymes and substrates are needed to break the stronger chemical bonds at the atomic level, by shifting electrons around in the nucleotides. However, the weak hydrogen bond extends for the length of genes as all bases are held together by hydrogen bonds. Genes can be expressed or duplicated as units by insertion of a ionic field through the desired length of the genes or chromosomes. The length of the molecular bond forming chromosomes does not matter if an ionic field is used to control separation of chromosomes.

The input of the current of injury, being a more powerful ionic field than the hydrogen bonding, disrupts hydrogen bonds allowing the DNA nucleotides to separate, while remaining attached to the deoxyribonucleic chain of sugar molecules joined by the more powerful ionic and molecular bonds. The highly energized cytoplasm with its population of atoms and nucleotides along with electrostatic forces in molecules causes the growth of new nucleotides to result in replication of the DNA chains.

Since ionic bonds are electrostatic, or magnetic, it follows that electomedicine, or pulsed magnetic fields, light and sound therapies can play a role in medicine. It is important that we review this concept.

The hydrogen bond tends to break the rule that hydrogen forms only one type of bond because it has only one electron. The strong attraction of the oxygen bond can polarize the hydrogen atom so that an ionic field is created. The ionic field can be utilized to control body functions. Glues and paints are hydrogen bonds, as is the ionic layer making up a cell-wall membrane formed by layers of cells. Ionic bonds can be modified by an ionic field. The whole theory of the current of injury causing DNA replication rests on this principle.

To help understand the quotation that follows, the author calls the hydrogen bond a *"vestigal ionic bond."* The word *vestige* meaning a visible trace, comes from the Latin word for footprints. A vestigal bond is identified by its footprint or function. Diagrams of molecules in chemistry indicate the hydrogen bond by a series of dots whereas molecular and ionic bonds are indicated by a solid line.

Let's review the explanation of hydrogen bonds as expressed in the book by P. W. Atkins called ***Molecules*** (Page 11):

> The bond is formed because the oxygen in A—O—H *(hypothetical generalized molecules)* attracts electrons so strongly that it draws the shared electron pair in its own O—H bond toward itself, leaving the positive charge of the hydrogen nucleus almost fully exposed. ***That exposed positive charge is strongly attracted to other electrons nearby,*** particularly those of another oxygen atom, as in the molecule O—B *(another hypothetical molecule)*. The hydrogen bond is therefore a *vestigial ionic bond* between two molecules. It can occur only between atoms that can attract electrons strongly, which for our limited palette of elements include: O—H...O; O—H...N; N—H...O and N—H...N
>
> *(Fluorine, is the only other element for which hydrogen bonding is important.)* As you see, hydrogen bonding is of enormous importance in the world, for among numerous other things, it accounts for the existence of oceans and the strength of wood.

In diagrams on DNA, we see that T-A bonds (thymine pairs with adenine) contain two hydrogen bonds; namely, O...H—N and N—H...N. Please note that these bonds are 50% nitrogen-nitrogen based, and 50% oxygen-hydrogen based.

In C-G bonds (cytosine pairs with guanine) there are three hydrogen bonds; namely, N—H...O; N...H —N; and O...H—H. Please note that these bonds are 33% nitrogen-nitrogen based and 66% oxygen-hydrogen based. These bonds strengths are not equal.

Based on the content of oxygen, hydrogen and nitrogen in these bonds, there are three different types of vestigal bonds presenting the possibility of three different bonding strengths. In addition nucleotides A-T bond with two bonds whereas nucleotides of C-G bond with three bonds, thereby giving C-G bonds more stability. In long rows of DNA bases, every combination presents a unique bonding force.

The quantum theory would suggest that three different energy levels would be required to initiate breaking of these bonds. As a result, the selection of a gene to produce functional parts can be made by providing the precise quantum of energy for that particular gene. Similarly, the reduction and assembly of DNA can proceed in an orderly and repetitive manner by controlling the strength of the ionic field.

If you do an Internet search for "vestigal bonds in DNA" in Alta-Vista, you will be promptly rewarded with about one million web pages of data. In these pages, you will find numerous color-coded descriptions of these bonds along with animated videos of the DNA replication process. Similarly, numerous books and texts give detailed descriptions of these bonds. With such a wealth of material at your fingertips, if you need diagrams to picture the genetic structure, please access these in reference material. You will also find proof that DNA is formed with weak hydrogen bonds.

For example, we read in http//wakesman.rutgers.edu…

Hydrogen Bonding

Hydrogen may covalently bond to F, N or O. These atoms are very electronegative and prefer to have much electron density around them. The electron pair is unequally shared with hydrogen being left with a slight positive charge and the other atom with a slight negative charge. The positive charge on hydrogen will attract another electronegative atom from a second molecule. This strong attraction results in molecules being held together much more tightly than might be expected.

The strongest hydrogen bonds are between the electronegative atoms of F, N, or O. In a water molecule, for example, the slight negative charge around oxygen will attract a slightly positive hydrogen from a second molecule of water.

DNA uses hydrogen bonding to hold the two strands of the double helix together. The hydrogen bonds are strong enough to hold DNA together since there are so many in each strand. Hydrogen bonds are weaker (~5kcal/mole) than a covalent bond (~100kcal/mole), so easier to break and reform. The ease of breaking and forming H-bonds in DNA allows for replication and protein formation.

In the above quotation, there is no mention of an ionic field being used to initiate DNA replication but it does state that these bonds are only 5% as strong as chemical bonds. The attraction is molecule to molecule. It follows that this bond is not a chemical bond that is enzyme controlled. A modest ionic field is all that is required to disrupt this weak ionic bond. The amount of energy required to initiate replication varies with the combination of bases.

The bond in G-C pairs are 66.6% oxygen to hydrogen bonds, and 33.3% nitrogen to nitrogen bonds. Bacteria from thermal hot pools have more G-C bonds and have greater heat tolerance for this reason. It follows that anaerobic bacteria, with more of the A-T base pairs, containing only 50% oxygen-hydrogen bonds and 50% nitrogen-nitrogen bonds would be less heat stable than human DNA. The capacity of a high fever to destroy microbial infection is probably based on this phenomenon. Increasing the temperature of infected cells will also help destroy the infection. Control of body temperature is important for control of DNA assembly and curing cancer.

Knowing that the DNA nucleotides are based on a variety of weak vestigal ionic bonds is important for an understanding of DNA function and replication. The life-force can express genes, as desired, and the life force can produce a current of injury capable of initiating DNA replication.

Genes come in long strings with terminator points at each end. These terminator points are simply strings of genes with a very low bonding strength. In the process of replication, these terminator bonds are the first to come apart, allowing the gene to be duplicated as a manageable unit. That is why the theories of controller genes and defective controller genes, or over expression of controller genes are false theories. There are no controller genes that initiate DNA replication. The genetic structure allows for energy fields to control genetic function and replication.

The above statement that hydrogen bonding "accounts for the existence of oceans and the strength of wood" is also quite significant. Wood is a *diamagnetic material*. Wood is repelled by both the north and south pole of a magnet. It follows that the strands of DNA, being held together by hydrogen bonds, would separate due to a magnetic field, just as wood is repelled by magnetic fields. An ionic field or force that repels molecules would be far more functional for causing DNA, genes, and chromosomes to separate than would be chemical bonds that can only attract and bond by sharing electrons.

What is diamagnetism?

Diamagnetism causes DNA strands to separate

Author Philip Callahan, Ph.D., in his book *Paramagnetism,* writes about the phenomenon of diamagnetic materials (Page 46):

> ... Diamagnetism is the magnetization in the opposite direction to that of the applied magnetic field, e.g., the susceptibility is negative away from the magnetic field...Diamagnetism results

from changes induced in the torque by bits of electrons that oppose the applied magnetic flux. There is thus a weak negative susceptibility to the magnet. Most organic compounds, including all plants, are diamagnetic.

The concept that organic compounds such as plants and DNA are repelled by a magnetic field is rather exciting. Enzymes, which modify a chemical reaction without entering into the chemical action could do so by repelling, or pushing around, so to speak, the atoms in the reaction. Nucleotides of DNA such as guanine and cytosine can be pushed apart for replication. Strands of DNA can be pushed apart for expression of genes. Chromosomes could be made to unwind and wind simply by polarization and depolarization, similar to the autonomic function of increasing or decreasing the rate of our heartbeat.

It follows that a polarized ionic field, creating a north or south polar magnet, could disrupt these ionic bonds and do so in a specific order based on the differences in bond strength. This would help account for the capacity of genes to separate one from another, and reform in the reverse manner as soon as the polarization is reduced.

It is reasonable to conclude that the signal for DNA replication for growth and repair—the current of injury—is a function of the life form that initiates chromosome, gene strand, and DNA base separation. It is based entirely on variations in ionic energy. Initiating replication has nothing to do with controller genes, defective genes, or enzymes.

Enzymes only control the stable chemical bonds in which electron orbits are shared and these chemical bonds are based on the forces within atoms and the quantum theory. DNA pairs, bonded with vestigal hydrogen bonds, are diamagnetic molecules, similar to that which gives strength to wood. To initiate replication and express genes, strands of DNA are pushed apart because they are diamagnetic molecules.

Life is an electromagnetic phenomenon. The life force, emotions, thoughts, fears and desires create waves and these waves act directly on the genes to control life functions.

The construction of DNA as liquid crystals gives life to DNA. The earth is a giant resonating magnetic field due to the spin of the earth. The movement of molecules of DNA through the sun's magnetic lines of force, due to the spin of the earth, would cause diamagnetic molecules to vibrate and resonate with the frequency of this vibration. Energy receptors, such as phosphate molecules could absorb this energy and form electron that energize ATP and pentose phosphate in DNA.

The internal structure of the energy producing mitochondria shows a series of plates extending from the cell wall into the cell. These plates could vibrate due to resonance with the earth and absorb this vibration to produce useful energy. The concept is similar to the hairs in the middle ear forming our balance mechanism that is energized by vestigal energy.

The energy source can be seen in the highly energetic tumbling motion of colloids in water, known as the Brownian movement. This movement is caused by the magnetic field moving past polar molecules.

To assist further understanding of energy production, let's review the concept of ions and ionic energy. You are familiar with ionic energy fields through static electricity when you walk across a carpet and get a shock upon touching a doorknob.

Ionic energy explained

An ion is an atom that has lost or gained an electron, and therefore has a positive or negative charge. An atom that loses an electron is said to be positively charged and is called a *cation*. An atom that gains an electron is said to be negatively charged and is called an *anion*. These atoms have magnetic fields and form molecules by electrostatic charges. Just as electrons can flow down a wire as particles, ionic energy can flow down nerves as waves, and flowing ions create an ionic field. Static electricity that attracts hair and dust is an ionic field. We can also have positive and negative ionic fields. Ionic fields are a wave from of energy. Wood is slightly diamagnetic, which means it is repelled by both poles of a magnet. Wood, being a crystalline structure, appears to produce or contain residual ionic energy that is repelled by a magnetic field. I believe organic crystals in wood generate the ionic energy that appears to be residual, just as the electron continues to circulate around the nucleus of an atom without ever running down.

Use of ionic energy in living systems

There is evidence in medical texts that the body uses ionic energy for maintaining bodily functions of the autonomic nervous system. Replication of DNA is only one of these autonomic functions.

In Dr. Guyton's Textbook of Medical Physiology Chapter 52 is called *Motor functions of the brainstem and basal ganglia*. One unique group of nerve cells and nerves are called the *vestibular* nucleus and *vestibular* nerves. On Page 641 we read about these nerves:

> In general, these specific nuclei are not considered to be part of the reticular formation (collective term for the nervous system) per se, even though they do operate in association with it. In most

instances, they are the loci of 'preprogrammed' control of stereotyped movements.

The text goes on to describe how the balance mechanism in the inner ear uses tiny hairs to produce *vestibular energy signals* that control balance without conscious input from the brain. These hairs have a specific gravity 3 times that of normal tissue and are the first to respond to movement of the body. Just imagine breezes blowing patterns in a field of grain, or ripples on a quiet pond, and you can picture the mechanics of balance. As hairs bend to gravity and movement, they touch one another, creating electrical circuits that the body interprets as movement. The energy impulses could be created by the piezoelectric generation through bending of hairs in the inner ear region of the head. Electrons are captured between hairs and bending the hairs forces them out. Alternately, since these hairs are connected to *vestibular axons* at the base, the energy could flow outward from the nerves to energize the hairs. The waving motions short circuit those hairs that contact one another enabling the body to sense direction and orientate itself upright.

What is piezoelectric energy? If you use a B.B.Q. lighter that generates a small spark when you pull the trigger, this spark is generated by the piezoelectric method. Layers of metal will retain free electrons between the layers. Bending the layers of metal force electrons out of resting areas between the layers, much like wringing a floor mop forces water out of the strands.

Robert Becker describes how the normal use of arms and legs causes bones to flex, and this produces energy through the piezoelectric method of electron production. This energy initiates growth. That's why physical effort and weight lifting increases bone and muscle mass. Weightlifting and training is an application of ionic energy to cause increased growth.

The same phenomenon is recorded in tree growth where branches have their center ring close to the top edge of the branch. Due to twisting and swaying of the branch by the wind, the growth of the branch is in direct proportion to the amount of bending produced on the branch. Growth occurs where it is needed most at the bottom of the branch. Anytime you find a round piece of wood with the center of the rings near one edge, rather than the middle, you know you are holding wood that came from a branch of a tree. To observe this effect for yourself, check the growth rings from the branch of a tree.

Concerning vestibular energy signals, Guyton's text goes on to state: "*The base and sides of the hair cells synapse with sensory axons of the vestibular nerve.*"

Although it doesn't say how energy is transmitted, I suspect energy is transmitted as a wave, not as the flow of electrons. In engineering of tiny microchips, called nanoengineering, it has been found that confining electrons to a field smaller than their required orbit results in electrons existing as waves instead of particles. The bizarre changes in electrical properties of atoms at absolute zero can be attributed to switching electrons from particles to waves. Ionic fields exist as energy below the electron level and therefore function as wave energy in nanoengineering. Human energy is not limited to electrical energy. The life force operates at the wave energy level known as ionic field energy.

Perhaps the vestibular energy of the balance mechanism explains why medicine cannot determine the physical problem that causes ringing in the ears. The problem is not measurable as a nerve or electrical fault because it is an imbalance or polarization of the vestibular energy fields. Many common ear problems result from drugs and chemicals that poison the ear, causing problems with the vestibular nerves sending confusing signals to the brain. When we take drugs, movement causes dizziness because the eyes are connected to the balance mechanism and eye focus shifts automatically upon movement of the head. By disturbing this mechanism with drugs, one becomes dizzy through any motion.

Although I researched this problem quite thoroughly, I have not seen any mention of vestibular energy as a cause of disease in any of the medical literature. I have never seen any mention of vestibular energy or hydrogen bonds in relation to health problems or DNA replication. Have you?

It is scientifically reasonable to assume that the life-force communicates with the body through ionic wave energy. Thoughts are waves that originate in the brain, but can be measured outside of the brain as with a lie detector test. The process of thinking consumes vast amounts of oxygen therefore, it must produce significant amounts of energy. Thoughts exist and are conveyed as vestibular energy. Staring at the back of the neck of someone often causes that person to turn around and look back. Looking at a person, and thinking about where you are looking, sends a vestibular signal to that person, causing him or her to sense your attention. Vestibular energy plays a large part in the life of living things and probably accounts for mental telepathy and affects personal relationships in many ways. Various health benefits from massage and therapeutic touch could similarly be explained as stimulation of ionic energy fields. Obviously, ionic energy fields can affect the health and function of the body as well as initiate replication of DNA.

Is vestibular energy also produced by DNA? Let's assume for discussion purposes, that DNA crystals resonate to sunlight and the vibrational frequencies of the earth. DNA crystals produce vestibular energy, in much the same way as chlorophyll in plants converts sunlight into growth. The secret power of DNA molecules and bases is the frequency of vestibular waves produced by the unique crystals that make up the 64 bases in the Universal Genetic Code. Every change in the crystal form of DNA bases results in a change of vestibular energy wave frequency, and therefore a change in function.

In chemistry, the symmetrical pattern of atoms, molecules, and ions is referred to as the crystal lattice. Just as we tune in to radio stations (originally called a crystal) by a change in frequency of the signals, the life-force uses different frequencies of vestibular energy from different crystal lattices for different functions in DNA.

Perhaps too, the power of suggestion and subliminal advertising follows from thoughts effecting output of vestibular energy and DNA function.

The major point of the above reference concerning cancer is that the body uses ionic energy for control of primitive life functions. This energy is communicated by very tiny nerves for balance and orientation, or along the cell-wall membranes in invisible meridians that connect all parts of the body. When a membrane forming a storage vessel or duct is broken, the ionic energy being stored in adjacent membrane flows to the injury. The resulting current of injury used to repair damaged cells is a basic life function. This explains why the strength of the ionic field produced by an injury is dependent on oxygen levels, or vitality of the body, and is directly proportional to the extent of injury.

Perhaps the physical connection between cancer and emotional and mental shock, as in the sense of trauma, is through disruption of vestibular energy. Cancer often occurs within a year or two of a physical or emotional trauma because it takes that long for the energy imbalances to result in microbial infection of cells, injury, and cancer. A severe trauma can modify all autonomic functions and cause shock to the entire system.

Injuries affect the alignment of the neck and back bones, which in turn affect the flow of energy through the body. Chiropractic adjustments, massages, and body toning all contribute to health by increasing the natural flow of energy in the body. Everyone with health problems should use these alternative health services to help prevent diseases of all kinds.

Magnets are formed when electrostatic charges in atoms or molecules are orientated in one direction or polarized. Similarly, the membrane of cell walls can be strengthened by the polarization of molecules in the membrane. Therapeutic touch can improve your health.

Paramagnetism, which plays such an important part in function of growth in plants and function of enzymes, is founded in the ionic bonds of atoms and molecules. Ionic charges can be instantly polarized, but lose polarization just as fast. The reason why oxygen is so vital to life is that oxygen in unsaturated fats creates the ionic hydrogen bond that serves as the electrical circuit in living things. Oxygen creates the *vestigal ionic hydrogen bonds* upon which life functions. Three of the four vestigal ionic bonds mentioned above contain oxygen. These are O—H...O; O—H...N; and N—H...O.

The forth ionic hydrogen bond is found as N—H...N. Ammonia is NH3 and ammonium is NH4. Ammonia can also form vestigal ionic hydrogen bonds and disturb the function of the autonomic nervous system. Ammonia has been indicated as the cause of Alzheimer's and ALS and other damaged nerve diseases for this reason. Ammonia disrupts the ionic energy system. In a cell lacking in nutrients or poisoned with toxins, ammonia could create the ionic energy, at the cellular level, to initiate replacement of the cell by mitosis. Ammonia could also disrupt the other oxygen based bonds to cause disease.

Vestibular energy flows in *vestibular nerves* and cell-wall membranes of living things. We die from lack of oxygen due to lack of vestibular energy. We also die from lack of water because water is the source of hydrogen atoms consumed in vestibular energy. The life-force relies on *vestigal hydrogen ionic energy*. This is the energy that bonds DNA nucleotides together and connects the life-force with DNA.

The cell-wall membrane of healthy cells is a polarized ionic field that bonds to other cells to form sheets of tissue we call membranes or skin. If the cell wall is mutated by microbial chitin, for example, the new cells do not connect to normal cells and are rejected for this reason. The cancer tumor membrane lacks this polarized ionic field as do cells that are constructed from hydrogenated fats and oils.

The basis for electrodermal-testing devices is based on this ionic energy phenomenon, as is Chinese treatment of illness through acupuncture. The ionic energy in cell-wall membranes can be located as trigger points or meridians of a high-energy concentration. A probe pressed against the skin at certain points will result in a current through the probe. Dr. Hulda Clark's syncrometer used to measure toxins and parasites in the body is based on this phenomenon. The syncrometer, with a test plate to hold a sample, creates resonance if the body and the test-plate contain the same vibrational frequency. A metal probe is held against a finger to pick up the resonant frequencies of the body. In acupuncture, needles placed in these meridians can block pain by serving as antennae to attract energy from the patient and the caregiver or from the ether.

Some creatures such as frogs and salamanders have the capacity to grow new legs after surgical removal or encounters with predators. It was determined that this unique capacity arises from the fact that amphibian red blood cells have DNA whereas adult mammal red blood cells do not have an active nucleus. Red blood cells in humans should be called corpuscles because they do not contain a nucleus and are not really a cell. In salamanders, the red blood cells contain expressed DNA nucleotides. These DNA bases are activated by the current of injury so that the red blood cells differentiate into normal bone and other tissue needed for replacement of lost parts.

In *Harper's Review of Biochemistry*, we have confirming evidence that the microbial DNA polymerase can influence the growth of a cell and the differentiation. In *Chapter 28, DNA Organization and Replication*, we read (Page 379):

> In mammalian cells, there is one class of DNA polymerase enzymes, called maxi (large) polymerase or polymerase alpha, which is present in the nucleus and responsible for chromosome replication. One polymerase alpha molecule is capable of polymerizing about 100 nucleotides per second, a rate 10-fold less than the rate of polymerization of deoxynucleotides by the bacterial DNA polymerase. The reduced rate almost certainly results from the interference by nucleosomes that do remain attached to DNA during its replication, perhaps all remaining attached to the leading strand.

If bacterial DNA polymerase is able to synthesize cell-wall nucleotides ten times faster than human DNA polymerase, it follows that DNA replicating in the cytoplasm of a cell infected with bacteria, could have the great majority of the protein molecules in the membrane wall assembled according to the microbial DNA template. Consequently, the new cells are mutated sufficiently to be rejected by the adjacent normal cells and the two do not knit together to heal the injury and shut down the current of injury. The glue that normally connects individual cells into a membrane are probably ionic hydrogen bonds as well. This allows cells to be flexible while still retaining their functions.

The 10 times faster rate of assembly explains why cancer cells can grow so much faster than normal cells. With each generation, there are fewer encumbrances as the cell mutates towards a more primitive embryonic cell. Cancer growth goes into high gear as the cells dedifferentiate and lose their similarity to normal human cells. The more times a cell multiplies and loses encumbrances, the faster it can multiply.

The significance of the fact that ammonia is closely related to cancer cells, fungi and bacteria, fermentation of protein, and that ammonia has the capacity to damage human tissue and form ionic hydrogen bonds, cannot be overestimated. Ammonia, secreted by tumors, may well be all that is needed to maintain the spread of cancer by damaging epithelial cells and arousing the current of injury in adjacent cells. The microbial infectious process follows ammonia toxicity and disruption of the immune system defenses in adjacent cells.

The most significant feature of mutated cells of the first generation is that these cells do not knit to human cells and repair the injury. Later generations of mutations lead to invasive protein-consuming cells, whereas the first generations appear to be more glucose dependent.

In chemical terms, the loss of biological function by a protein brought about by any disorganizing action is referred to as *denaturalization*. It is highly likely that most human degenerative diseases are the progressive denaturalization of cell-wall membranes due to pollutant or fungal contributions to the cytoplasm and cell wall of human cells. Other forces, such as evidenced by the aging of skin due to sunlight indicate another progressive change in cell wall lipid content.

Light energy and genetic changes

Numerous experiments implicate light as another cause of genetic changes and the cause of cancer. In a book by John N. Ott called *Light, Radiation and You,* we read about the influence on light on the ratio of male to female offspring in chinchillas. Information that follows only makes sense if we recognize the capacity of genes to respond to electromagnetic stimulus such as light. (Page 14):

> The lights were not installed until ten days after mating had occurred, and the same parent animals that had been consistently producing approximately 95% males in the litters under the regular incandescent bulbs now produced 95 per cent females, which is contrary to the long-established X-Y chromosome theory. Daylight incandescent bulbs are now in worldwide commercial use by chinchilla breeders to increase the number of females in the litters.

If the long established x-y chromosome theory can be challenged, perhaps defective genes can also be repaired. Genes appear to be responsive to the polarization of light because the ionic hydrogen bond is so weak. The capacity of light to cause cancer in animals has been established by a number of university studies. In John Ott's book, mentioned above, we read (Page 17):

The abnormal responses in the animals under the pink florescent consisted of excessive calcium deposits in the heart tissue, smaller numbers of young in the litters, with lower survival rates, significantly greater tumor development or cancer (which has now been confirmed by six major medical centers), and a strong tendency toward becoming irritable, aggressive—consistently fighting with one another—and cannibalistic

How does visible light energy cause cancer? Perhaps the frequency of the pink florescent light bulb disrupts the ionic hydrogen bond forming cell-wall membranes and initiates the current of injury. Perhaps too, the pink frequency imitates the effect of the current of injury. In any case, there is still more to learn about cancer and how artificial electro-magnetic fields turn replication on and off. However, there is sufficient proof and understanding to say that the signal for replication is a vibrational one from outside of the cell. The mechanical batteries that produced normal replication and growth in rats and electromagnetic devices to improve growth rate of bones proves the point. Life is an electrical phenomenon, and it follows that replication would be controlled by electrical stimuli.

The lipid content of membrane cells converts them into a structure closely similar to liquid crystals found in modern electronic devices. A liquid crystal is a substance that can flow like a liquid but has some physical properties normally associated with crystals, such as the capacity to resonate. Ionic bonds in liquid crystals can be polarized by an electric current, as seen in digital displays.

If you go to the Internet and type in three words: *liquid crystal membranes* you will be rewarded with over 250 thousand pages in biology, osmosis, and electronics such as the liquid crystal devices in modern computers and read-out devices. Cell-wall membranes and all epithelial tissues are polarized liquid crystals. It is incredible that mainstream medicine continues to reject electromedicine for treatment of disease and the cure of cancer.

I believe that DNA is a liquid crystal that resonates with the frequency of light. The sun's energy is converted by DNA resonance into chemicals such as vitamin D. The DNA structure, you will recall, is a combination of six-sided molecules called pyridines and purines. Every atom creates a tiny ionic/magnetic field. Molecules formed in a ring-structure form a more rigid or stable molecule than any other form because the magnetic field reaches across the ring. The stability of DNA is based on the magnetic stability of the structure. This six-sided crystal-like structure resonates with magnetic energies surrounding it. That is how the current of injury is able to polarize DNA molecules and initiate DNA replication without disrupting DNA structure.

In Sharon Mcgraynes book, *365 Surprising Scientific Facts, Breakthroughs and Discoveries* we read (Page 14):

> In conventional transistors, electrons behave like particles. But in nanoengineering, dimensions are comparable to electron wavelengths. And when electrons are confined to regions the size of their own wavelengths, they behave like waves.

It is well known that light is both a wave and a particle, depending only on the device used to measure it. Perhaps photons become ionic energy when confined to the diameters found in pentose phosphate rings. Plants produce pentose phosphate molecules and animals take these molecules from plants to form and energize DNA.

Perhaps DNA nucleotides accept wave energy and concentrate it to form chemical energy. Thought is a wave. Thought waves explain why a life-force, sensing sights, smells, and sounds can affect the expression of DNA and functional genetic products. It also explains why mental and emotional states influence health. But most of all, it explains why those with a deep religious faith and a will to live survive seemingly against all odds, when those who give up do not survive.

One of the great mysteries of life can be found in a book by Jess Stearn called *Edgar Cayce, The Sleeping Prophet.* In case you are not familiar with Edgar Cayce, he is considered America's foremost mystic, and predicted many events that happened years later. He also did readings to help cure people of many different poor-health conditions. He died in 1944. Science cannot explain how he connected with events and places far outside of his physical being.

How did Cayce connect with other beings and identify their health problem? Perhaps it was through DNA and a transfer of his thoughts into their DNA. The whole concept that electrons behave as waves in confined crystals such as DNA, and that thought is a wave-energy is intriguing. The mystery of the hypnotic state becomes understandable. Allowing yourself to be put into a hypnotic trance allows the hypnotist to control your body through his thoughts. All of the mysteries of hypnotism, precognition, dreams, visions, messages, etc., may someday be explained. The close mental connection between identical twins is a thought-wave connection.

Cayce made one interesting statement on the cause of cancer that confirms my theory on the cause of cancer. I did not read this information until after I had worked out the cause of cancer from research. Indeed, one can not even understand what Cayce meant until after one has the background presented in this report. In Stern's book we read about one of Cayce's readings on the cause of cancer (Page 162):

> Long before the modern concept of cancer, he described the difference between benign and malignant growths. "Ulcer is rather that of flesh being proud of infectious, while cancer is that which lives upon the cellular force by the growth of itself." The dreaded sarcoma, he said, was "caused by breaking of tissue internally which was not covered sufficiently by the leukocyte [germ-killing white corpuscles] due to the low vitality in the system.

If one were to paraphrase the above reading, one could say that cancer is caused by injury to internal tissues due to uncontrolled infection and the current of injury to repair the injury. That cellular force is now known to be the current of injury and the low vitality is the incapacity to produce ATP. Amazingly, every phrase in Cayce's statement is now understandable and conforms to my observations and conclusions. *Cancer is that which lives upon the cellular force by the growth of itself caused by a breaking of tissue and infection.*

How could Cayce know this from a dream-state reading?

I find it difficult to believe that thousands of dedicated cancer researchers could not connect these medical facts and 'discover' the cause of cancer. One could argue that anyone who discovered the cause of cancer would become rich and famous, but that is very questionable. Since known cancer cures are suppressed, and the system controls the media, how could any cancer researchers profit by going public with this information? They would just end up destroying their careers, along with the careers of friends and associates. CanCell is a good example of a cancer cure that has been developed, but cannot be used to benefit mankind and make a profit for the developer. The system does not allow it.

I must admit I have not found any one source of information to indicate that someone has connected the current of injury to the replication of infected cells as the cause of out-of-control multiplication of cells. Perhaps I did 'discover' the cause of cancer. However, due to the simplicity of the solution, I believe I have only *uncovered* and *disclosed it to the public* for the very first time. The obvious fact that numerous cancer cures are suppressed makes it highly unlikely anyone in the cancer industry would publicly announce membrane cell mutation and rejection of cells as the cause of cancer.

9. DNA polymerase chain reaction proves microbes cause cancer

The technique of DNA replication in test tubes provides another proof that medical science knows the cause of DNA replication. Let's look at the man-made and controlled cancer in a test tube known as the DNA polymerase chain reaction.

Law enforcement officers use a process called the *DNA Profiles* to prove people either innocent or guilty of crimes. A tiny sample of human DNA taken from their skin, hair, blood, or body fluids can be multiplied millions of times and observed for unique characteristics or *profile*. This process is considered reliable because it is based on fundamental laws of chemistry and biology. This process duplicates key steps in the biological process of DNA replication and normal growth. It also duplicates out-of-control cancer growth. We can understand the cancer process by comparing cancer to the DNA polymerase chain reaction. Instead of a current of injury, we probably have an artificial man-made current similar to that used by Robert Becker to stimulate growth of cells and regeneration of body parts.

Test tube DNA polymerase chain reaction explained

According to Levine and Suzuki in a book called *The Secret of Life,* scientists discovered that an enzyme called DNA polymerase under specific conditions in a test tube could be used to duplicate millions of copies of a single DNA strand. Hence, the name *DNA polymerase chain reaction* entered scientific journals.

Scientists found that gently heating and cooling DNA in a bath of nucleotides, with DNA polymerase, enabled the DNA to replicate in exactly the same process that accounts for growth. Unfortunately, the heating process destroyed the enzyme so the reaction stopped. Replacing the enzyme frequently became a costly procedure.

Turning to bacteria solved the problem of DNA polymerase enzymes being destroyed by heat. Since bacteria also use DNA polymerase enzyme to assemble their own DNA, this enzyme can be harvested from bacteria for industrial use. Some bacteria, such as *Thermus Aquanticus* thrive in hot water springs. By harvesting DNA polymerase less sensitive to heat, scientists obtained a source of polymerase, which could withstand the heating process needed for a continuous chain reaction. Consequently, scientists can now duplicate millions of copies of a single gene segment without replacing the enzymes.

By its very nature, the polymerase chain reaction proves that microbes can cause cancer.

The very foundation of the DNA polymerase chain reaction is the *incredible precision and power of DNA to replicate* exact duplicates of itself, and nothing but itself. The fact that a target gene can be replicated millions of times, without any defects resulting in cancer cells *establishes that errors during replication leading to cancer just don't happen.*

In the DNA polymerase chain reaction, we have a process similar to cancer because both processes use microbial DNA polymerase, and a primer. Four items are involved in the laboratory process.

1. Target DNA to be replicated taken from a criminal suspect, a victim, or a desired subject.

2. Two DNA primers *(details unknown in my source of information).*

3. A large supply of DNA nucleotide building blocks. In cloning, a similar process, 'Yeast Artificial Chromosome' is taken from the mycelia of yeast or fungi. Any source will do.

4. Bacterial hot-spring DNA polymerase.

The fact that primers must be added to the environment of the target DNA in test tubes is proof that the mysterious factor that initiates replication is not gene related. During DNA replication, ionic energy to mimic the current of injury will be needed. In addition, I suspect that a high-energy molecule capable of providing a quantum of energy sufficient to break the stability of the DNA nucleotides is required.

I find it difficult to believe that scientists can replicate DNA in a test tube but claim they do not know the cause of the identical process in living things. The close similarity of the two processes is so obvious.

Since special enzymes control assembly of cells and cell-wall membranes that cause cancer, let's review the functions of enzymes more fully than previously discussed earlier in this text.

Enzymes defined as protein catalysts

The following description of enzymes is taken from *Harper's Review of Biochemistry* (Page 51). This one definition contains almost all the references needed to explain how microbes cause cancer. It also explains why we have a defective gene theory for the cause of cancer. I have blocked the passage into sections to focus attention on significant points.

1. Enzymes were once thought to operate only within a cell, hence they were called "*en-zyme*" meaning "in yeast."

2. Catalysts are substances that accelerate chemical reactions. They undergo physical change during a reaction but revert to their original state when the reaction is complete.

3. Enzymes are protein catalysts for chemical reactions in biological systems.

4. Most chemical reactions of living cells would occur extremely slowly were it not for catalysis by enzymes. In contrast to non-protein catalysts *(acids, bases, metal ions)*, each enzyme catalyses a small number of reactions, frequently only one.

5. Enzymes are thus reaction-specific catalysts.

6. *Essentially all biochemical reactions are enzyme catalyzed.*

7. The production of human energy in the form of ATP through oxidation requires a specific group of enzymes following one after another in what is termed the citric acid cycle.

8. Enzymes may be extracted from cells without loss of their catalytic activity. An enzyme called DNA polymerase is extracted from bacteria and used in the DNA Polymerase Chain Reaction that enables scientists to duplicate tiny samples of DNA.

9. Coenzymes: Many enzymes catalyze reactions only in the presence of another enzyme…they are thus called coenzymes.

The most significant points about the function of enzymes relating to cancer are numbers 6 and 7. The sixth point "*essentially all biochemical reactions are enzyme catalyzed*" is the basis for the mistaken belief that DNA replication is controlled by enzyme catalysts. This statement ignores the fact that the autonomic nervous system is controlled by wave energy and the life-force.

The fact that DNA bonds are ionic hydrogen bonds means that division of DNA is a *bioelectric reaction*. Division of DNA is controlled by bioelectric energy of the autonomic nervous system. *Biochemical reactions* relate to exchange of electrons and electrostatic charges. The initiation of cell division is not a biochemical reaction, and is therefore not gene related.

Enzymes function by combining with substrates

We are still left without a clear understanding of how enzymes such as DNA polymerase function to assist in cell division. The best explanation I could find is that enzymes modify substrates via magnetic fields and thereby modify the chemical reaction.

Isaac Asimov compares enzymes to a knife with a wooden handle. We can remove sections of the handle, without damaging the cutting action, but we cannot remove sections from the blade without damaging the cutting action.

He writes in *The New Guide to Science* (Page 577):

A case in point is the hormone called ACTH (adrenocorticotropic hormone). This is a peptide chain made up of thirty-nine amino acids, whose order has now been fully determined. Up to fifteen of the amino acids have been removed from the C-terminal without destroying the hormones' activity.

The same sort of thing has been done with an enzyme called *papain*, from the fruit and sap of the papaya tree. Its enzymatic action is similar to that of pepsin. Removal of the pepsin molecule's 180 amino acids from the N-terminal end does not reduce its activity to any detectable extent.

Isaac Asimov's summary of scientific research establishes an essential difference between proteins and enzymes. It appears that the protein is more likely an enzyme carrier since large portions of the protein molecule can be removed from one end without damage to the enzymatic activity. Based on the work of the 1999 Nobel Prize winner Guenther Blobel on protein distribution within cells, one can safely assume that the protein portion delivers the active enzyme portion to the right location in the cell. The protein portion contains the postal-code for delivery so that the enzyme portion is delivered to the correct location.

From this, one could assume that the enzymes required to assemble cell wall components are connected with a protein delivery system. Fungi and bacteria present in the cell have equal access to contributing cell-wall components to the membrane. The contribution of other pollutants and the lack of essential fatty acids would also contribute to the defects in the completed cell-wall membrane.

DNA profile cannot find cancer-causing genes

If defective genes cause cancer, one could take a target sample of DNA from a cancerous cell, and replicate the genes suspected of causing cancer. By replicating genes from normal cells of the same tissue and comparing the two profiles, one could identify the cancer causing genes. Since cancer is considered hereditary, genes from different family members could be duplicated and studied to find the common defective gene that causes cancer. **Any identical genes from cancer cells found in other members of the family with cancer would be the defective cancer genes.** Identifying the cancer gene would be no different than proving someone innocent or guilty of a crime by comparing the DNA profile in target DNA (the cancer cell) to normal DNA through the DNA polymerase chain reaction.

Why hasn't the defective cancer gene been isolated and the results made public? The obvious reason is that defective genes do not cause cancer *(assuming researchers are looking for the cause)*. The defective gene concept is a medical myth.

DNA cloning with Yeast Artificial Chromosome mimics cancer.

DNA cloning also proves that mainstream medicine knows what causes DNA replication. From the Internet under Biochemistry, Genetics, and Molecular Biology, there is a section on *DNA CLONING*.

The enzymes required to cut genes into manageable units come from bacteria, which normally use this enzyme to cut and destroy invading viral genes. In addition, the most commonly used source of chromosome material comes from yeast. It is referred to as *Yeast Artificial Chromosome* because it has all the information needed to make up complete human chromosomes.

I was amazed to learn that DNA engineering uses both microbial enzymes and fungal nucleotides for cloning DNA. Genetic cloning parallels the cancer process!

In a human body, with fermentation of blood sugars and blood proteins in the lymphatic system (a source of *Yeast Artificial Chromosome)*, and bacteria resident in the cell to provide enzymes and cell-wall material, we have all of the ingredients for an uncontrolled DNA polymerase chain reaction. We have all that is necessary for cancer.

There are many ways to prevent and cure cancer

The major difference between the test tube DNA polymerase chain reaction and cancer is that *microbes in living cells provide the growth factors that make the replicating genes continue to grow and differentiate*. Since the growth factors originate from an anaerobic life form which has created an anaerobic microsphere filled with carbon dioxide and ammonia, newly multiplied cells express genes to support fermentation. Cells which multiply and mature within an aerobic microbial environment become dedicated cancer cells because after one or two generations these cells lose the capacity in expressed genes to maintain oxidation of glucose. Cancer cells lose the capacity to produce enzymes to handle oxygen and can therefore be destroyed by oxygen therapies.

That is also why effective natural products such as oxygen, colloidal silver, magnets, electrical or magnetic impulses, or herbal combinations are capable of killing cancer cells. Colloidal silver kills over 600 known microorganisms probably by coating the cell wall with electrical properties. A colloidal dispersion such as colloidal silver is a mixture with particles smaller than those in suspension, but larger than those in solution, having one dimension of 1 to 10 nm (nanometers). Existing cancer cells can be killed with natural methods. We don't need toxic drugs with side effects that also kill all rapidly growing human cells. Just kill the parasites that infect the cells and kill the cancer cells with natural oxygen rich products, and cancer growth will stop.

Breaking free of indoctrination and propaganda

In conclusion to this section, the DNA profile proves that replication of genes does not cause defects in genes. There are no genes that control replication of other genes and thereby cause cancer. There are no suppressor genes that fail to stop microbial DNA polymerase enzymes from causing replication of human cells. There are no mutated or defective genes that cause cancer, no oncogenes, no protein oncogenes, and no proto-oncogenes. There are no cell cycles and cell-cycle clocks. There are no viral oncogenes that cause cancer by producing genetic faults in the DNA nucleotide structure.

In addition, there are no hereditary genetic liabilities that cause cancer directly. Hereditary defects related to cancer are also related to metabolism and assimilation of food or a weak immune system response. Defective genes may result in impaired metabolism, reduced respiration, loss of oxidation, impaired immune system function, and increased frequency of internal bleeding with trapped blood proteins. These conditions lead to microbial infection and replication of infected cells.

Have you ever wrestled with a personal or business problem with a feeling that you were missing something right before your eyes? Then suddenly, a thought flashed into your mind, when you were not even thinking about your problem and you knew you had the answer. I had such an experience in researching the cause of cancer. All the medical books I read at the beginning of my research stated cancer must be a genetic disease. After researching defective genes as the cause of cancer, I sensed something was wrong. Far too many observations could not be explained.

What was I missing? One day, rather suddenly I realized defective genes had nothing to do with cancer. Suddenly, everything started falling into place. Medical textbooks, journals, publicity TV commercials and TV interviews are all used to indoctrinate the public, politicians and the health care industry about the importance of drugs and genetic therapy to treat cancer. This is indoctrination with false information.

I gave up looking for something I might have missed. I also gave up interpreting written medical information as true and unbiased. I knew without a doubt, that genes do not possibly cause cancer. From this, I realized that most mainstream medical information could not be trusted. From that point onward, everything I had researched about cancer fell into place or into the circular file where it belongs.

If you were taught to believe in the defective gene theory, I hope that by this chapter you have had that 'sudden insight' or mental realization to question your indoctrination. Let go of any confidence you may have about defective genes causing cancer. Let go of any confidence you may have in medical propaganda and promises for new cancer cures. All effective cures available now are being suppressed. How is a new cure for cancer possible? Multiplication of cells is based on the atomic structure of genes. The process is at least one billion years old and very reliable. Cancer cells do not have defective genes, they have a defective cell-wall membrane. Cancer is cured and prevented by controlling the cellular environment and eliminating the microbial growth factors that cause cell-wall mutation and rejection by adjacent membrane cells. Cancer is cured by growing healthy cells capable of repairing an injury. There is no other way for a permanent cure.

In the next section of this book, let's look at examples of *alternative health therapies* that cure infectious microbial diseases such as cancer.

Section TWO:

The prevention of and cure for cancer

10. Restore electrolyte balance to help cure cancer

In this section, we will deal with secondary causes that lead to cancer and how to eliminate them. We will first focus on mineral imbalances leading to loss of vital enzymes required for metabolism, and removal of waste products. Equally important, we will deal with cleansing the lymphatic system and eliminating pockets of fermentation that can lead to cancer. Essential minerals and trace minerals called electrolytes are of primary importance for maintaining healthy cells.

Silica helps prevent internal bleeding that could lead to cancer

Silica is one of the most important minerals to stop blood from being trapped in ducts and storage vessels. It is needed to maintain the flexibility of arteries and plays a major role in preventing both cardiovascular disease and cancer. This vital mineral is also necessary for the formation of connective tissues, healthy skin, and hair. Lack of silica in the diet leads to reduced flexibility in arteries and cell walls, with the increased possibility of blood leaking directly into storage areas, where it can ferment and start the cancer process.

Klaus Kaufmann, author of the book *Silica, The Forgotten Nutrient,* writes (Page 66):

In the area of Daun in West Germany there is an extremely low incidence of cancer. In searching out the reasons why the locals should be more fortunate than folks elsewhere, it was discovered that their local Dunmaris water well is unusually high in silica. **The organism of cancer patients often presents mineral imbalance. The most prominent losses suffered are silica, magnesium, calcium and iron.** Even benign tumors such as warts are known to develop mainly during periods of bodily demineralization or shortage of these minerals, and sometimes disappear spontaneously when the mineral imbalance has been corrected.

Make a mental note of the four minerals mentioned in the Dumaris water supply: *silica, magnesium, calcium* and *iron*. Watch for references to these minerals in information on cancer. Lack of these minerals leads to warts and benign growths that rupture and cause a current of injury in infected cells. Lack of magnesium minerals leads to lack of enzymes for efficient metabolism and energy production. Minerals are needed for enzymes for transfer of oxygen and carbon dioxide. These are four vital minerals required in the proper ratios to prevent and cure cancer. Curing cancer starts with curing the mineral imbalances in your body.

Valuable minerals are found in drinking water providing it has not been distilled or processed through reverse osmoses.

It should be obvious to people that drinking distilled water will deprive them of valuable minerals that are normally dissolved in the water. Distilled water is mineral free. Though your local water is not mineral rich, it is more conducive to better health than is distilled water. Reverse osmoses leaves some minerals in water, but the process also removes most minerals. A simple conductivity test demonstrates the loss of minerals from tap water compared to reverse osmoses.

Water should be filtered through a solid carbon block or ceramic filter because these filters do not support microbial growth within a powdered base.

Water is a source of ionic energy

Have you ever heard about places on earth where people live long healthy robust lives such as the Hunzas? People who researched this phenomenon attribute longevity to the highly energized glacial water they drink.

On the other hand, have you ever heard of a group of people who drank distilled water and lived long and healthy lives? I know I haven't. Has anyone ever proven distilled water beneficial to our health?

Drinking distilled water eliminates the opportunity to ingest dissolved minerals from the soil. Distilled water is commonly referred to as 'dead' water.

I could never figure out what that meant. What makes water dead, alive, or whatever is meant by these terms? Obviously, water is never alive.

Water is a dipole molecule, meaning it has both a positive and negative terminal. The two atoms of hydrogen are bonded on one side, at 120 degrees, rather than opposite each other at 180 degrees as might be expected. We learned that the vestigal ionic bond always occurs with one-sided bonds such as oxygen and hydrogen because the stronger oxygen nucleus captures the electron of the weaker nucleus and exposes the hydrogen proton to attract other electrons lightly. Other atoms or molecules are attracted to the exposed nucleus to form an ionic hydrogen bond. Water forms two vestigal ionic bonds with other water molecules and water molecules becomes a liquid in which each molecule of water is ionically bonded or attracted to two other molecules of water. Water forms drops because of these forces, and water boils at a higher temperature than it should, (based on molecular weight) because of these forces.

Back in 1827, the Scottish botanist Robert Brown discovered that particles in water quiver and move around incessantly due to a bombardment from the water molecules. This phenomenon is now known as Brownian motion of colloids. Water is a highly energized liquid because the spin of the earth carries water through the earth's magnetic fields, resulting in a continuous tumbling action of water molecules. Water is said to be alive when the tumbling motion is high, or dead when the tumbling motion is reduced. Distilled water without minerals is low in magnetic energy and Brownian movement. Water molecules can be energized by spinning them rapidly. Water molecules can be made to spin in either direction, and be sorted by this spin force into positive or negative water. The body can use these energies for life functions.

Sunlight and magnetic fields can increase the energy levels in water and distilling it can reduce the energy levels. All waters are not equal. Water can be polarized into a positive or negative force, neutralized, energized with magnets, light, and sound, oxygenated with ozone and hydrogen peroxide, deoxygenated by boiling and evaporation, or neutralized by addition of chemicals. Juices from freshly made vegetables and fruit contain a wealth of energized molecules. Different colors in food and juices provide different energies used by the body.

We cannot expect to be healthy without drinking active water. Soft drinks and bottled drinks do not equal fresh juices or pure water. In order for the body to create the vestigal ionic bonds that sustains the life-force, the body needs energized water. The vestigal ionic bond responds to plasma and the life-force is plasma. Water gives life to living things, and living things are mostly water, because the two go hand in hand.

Have you ever wondered why mammals die in four or five minutes if deprived of oxygen? What are the mechanics of asphyxiation? Why does the brain go first? What is it about oxygen that cannot be replaced?

Perhaps the vital life-force in oxygen is production of the vestigal ionic bond that bonds DNA molecules and gives life to living things. Increasing oxygen levels in the body increases vitality by increasing ionic vestigal bonds. Have you ever wondered why you can do physical work, golf, or do a workout, expend tons of ATP, so to speak, and feel refreshed and energized? With the loss of ATP, you should be more tired. You feel better because exercise, fresh air, and exertion have increased the ionic energy in your body.

The air we breathe, energized by the sun, is another source of ionic energy. Spending winters in the South, or Arizona have significant health benefits for older people because they absorb ionic energy from the sun through the air they breathe and water they drink. They spend more time out doors. Some of these health benefits can be duplicated during the winter months in northern areas by using ionized air devices, room ozonators, ozonated water, mineralized baths, vitamin D supplements and magnetically energized water.

In the book *The Ion Effect* by Fred Soyka we learn how important it is to have ionized air and water. Ions are absorbed through the skin and air we breathe. A researcher tried raising mice, rats, guinea pigs, and rabbits in totally de-ionized air. Within two weeks almost all of them died. Despite the fact that autopsies proved they had died for a variety of reasons—fatty liver, kidney failure, heart degeneration, and, among other ills, anemia—the researcher concluded that the real cause of death was the animal's inability to utilize oxygen properly (Page 52). One of the major pathways to disease is a life-style lacking in negative ions. The pathway includes lack of essential trace minerals, lack of essential fatty acids, and too many toxins and pollutants in the body.

Drinking distilled water is not recommended because it is low in negative ions. It strips your body of ionic energy. Distilled water stored in plastic containers will absorb toxic chemicals from the container. I learned this by having distilled water tested for chemicals after we noticed a taste in the water. Distilled water absorbs carbon dioxide from the air and becomes acidic. You can prove this by testing freshly distilled water in a container. Test and record the acidity level, blow on the surface of the water several times, and retest it. You will be surprised by the increased acidity. The water absorbed carbon dioxide from the air. If you make your own distilled water, try adding some liquid mineral supplements to the empty container before you collect the distilled water. Willard water, Trace-Lytes or any good colloidal mineral supplement will help.

Distilled water will help flush toxic waste from your body, but it also destroys the enzymes needed to convert waste into a form suitable for removal. Distilled water also flushes good minerals from your body. The advantages of distilled water to avoid microbes and pollutants are lost by the disadvantages through loss of dissolved minerals and increased susceptibility to infection.

Mineral imbalance is clearly associated with cancer. Dr. Johannes Fibiger found mice with stomach cancer living in a sugar storage warehouse. These mice developed a mineral imbalance from excess sugar consumption, resulting in immune system dysfunction. Pets fed human food and processed pet food develop disease and cancer for the same reasons. Heating and processing food destroys bioactive enzymes and removes minerals.

Production of enzymes in the cells is temperature sensitive. If the body can maintain the oxygenation process, the body temperature remains higher and more enzymes are produced. If body temperature drops, fewer enzymes are produced. Continuous metabolism of glycogen and production of ATP are required to maintain a strong immune system. The capacity to maintain body temperature and produce a fever when necessary is part of the immune system defense.

Dr Stephen Langer, M.D. and James F. Scheer, authors of *Solved: The Riddle of Illness*, give us a plausible explanation of the cause for human diseases. Their concept is that all diseases result from a slight loss of body temperature that restricts the formation of vital enzymes. In Chapter 15, *Guard Yourself Against Cancer*, we read:

> Subnormal thyroid function appears to invite cancer. This has been shown clinically in numerous animal experiments. Malignant tissue from rats grafted onto other rats took hold readily in those animals whose thyroid glands had been removed, but rarely in those with normal thyroid function.

> Dr. Eskin discovered that the highest incidence of breast cancer and deaths from it are in the goiter belts of Poland, Switzerland, Austria and the United States. The iodine-impoverished Great Lakes region of the coast-to-coast goiter belt shows the highest rate of breast cancer in the United States.

Some sixty-four different symptoms are associated with one root cause: hypothyroidism, an ailment so widespread and sometimes so difficult to detect that a vast percentage of the population unknowingly suffers from it.

Some cancer support groups make and donate blankets and comforters to cancer hospitals. It is a well-known fact that cancer patients often feel cold at normally comfortable room temperatures. Their mechanism for body heat control is not effective and their body does not produce sufficient heat for comfort. More significantly, the body temperature is not sufficient to form vital enzymes or create a fever to destroy parasitic microbial enzymes such as DNA polymerase that control assembly of genes.

When parasites invade the organs that produce enzymes for control of body temperature, such as the thyroid and pancreas, they can cause illness everywhere in the body by destroying the ability of other organs to produce enzymes. *Solved: The Riddle of Illness* presents a good case for saying that all illnesses start with a metabolic deficiency and mineral imbalance. Treating ill people with thyroid supplement is a good first step towards better health. Iodine deficiency is often the major cause for low body temperature. Dr. Hulda Clark has published a 20-day tumor reduction program in her book called *The Cure for All Advanced Cancers*. In the 20-day program of parasite cleansing and nutritional supplements, we find a two grains of thyroid supplement daily as part of the program.

The medical advice to go to bed and rest at the first sign of a cold or flu makes sense. If you use extra blankets and create fever-like temperatures, along with taking thyroid and oxygen supplements, you can help your body fight viral infections.

Magnesium required in enzymes to digest protein

In the book *Healing with Amino Acids*, by B.J. Sahley, Ph.D., and K.M. Birknew, C.R.N.A., Ph.D., we find the following reference to magnesium (Page 61):

> The absorption and assimilation of all amino acids are dependent on the presence of B6 and magnesium. Magnesium is deficient in 60% of American diets. Yet magnesium is the number-one stress mineral. It is needed by the body and brain for proper functioning, and is involved in over 300 biochemical reactions in the body. Food processing deletes over 75% of the magnesium in foods. Diets high in sugar, soda intake (high in phosphates), alcohol, food processing and high fat consumption along with stress, chronic illness and chemicals promote the exhaustion of magnesium supplies.

The above quotation supports three conclusions:

1) Sugars high in phosphates deplete the body of magnesium.

2) The assimilation of all amino acids is dependent on magnesium and Vitamin B6. Without magnesium, proteins cannot be assimilated and this will lead to fermentation in the cells

3) Fermentation of proteins leads to production of toxic ammonia and high-energy primers to initiate chromosome replication. It all starts with too much sugar in the diet. That's why Dr. Fibiger could find mice with cancer only in a sugar storage warehouse. It is also probably why some researchers were unable to repeat Dr. Fibiger's research by using healthy laboratory mice and rats.

Trace elements lost by food processing

Chromium has a unique position in the cancer story because it is vital for enzyme production. Several books have been written extolling the benefits of bioactive chromium supplements such as chromium picolinate for diabetes and cancer. As a result of these "so-called drug claims", the Health Protection Branch regulated these essential nutrients as drugs. Now, chromium picolinate requires a Drug Identification Number in order to be imported into Canada. Rather than encourage use and distribution of this valuable food supplement, regulations are in place to control and reduce availability to the public.

Author Henry A. Schroeder M.D., in his book *The Trace Elements and Man,* cites the lack of chromium required to produce vital food enzymes as the cause of disease. The lack of chromium in our diet results from crops grown in mineral-depleted soils, processed foods, and excess sugar. He writes (Page 78):

Therefore, the typical American diet, with about 60 per cent of its calories from refined sugar, refined flour, and fat, most of which is saturated, was apparently designed not only to provide as little chromium as feasible, but to cause depletion of body stores of chromium by not replacing urinary losses. Again, the 'article of faith based on reason' stated previously, that whole foods contain the micronutrients necessary for their metabolism, has been shown to hold true, and the refining of these foods based on custom, habit, preference and industrial practices has been shown to provide foods lacking in sufficient amount of a micronutrient necessary for their metabolism.

One of the most valuable trace mineral supplements that I have found is Trace-Lytes by Natures Path of Venice, Florida. Each teaspoon contains organic copper, iodine, manganese, zinc, potassium, cobalt, sodium, selenium, chromium, silica and boron in trace amounts. All of these minerals are vital parts of enzyme complexes in our body. Minerals such as these are normally found in fresh fruits and vegetables as food. However, due to our depleted soils and harvesting methods, it is now generally believed that mineral levels are no longer adequate for human nutrition.

A recent study on zinc co-authored by Robert Black chairman of the John Hopkins School of Public Health in Baltimore found zinc supplements of 5 to 20 milligrams per day had substantial benefits to prevention of diarrhea and pneumonia. The report goes on to say that zinc is a mineral "...essential in the synthesis of RNA and DNA, the genetic material that controls cell growth, division, and function. Zinc contributes to bone development, energy metabolism, wound healing, the liver's ability to remove toxic substances from the body, immune function, and regulation of heart and blood pressure."

As you see, several of the steps in the process of cancer, including wound healing, cell division, energy metabolism and cell function are mentioned as dependent on zinc. What happens to your metabolic system if your body is short of zinc? According to Dr. Hulda Clark, all cases of prostrate cancer show a zinc deficiency with excess nickel. It appears that the body will substitute one mineral for another in the absence of the mineral it normally uses. This leads to benign growths because new cells are rejected, not because of microbial infection, but because of mineral and cell-wall trait deficiencies.

Chromium is especially valuable for fighting cancer because it is so essential in the process of food metabolism. Taking chromium supplements is highly recommended. However, do not take the metallic type, as the body cannot produce enzymes to assimilate it. Lack of chromium also leads to diabetes.

Chromium essential for enzymes is depleted by sugar

In her book *The CHROMIUM Diet, Supplement and Exercise Strategy*, author Betty Kamen, Ph.D. informs her readers about chromium supplements. Chromium bound to niacin becomes chromium polynicotinate. Niacin assists in the breakdown and utilization of fats, proteins, and carbohydrates as well as the oxidation of sugars. Inorganic chromium is not absorbed by the body. We read (Pages 181-182):

THE REASON FOR CHROMIUM POLYNICOTINATE

Niacin, part of the B complex (B3) assists in the breakdown and utilization of fats, proteins, and carbohydrates. In its role as coenzyme, niacin helps the oxidation of sugars and is essential to proper brain metabolism. By potentiating insulin, it also helps regulate blood sugar levels.

Recall that niacin, the common name for nicotinic acid, has been identified by D. Murtz as the compound associated with GTF (*glucose tolerance factor*) chromium biological activity. Apparently, niacin is crucial for the formation of the proper molecular structure of GTF that facilitates insulin binding to cell membrane receptor sites. In other words, niacin-bound chromium, or chromium polynicotinate, provides the correct key to unlocking insulin's powerful effects in your body.

Hardly any uncomplexed chromium compounds can be found in natural sources, not even in water. Only one half to one per cent of ingested inorganic chromium is absorbed.

Studies which demonstrate a lack of effect on glucose metabolism after chromium supplementation are almost always conducted with inorganic chromium.

Chromium polynicotinate has been tested extensively in animals and on humans for five years before being marketed to consumers. After that, it was available strictly through doctors until its safety and efficacy were well established.

Chromium polynicotinate is now sold in U.S. health food stores without special regulations. However, in Canada it is still sold only with a drug identification number. This policy restricts one of the most valuable cancer prevention minerals from the public even though it has been proven safe in the U.S. market.

Mothers with children and infants who have colic or digestive problems find that feeding organic chromium supplements to children is immensely beneficial for clearing up these problems.

Please note the subtitle of Kamen's book: *Supplement and Exercise Strategy*. **Supplements and exercise** go hand in hand as a successful health strategy. Supplements will chemically help the body cleanse cells of toxins and pollutants, but exercise is needed to physically move pollutants out of the system. Exercising until you perspire ensures your cells have an opportunity to flush out toxins. Don't block your perspiration. Perspiring is one of the most effective ways to cleanse your body of toxins. If your perspiration has an odor, you know your body is toxic. Keep at it until perspiration is normal.

Supplementing the body with minerals is highly recommended, but choosing the best mineral supplements is very confusing. Many available supplements are not what they seem to be. Chromium, for example, is available in different forms. What should we use?

In a booklet called *The Power of Minerals,* Elmer G. Heinrich tells us that chromium can be found in grapes and almonds. Almonds are often recommended for curing cancer because of their chromium content. Then he describes the significant difference between minerals derived from rocks, and mineral from plants as found in his food supplement 'Body Booster' (Page 17):

> We must remember that the minerals found in these foods are no longer metallic minerals.
>
> According to food chemistry, plant-derived colloidal minerals are 100% absorbable, so comparing metallic minerals to plant-derived minerals would be like comparing sawdust to oatmeal. Plant-derived colloidal minerals are the result of plants converting metallic minerals to colloidal minerals through the root system by a process known to science as assimilation through plant syntheses. By the process the metallic mineral is assimilated or digested by the plant, therefore it can be more easily assimilated by the human body. This sidesteps the normal digestive time of from 15 to 21 hours as required for the small amount of metallic minerals utilized. A plant mineral is as much as several hundred to as much as a thousand times smaller than the smallest metallic mineral. This makes it colloidal in nature. A plant-derived mineral is less than 0.001 micron in size, which is approximately 1/6000 the size of a red blood cells. The small size gives them an enormous surface area. It has been calculated that the plant derived colloidal minerals in one teaspoon of Body Booster would have a total surface area of approximately 55 acres.

Bioactive chromium is also found in brewer's yeast. A dietary supplement of 200 to 500 micrograms of chromium has resulted in dramatic reduction in cholesterol and triglyceride levels. Twin Laboratories offers an organic, grain-grown type, as well as one called Nutritional Yeast, which is perhaps the best tasting of them all. Many other sources are also available.

An inverse relationship exists between chromium deficiency and sugar intake. If we are chromium-deficient, we crave more sugar, because there is not sufficient blood sugar in our system. If we have an adequate amount of chromium, our body produces an adequate amount of insulin to control blood sugar levels. Consequently, we do not crave sugar. When we have a craving for sugar, we should first reach for a chromium supplement and if we over-indulge in sugar, we should increase our chromium supplementation.

Everyone with health concerns should make an effort to study the importance of bioactive minerals in the diet and how they interact. Included in this study should be a careful analysis of processed white sugar and its damage to the system. Sugar and glucose should be tested as a carcinogen because it upsets our mineral balance and promotes fungal growth. In addition, sugar is processed from sugar cane and sugar beets that are exposed to fungal growth in open fields and storage. Sugar may contain fungal residue and mycotoxins.

Magnesium in enzymes for a carbon dioxide substrate

The geology text *Oxford Guide to the Elements*, helps explain why magnesium is so vital to living things (Page 57):

> Magnesium is the seventh most abundant element in the Earth's crust and is present in such large quantities in seawater that the world's oceans contain an almost unlimited supply of the dissolved metal ...Interestingly, magnesium will burn in carbon dioxide...

The capacity of magnesium to burn in carbon dioxide, just like iron rusts in oxygen, gives magnesium in plants the capacity to use carbon dioxide as a substrate for photosynthesis of carbohydrates, and for human cells to control carbon dioxide in metabolism. Lack of magnesium in cancer patients is well documented, and the incapacity to control carbon dioxide build-up leads to reduced oxygen levels.

In the 1930s, it was discovered that red blood cells were very similar to chlorophyll in plants. The essential chemical difference is that chlorophyll has an atom of magnesium whereas red blood cells have an atom of iron. The difference of that one atom directs whether the life form functions through respiration of carbon dioxide as a plant, or respiration of oxygen as an animal. It follows that enzymes containing magnesium found in plants can be used directly by the human body. We can supplement our enzyme capacity by eating fresh and raw plant-based foods and herbal remedies. We can also maintain a healthy acid-alkaline balance by doing so. On the other hand, by eating only processed grains and starches, we destroy our acid-alkaline balance

The significance of magnesium to the metabolic process can be found in *Harper's Review of Biochemistry* (Page 577).

> **Magnesium ions are present in all cells. In essentially all reactions for which ATP is a substrate, the true substrate is magnesium ... Thus, the synthesis of all proteins, nucleic acids, nucleotides, lipids, and carbohydrates and the activation of muscle contraction requires magnesium.**

If magnesium is required for all metabolic functions, and if we refine magnesium out of our grains, sugar, and oils, we are going to lack magnesium in our food. Our modern diets do not provide the essential minimum nutrition for good health. It follows that taking mineral supplements is a good choice.

Millions of people suffer from respiratory problems, due to toxins in the air, household chemicals, smoking, and a lack of minerals in their bodies. Minerals that increase the capacity to oxidize food nutrients are also vital to curing cancer.

A mineral-rich cocktail exists that is capable of killing cancer cells.

The fact that cancer cells function in reduced oxygen levels, but still require some oxygen has created a unique opportunity to isolate them from normal cells and destroy them. By reducing cancer cell respiration below what is needed for fermentation of glucose, cancer cells can be killed. One of the most promising cures for cancer, called CanCell, is based on this asphyxiated. We will read more about CanCell, the magic bullet for cancer, in Chapter 22, *The Ruthless Suppression of Cancer Cures.*

Food processing eliminates minerals and enzymes

In the book *Trace Elements and Man* by Henry Schroeder (Page 152), we find a summary of how refining destroys mineral values in food and makes processed foods a cause of disease.

The milling of wheat into refined flour removes 40% of the chromium, 86% of the manganese, 76% of the iron, 89% of the cobalt, 68% of the copper, 78% of the zinc, and 48% of the molybdenum, all trace elements essential for life or health. Refining of sugar removes most (93%) of the ash, and with it go the trace elements necessary for metabolism of the sugar: 93% of the chromium, 89% of the manganese, 98% of the cobalt, 83% of the copper, 98% of the zinc, and 98% of the magnesium. The essential elements are in the residue molasses, which is fed to cattle.

All of the above quotations support statements saying that the cause of the present cancer epidemic is directly related to the excess consumption of sugar and refined foods which cannot be metabolized due to lack of essential minerals and digestive enzymes. Food nutrients that cannot be metabolized result in fermentation and increased production of microbial enzymes and toxins in the body.

Cancer and aging due to metabolic problems

Cancer occurs with aging primarily because aging often results in impaired nutrition, digestion and assimilation. Lack of digestive enzymes leads to increased trapped blood proteins, increased fermentation, and more fungal mycotoxins. A lack of physical activity and development of bowel problems leads to increased toxicity. In addition, the lure of convenience foods, already cooked and packaged for individual servings, leads older people away from meals made of fresh and raw fruits and vegetables. Cancer arises in older people, not because they are old, but because they no longer maintain an adequate oxidative metabolism.

Cancer Society advises against mineral supplements for energy

While visiting a Canadian hospital specializing in cancer, I reviewed cancer information available to cancer patients. One interesting booklet is called *Nutrition Guide for People with Cancer*, as prepared by the Canadian Cancer Society.

The only recommendation concerning mineral supplements for people with cancer reads as follows (My italics added):

> Nothing about nutrition is more misunderstood than vitamins and minerals. *Contrary to popular belief, they do not provide energy, and cannot substitute for a well-balanced diet. In fact, large amounts of vitamins and minerals can be harmful.* If you are concerned about the vitamin and mineral content of your diet, please discuss it with your doctor or dietitian. They can tell you whether you need vitamin or mineral supplements.

The Canadian Cancer Society doesn't help people with cancer by advising them that vitamins and minerals do not provide energy. The statement is true but it ignores the importance of taking supplements for other reasons. Obviously, a well balanced diet will provide more energy than taking vitamins or minerals. Energy comes from eating food, not vitamins, and minerals.

What they say has the effect of telling people with cancer that they do not need vitamin and mineral supplementation because a well-balanced diet provides all the minerals and vitamins they need. If their diet provides all the minerals and vitamins they need, why do they have cancer? Why do they not advise cancer victims to supplement their diets, not for more energy, but for increased electrolytes, magnesium, tissue health, and improved immune system function? Do you suppose that they don't know such basic facts? Why focus the criticism on saying minerals do not provide energy?

Minerals are essential for digestive enzymes and metabolism drops with a lack of these minerals. Chromium, for example, is required to metabolize sugar. Without minerals cellular functions stop. The problem is that people who eat mainly processed foods do not have a well-balanced diet. Processing of food destroys the mineral value. Our depleted soils do not provide adequate levels of minerals in food to start with. Few people, if any, gain an adequate supply of minerals for optimum health from the modern diet. Cancer patients need mineral supplements of bioactive minerals more than they need food for energy. They need the minerals so that they can get energy from food.

Where can you find reliable advice on mineral supplements? The Cancer Society suggests: *"...please discuss it with your doctor or dietitian."* How many doctors will take the time to educate you about minerals? How many have ever studied the effect of minerals in the body? I haven't found any information of mineral supplementation in my set of medical textbooks. The information in the nutrition guide for people with cancer is woefully lacking in useful information on minerals.

I believe you will find much better advice by purchasing small booklets or books on minerals at health food stores and reading about them. Learn the name, function, and food sources of about 22 minerals and you will have valuable knowledge to take control of your health. Put concern about vitamins, cholesterol and antioxidants on the back burner until you complete a study of bulk minerals, trace minerals, and cell salts. Cell salts are oxides of minerals found inside cell tissue. Various formulations of these cell-salt minerals as homeopathic supplements have powerful health benefits.

Take the right kind of mineral supplements (not metallic)

The previous reference from The Canadian Cancer Society stating that nothing is misunderstood as much as vitamin and mineral supplements is certainly true. Why are mineral supplements so badly misunderstood?

It seems to me that a lot of hype and promotion goes into promoting the wrong type of vitamins and minerals for business profits. Misunderstanding of minerals is highly promoted for economic reasons.

Pick up any bottle of mineral supplements. The label will probably list the mineral contents as USP or United States Pharmacopoeia. This indicates that THESE ARE CHEMICALS manufactured according to standards set out by the U.S. Government. You don't want chemicals for supplements. Look for supplements from natural sources, preferably in liquid form.

For millions of years our digestive system has produced enzymes to digest food from plants or food from animals that eat plants. Human metabolism is based on foods. Chemicals are not foods. We do not assimilate chemicals and rocks even if the label says: "made according to standards of U.S. Pharmacopoeia." Perhaps friendly bacteria in our colon can assimilate some of it for us, but most is wasted as expensive urine. DNA bases and nucleotides are absorbed intact from the digestive system because the digestive enzymes and acids do not break down these chemical bonds.

DNA bases, are stable, ring-shaped molecules of carbon, hydrogen, oxygen and nitrogen that do not disperse in water. These molecules assemble like crystals due to the atomic forces within the atoms. Since they do not break up in water, these crystal-like non-metallic molecules become *crystalloid* in solution. Minerals in the structure of these crystals are the most effective mineral supplements available. Crystalloid minerals pass through cell membranes to provide essential minerals inside cells. Nothing is wasted due to lack of assimilation and small amounts like a few teaspoons per day are all we need. Taking more doesn't help because the body only takes what it needs for mineral balance. The ocean contains vast amounts of minerals in solution that can be structured into crystalloids. The bounty of the sea is a crystalloid harvest. Whales are the earth's largest mammals because of this bounty.

In comparison to crystalloid solutions, let's look at calcium supplements, for example. If the label on your bottle of mineral supplements says:

• calcium carbonate: you are eating finely ground limestone

• calcium phosphate: you are eating finely ground chalk

• Calcium sulfate: you are eating plaster of Paris

Drinking milk is recommended as a source of calcium. Where do cows get their calcium? You can be sure it is not from calcium supplements or milk. Plants are our best source of calcium because it is bioactive and balanced with other minerals.

Taking too much calcium without a balance of magnesium and phosphorus, or consuming calcium in the metallic form the body cannot use, results in calcium toxicity. The logical answer for calcium toxicity is to take the proper form of calcium and increase the ratio of magnesium and phosphorus. .

Nancy Appleton has written a valuable book called *Lick the Sugar Habit* and prepared a 21-day healing program complete with eight one-hour cassettes to teach us about minerals and vitamins. Appleton suffered from ill health for most of her life until she eliminated sugar from her diet and balanced her mineral base.

She points out that the proper balance (homeostasis) between calcium and phosphorus is exactly 10 ppm (parts per million) calcium to 4 ppm phosphorus. After eating sugar, the phosphorus levels go down. If the phosphorus levels were to fall to 2 ppm, for example, the proper calcium level would be 5, maintaining a ratio of 10 to 4. After taking sugar, the body experiences calcium toxicity, not because it has increased the amount of calcium, but because it has reduced the levels of phosphorus and destroyed the essential balance. Calcium levels can be low and toxic at the same time if one is lacking the other minerals required for balance of other minerals. The same principle applies to all minerals.

Minerals must be taken only in proper proportions. If you find a specific mineral supplement such as calcium does not appear to help, and gives you colored urine, you are probably not consuming the proper balance for homeostasis. Any excess is waste and toxic to the system.

Many of the diseases related to aging, fragile bones, loss of teeth, and so on follow from lack of proper mineral balance. Sugar addiction of any kind upsets your whole body chemistry. In her book, Appleton discusses the effect sugar has on 20 common diseases. Everyone with cancer or any serious disease or calcium toxicity should focus on elimination of sugars from the diet. Even fresh fruit should be consumed in moderation.

Toxic levels of calcium are often treated with drugs called calcium blockers.

The U.S. publication *Townsend Letter for Doctors and Patients*, Oct. 1998 reveals the scope of drug profits related to the sale of calcium blockers to suppress symptoms of calcium toxicity. In 1996 there were more than 64 million prescriptions in the USA sold for calcium blockers, worth an estimated $2.5 billion U.S.

Consumption of sugar and metallic mineral leads to calcium toxicity and huge drug profits for sale of antidotes or calcium blockers. We feed our children with enriched bread and enriched breakfast cereals. These enrichments are only beneficial to manufacturers. They increase the appearance of value, increase sales, and develop an addiction to sugarcoated products. These enrichments enrich the seller, not the buyer. They are not bioactive supplements and do not add significant food value to the product.

There are only a few original sources for the majority of vitamins and mineral supplements. The major sources mine metallic minerals and produce chemical vitamins rather than using bioactive sources such as plants or animals. Blue-green algae, brewer's yeast, and chlorophyll are examples of supplements derived from natural sources. Kelp products derived from ocean water are sources of minerals that can be used immediately by the body. Deep-rooted plants such as alfalfa and tree products such as nuts are rich in natural minerals. Coconuts, for example, are a natural source of selenium and other minerals. Herbs are frequently rich in minerals and provide bioactive minerals for better health. Green drinks made from fresh plants provide an excellent source and balance of minerals. Trace-Lytes produced through a process of microbial engineering is also an excellent source of these minerals. Chemicals and rocks do not provide an effective supplement for most minerals and vitamins as well.

The U.S. Government recently won a court case against Hoffman LaRoche Ltd., a Swiss pharmaceutical company, and BASF AG, a German-based pharmaceutical company, for price fixing the cost of Vitamins A, B2, B5, C, E, and beta carotene. Some of these *chemicals* are added to enrich processed foods. They can be found in food items such as bread, milk, orange juice and breakfast cereal. Obviously, if major customers had alternative sources, they could have purchased them from other suppliers. Price fixing was made possible because they are the only two major manufacturers. These supplements are all man-made chemicals. They are not food for the cells nor are they healthy choices.

The first misconception about chemical supplements is that we can feed ourselves effectively with "enriched" white bread and processed cereals because the essential vitamins and minerals have been replaced. We can feed ourselves until we are overweight and undernourished. The enrichment process does not return important vitamins and minerals lost in the processing of food. The second misconception is that we can supplement our diet by taking these chemicals and rocks. Human genes do not have the capacity to transcribe enzymes to digest chemicals and powdered rock.

Crystalloid minerals are our best source of supplements

Mineral supplements are available in three types, based on the size of the particles we ingest. These are *metallic, colloidal* and *crystalloid.*

1. Metallic minerals (as mined from the earth) are still rocks

'Metallic minerals' are ores found in deposits within the earth's crust such as salt in ancient seabeds. Lumps are mined and ground to a fine powder and added to food as a supplement or served as tablets and capsules. These are significantly different from minerals in solution, or minerals, which have been modified by soil bacteria and taken up into plants for cell-wall structure, protein, and ATP. Plants produce ATP, which is the major source of energy for plant-eating animals. Phosphorus in ATP is far better for assimilation and health than phosphorus in rock-dust or 'metallic' capsules. Mineral oxides in crystalloid molecules that we call electrolytes are more bioactive that the ores.

Metallic particles are too large for absorption into cell walls. The human physiology does not contain enzymes or substrates suitable for metabolism of metallic minerals. Most of these so-called supplements become toxins in the body and are excreted as expensive urine. Salt goes into solution, but most metallic minerals do not.

Chelated minerals are metallic minerals bonded to amino acids. Other mineral supplements marketed as being in a food base are mixtures of metallic minerals in dried plant material. These mineral particles are still too large to pass through cell-wall membranes in order to serve useful functions in enzymes.

If your mineral supplement gives you colored urine, assume that your body is not able to use it. If your body could use it, or needed it, it would not be excreted as waste. In the process of eliminating these toxic minerals as waste, your body excretes valuable minerals already absorbed from your food. It is a lose-lose activity.

2. Colloidal minerals (particles stay in suspension in liquids)

Metallic mineral particles are ground to a fine powder and mixed with water or alcohol, but particles do not dissolve. Particles stay in suspension due to inherent movement of liquid molecules known as the Brownian movement. Particles are too large to pass through a parchment or collodion membrane. Colloidal metallic particles are still too large to pass through cell-wall membranes and cannot enter the cell wall without further metabolism.

Colloidal minerals mined from ancient forests and coal deposits and in various liquid tonics have some particles that go into solution in water. These supplements provide a source for bioactive minerals because they were incorporated into living things millions of years ago. In most samples that I have studied, these solutions also contain numerous minerals that are known to be toxic to human systems, or of unknown value. In addition, there is not likely going to be the correct balance of trace minerals, so mineral imbalance at the cellular level becomes a very serious problem.

Minerals are said to be ionic. What does that mean? Ionic refers to any substance that is electrically charged or has the capacity to take on or give off electrons readily. An ionic mineral is one in which the number of protons in the nucleus is not balanced by an equal number of electrons in the outer orbits. There is a net negative or positive ionic field or charge surrounding the atom or molecule. Positive charged ions, such as sodium, potassium, hydrogen and calcium are called cations. Negatively charged ions such as bicarbonate, chloride and phosphate are called anions. Many of our body's processes depend upon the movement of these ions across cell membranes. Ionic minerals function because they are highly active as electrical conductors in the body.

It seems to me that "highly reactive molecules" are words used to describe both beneficial ionic minerals and dangerous free radicals. What's the difference? I really do not know. Perhaps the only dangerous free radicals are manufactured chemicals that the body cannot use or an excessive amount of some minerals.

Ionic minerals in the proper proportions that the body uses are not dangerous free radicals. Like oxygen, these minerals are controlled by enzymes and substrates to render them harmless. However, if we have a large excess of any ionic mineral, it can become a dangerous free radical. Salt, for example, is essential for life but excess salt is harmful and may lead to conditions such as excess water retention within cells. Lack of water increases the concentration of ions and the parts per million in solutions. Drinking an adequate daily amount of water is essential for minerals to function in the body. Consuming mineral supplements, as mined from the earth, without first having these minerals converted by bacteria into a bioactive form, is probably not a wise choice. Consider your saltshaker as a container of two mineral supplements— sodium and chloride. Perhaps we should have a magnesium shaker on our table along with salt and pepper.

Some ionic minerals are colloidal sized particles that come from coal or other previous plant matter. Bottles of liquid ionic minerals often contain numerous toxic minerals not needed in the body. Be sure to read the label carefully and review the list of minerals. Bottles of colloidal minerals with more than 20 minerals probably contain many dangerous free radicals.

Minerals become functional in the body when individual atoms are combined with oxygen in proteins to make enzymes and cellular structures. Oxides of minerals impart paramagnetic qualities to proteins, making them more functional. Lumps of minerals, regardless how finely ground, are still too large for function in the body without further separation. Our minerals should come from living sources such as plants and animals, blue-green algae and the like. Ocean fish are an excellent source. We need minerals in solution and minerals in molecules with other atoms forming stable crystal-like molecules called crystalloids. Crystalloids are called the spark of life because they give cells the capacity to produce energy and crystalloid solutions conduct electrical energy in the body.

3. Crystalloid minerals (minerals in solution in water)

Crystalloid minerals are capable of passing through a cell-wall membrane. Seawater is loaded with minerals in solution, as is most natural spring and well water from underground streams and aquifers. All of the places on earth where humans are known to live long healthy lives have only one thing in common. They all drink water filled with minerals and life-giving energy. Numerous healing springs around the world, often associated with thermal hot spots, provide minerals in solution.

There is only one common denominator in all diseases: namely, mineral imbalance. Trace minerals are the spark of life that gives energy to our cells. Enzymes defend the body against microbes, and crystalloid minerals are required in all enzymes used in the metabolic process and immune system. The lack of minerals, or the imbalance of minerals, leads to the lack of corresponding enzymes and a strong immune system. These lead to cellular infection, parasites, and tissue weakness.

Author Bill Lane has written a best-seller in the health field entitled *Sharks don't get Cancer*, as well as a sequel called *Sharks Still Don't Get Cancer*. Why don't sharks get cancer?

Sharks live in seawater that is filled with trace minerals in crystalloid form. Sharks cannot experience a mineral imbalance because their environment provides them with the minerals they need, and they do not have an opportunity to disturb this mineral balance. Do otters, sea lions, and whales get cancer? No.

According to Ed McCabe in his book *Oxygen Therapies*, a Dr. Murray worked on a whaleboat. He observed the dissection of 964 whales and never found one with cancer. They had none of the systemic diseases or autoimmune diseases. When you consider that whales are mammals, they should experience some defective gene or autoimmune diseases. The reason sharks and whales do not get cancer is probably due to their ocean water environment of minerals in solution or in crystalloid form.

Numerous books have been written about the essential trace minerals, acid and alkaline balance, and minerals in general. It is not the purpose of this book to discuss minerals fully. This vital subject requires a special study of its own and application to your daily lifestyle. Perhaps the easiest way to educate yourself on minerals is to read a booklet called *ELECTROLYTES, The Spark of Life*, by Gillian Martlew, N.D. A person who specializes in the use of natural remedies for health care receives a Naturopathy Degree and uses the initials N.D. to signify this education.

Another excellent booklet is *Fire in the Water, How Minerals Become Biology,* by David Yarrow. This booklet describes the development in the 1930s of trace mineral electrolytes in liquid crystalloid form, by the New Jersey scientist George Earp-Thomas. Thomas realized the proper nutrition for bacteria are minerals. You may have heard about researchers finding bacteria thriving in rock miles below the surface of the earth. Bacteria in the soil modify minerals making them bioactive. Chemicals sprayed on crops reduce bacterial populations and thereby reduce bioactive minerals in the soil. This process results in fewer minerals in our food chain.

Thomas also realized that cells without minerals cannot maintain cell-wall pressure and a high-energy charge. Cells lacking minerals become weak and susceptible to infection and disease. This vital observation helps explain why nutrition plays such a vital part in health and why viruses cannot invade healthy cells. Mineral supplements added to a mineral deficient diet rapidly restore cell membranes, disrupt pathogenic bacteria in the lymphatic fluids, and restores infected tissues to health. Bioactive minerals supplements, complexed with water molecules as crystalloids, are liquid crystals. These are the key to preventing and curing infection, thereby preventing and curing cancer.

According to David Yarrow's book, Earp-Thomas worked with physicians at the Virginia cancer hospital in the 1930s and they had an 80% success rate against cancer, unheard of then or now. Earp-Thomas continued to distribute information of the importance of bioactive mineral supplements due to lack of minerals in the soil and food chain. In 1948, the FDA forced him to stop distributing 'medical advice' on the basis that he was not a medical doctor. Although he won the court case, it destroyed his financial base. That winter his lab burned down due to a mysterious fire, and his spirit was broken by the loss.

Yarrow goes on to say: "Another great American scientist surrendered broken-hearted to the dark, fearful forces haunting mainstream medicine in America." There is no doubt in my mind, from observing the beneficial results of TraceLytes and other mineral supplements, that all diseases have a mineral deficiency involved at the start.

Under a heading called *Resurrection,* Yarrow writes (Page 47):

We need to heed Earp-Thomas' warning that the loss of trace elements from topsoil, food, and water will promote a plague of degenerative diseases. We need to feed a full spectrum of minerals —including essential trace elements to our topsoil, and wean agriculture off its chemical dependent monocultures. And we must explore trace element electrolytes' medical application to not only treat, but prevent, disease.

As enzyme-catalysts, minerals regulate our body processes and supply us with energy. A loss of one mineral or an excess of another may upset the vital balance of the electrolytic system of the cells. Enzymes from the pancreas, for example, are essential for digestion of proteins and sugars. Without these enzymes, protein in the lymphatic system cannot be utilized, and protein molecules are attacked by the immune system as foreign invaders. Food allergies, allergic reactions, and so-called autoimmune disease result from mineral imbalance.

The major minerals in order of percentage of body weight include calcium, phosphorous, potassium, sodium, sulfur, chlorine, and magnesium. Minerals such as magnesium are extremely light, so the body weight concept is misleading. In order of importance, magnesium should be near the top of the list. Trying to identify minerals by importance is like trying to determine the most important leg of a three-legged stool. In the final analysis, any one mineral, if deficient, may reduce the capacity of the body to use other minerals, making them toxic to the system.

The essential trace minerals, according to David Yarrow, are only 15 in number. These are iron, iodine, silicon, fluorine, copper, manganese, zinc, selenium, cobalt, molybdenum, chromium, tin boron, nickel and vanadium. Each of these has been identified as essential for an enzyme or function in the body. Obviously, ionic mineral supplements containing more than these minerals probably contain toxins and contaminants.

I believe minerals should be taken from natural sources in foods as well as in food supplements such as the Master Formula, Green Alive, Greens Plus and any of the green powder or liquid-based mineral supplements. Synthetic chemicals and metallic minerals should be avoided.

The immune system and autonomic functions of the body are controlled by the primitive brain stem using direct current ionic energy connecting all parts of the body. Body fluids containing electrolytes and membranes containing phosphorus provide ion-transport meridians that are essential for health and a strong immune system. Minerals are the key to health.

11. Cleanse the lymphatic system to help prevent and cure cancer

Let's look now at how parasites initiate the cancer process in a body that is lacking in vitamins, minerals and enzymes required for a strong immune system response.

In the introduction to the textbook, *Hidden Killers, The Revolutionary Medical Discoveries of Professor Guenther Enderlein*, we find medical recognition that cancer is primarily a lymphatic disease.

What Dr. Enderlein found in the body fluids of human beings – as well as the tissue and fluids of plants and animals – made him one of the most prominent microbiologists of this century. He managed to explain that certain disease processes are caused by different kinds of microbial growth in the body fluids and cell tissues.

Microbial growth in the body fluids and cell tissues

Have you ever thought that cancer spreads mainly through the body fluids, ducts, and fluid storage vessels? When I first started my research on cancer, I was led to believe that cancer was a cell-based disease caused by defective genes going awry. When I looked at a piece of steak or organ meat, I imagined cancer starting in cells forming muscles and organ tissues of the body. One cell went bad, due to a defective gene, and commenced doubling repeatedly for several years until a tumor was formed. Numerous books on cancer show the gradual increase in size of a tumor and the years required for cells to double often enough to produce an egg-sized tumor. In addition, I also believed cancer spreads from cell to cell like one bad apple spoiling all apples in contact with it. Neither of these concepts is correct.

It is obvious to me now that cancer is a microbial disease of membrane cells in the lymphatic system, liquid storage vessels, and ducts. Cancer starts with fermentation of glucose and blood proteins. The reason why the vast majority of cancer occurs in skin tissue is that mycelia from fungi can grow unimpeded within body fluids that nourish our cells, within the lymphatic system veins and nodes as well as within storage vessels and ducts. Mycelia invade thousands of adjacent epithelial cells simultaneously and provide the nucleotides required for rapid cancer growth. Cancer cannot start one cell at a time, because the adjacent oxidative cells will eliminate the small quantity of toxins produced by a single cell. Cancer can only start when a large quantity of cells is invaded and a mass of tissue switches from aerobic to anaerobic metabolism simultaneously. Cancer can start only after cells lose the oxidative process due to contamination of ammonia or carbon dioxide.

Cancer growth is not limited to a doubling of cells taking many years to develop. Rather, millions of cells can be invaded simultaneously by fungal mycelia and a tumor developed in a brief period. A quantity of trapped blood proteins provides the energy base. That's why children a few months old develop tumors containing the equivalent of some 10 or more years of cellular-doubling. Cancer most often starts when parasites large enough to damage epithelial cells forming these vessels and ducts damage sufficient epithelial cells to cause internal bleeding.

Let's take a closer look at the lymphatic system as it relates to cancer.

Dr. Guyton on importance of lymphatic circulation

According to Dr. Arthur Guyton's *Textbook of Medical Physiology* (Page 362), about one-sixth of our body mass is made up of interstitial tissue forming spaces between the cells. A 200-pound person will have more than 30 pounds of tissue used by the body for structure and support. The structure supports other organ cells and allows for blood proteins, oxygen, and other nutrients to bathe the cells and remove wastes through the veins and lymphatic system. This tissue also keeps lymphatic liquids from running down to our feet when we stand up. Fermentation in this system leads to epithelial cancer, as does fermentation in ducts and storage vessels.

Dr. Guyton uses the first chapter of his massive text to give medical students a clear expression of the significance of the interstitial fluids. Chapter One is entitled: *Functional Organization of the Human Body and Control of the Internal Environment.* Understanding the human body starts with understanding the cell and the lymphatic system. The same principle applies to understanding cancer.

Dr. Guyton describes how blood sugars and proteins are continually fed from arteries into spaces between the cells to nourish human cells. Any unused material must be returned to the circulatory system within hours via the lymphatic system or it will deprive the cells of conditions required for life. Dr. Guyton writes:

> **If it were not for continual removal of proteins (by the lymphatic system), the dynamics of fluid exchange at the blood capillaries**

would become so abnormal within only a few hours that life could no longer continue.

Consider for a moment what would happen when internal bleeding or lymphatic fluids flow into a dead-end cavity such as a milk lobe or duct. Without continual removal and fluid exchange these carbon-rich fluids will ferment and support fungal growth. In time, the fungal mycelia from the fungal growth will invade vessel cell walls and cause cancer. In addition, new cells formed to repair the damage that allowed internal bleeding are forced into an environment controlled by microbial growth hormones and enzymes. Normal replication is not possible.

Dr. Guyton then goes on to describe the various control systems of the body. Control systems are based on enzymes. Cancer results when microbial enzymes disturb the control systems of the body by overriding the influence of human enzymes. That's why cancer should be considered a metabolic disease if viewed from how cancer cells function.

One-third of the human body is fluid in constant motion

In Dr. Guyton's text, we continue to read about the lymphatic system as being crucial for good health.

About 56 per cent of the adult human body is fluid. Though most of this fluid is inside the cells and is called intracellular fluid, about one-third of it is in the spaces outside the cells and is called extracellular fluid. *This extracellular fluid is in constant motion throughout the body.* It is rapidly mixed by the blood circulation and by diffusion between the blood and tissue fluids, and in the extracellular fluid are the ions and nutrients needed by the cells for maintenance of cellular function. Therefore, all cells live in essentially the same environment, the extracellular fluid, for which reason the extracellular fluid is often called the internal environment of the body, or the 'milieu interieur', a term introduced a hundred years ago by the great 19th century French physiologist, Claude Bernard.

Cells are capable of living, growing, and accomplishing their special functions so long as the proper concentrations of oxygen, glucose, the different ions, amino acids, and fatty substances are available in this internal environment.

Let's take a close look at the five items Dr. Guyton selected as most critical in the life of a cell. These same items are critical in curing and preventing cancer as well as all other diseases. Cancer occurs when constant motion of body fluids stops because lack of circulation fails to oxygenate the blood proteins.

Oxygen: in this case, the more the better

Glucose: for production of glycogen from carbohydrates

Different ions: from essential minerals and trace minerals

Amino acids: with all 22 essential amino acids

Fatty substances: natural oils and fats *(not hydrogenated)*

It follows that diseases stem from an imbalance in the lymphatic fluids that feed the cells and remove toxins. Dr. Guyton goes on to describe the differences between extracellular and intracellular fluids.

The extracellular fluid contains large amounts of sodium, chloride, and bicarbonate ions, plus nutrients for the cells, such as oxygen, glucose, fatty acids and amino acids. It also contains carbon dioxide, which is being transported from the cells to the lungs to be expelled as well as other cellular products, which are being transported to the kidneys for excretion.

The intracellular fluid differs significantly from the extracellular fluid; particularly, it contains large amounts of potassium, magnesium, and phosphate ions instead of the sodium and chloride ions found in the extracellular fluid. Special mechanisms for transporting ions through the cell membranes maintain these differences.

Let's take a moment now and review the above references. The cellular environment contains a group of minerals in specific ratios, as well as three important molecular groups.

1. The electrolytes are special compounds that conduct electricity, not like salty water or an acid, but as organic compounds with oxygen bonds that carry and produce ionic energy. Oxygen bonded to minerals such as silica, calcium, and chromium, produce unique bipolar molecules. Life energy flows through crystalloid compounds, and electrolytes are vital for life. Electrolytes are also essential for production and function of enzymes. Electrolytes are truly the spark of life.

2. Fatty acids are long-chained carboxylic acids produced by hydrolysis of lipids. A carboxylic acid means there are one or more oxygen molecules connected by double bonds. These bonds are unstable and allow water to hydrolyze or dissolve the long chain fat molecule into smaller segments and use them for energy and transfer of ionic

energy. Modern diets made up of saturated fatty acids have all of the oxygen molecules attached in stable single bonds with hydrogen. These cannot be dissolved in water. Filling your body with saturated fats and expecting good health is like trying to wash grease off your hands without soap. It doesn't happen.

3. Amino acids are combinations of nitrogen compounds and carbohydrates that are ready-to-serve food nutrients and building blocks for functional proteins. Eating mainly cooked and processed foods with a long shelf life does not provide ready-to-serve molecules the body needs for good health.

Minerals required for all metabolic processes

Minerals such as calcium, magnesium, and chromium are important for production of enzymes and substrates essential for metabolic processes.

We learned earlier that the synthesis of all proteins, nucleic acids, nucleotides, lipids, and carbohydrates and the activation of muscle contraction requires magnesium.

If intracellular fluid requires magnesium for all metabolic processes, including synthesis of all nutrients, what will happen to blood sugars and proteins in the lymphatic system when magnesium is missing in the cells? Answer: Nutrients in the lymphatic system will start to ferment within a few hours, if they are not circulated back through the body and eliminated or re-oxygenated.

Minerals such as magnesium, potassium, sodium and phosphorus in the intracellular fluid provide for the ion exchange and vibrational frequency of the cellular plasma. The electrical potential between a cell and the intracellular fluids influences health because this is the driving force to carry nutrients into the cell and waste products out of the cell.

The proper balance of minerals is essential for production of energy via the oxidative process. When we add chemicals, heavy metal toxins (lead and mercury from amalgams), microbial growth hormones and parasitic toxins to these fluids, we create disease. Vital minerals and nutrients are consumed and the essential balance destroyed. Without the proper balance, these protein-rich and glucose-rich liquids stagnate and ferment. Refined sugar, hydrogenated oils, and processed foods are the major cause of mineral deficiency and imbalance. Recreational and prescription drugs are similarly destructive of enzymes.

Lymphatic fluids found in three areas

The biology text *Human Physiology,* by E.B. Mason, teaches us there are three principal body fluids:

(1) the intracellular fluid, or fluid within the cells.

(2) the interstitial fluid, or fluid which surrounds the cells, also called the lymphatic fluids.

(3) the plasma, or fluid within the blood vessels that feed the cells. Together, the plasma and the interstitial fluids make up the extracellular fluid, or fluid outside the cells.

In an average 150-pound person, the interstitial fluid surrounding the cells measures about 11.2 litres in volume and makes up 16% of body weight. Lymphatic fluids transport carbohydrates (sugars) and other nutrients to the cells and remove wastes. Minerals in solution, or electrolytes, are required for this process. A young child demonstrates the immediate effect of consuming too much sugar by becoming hyperactive until the sugar is burned off. Older people, lacking in minerals, are unable to simply burn off excess sugar. The cancer process is fed by fermentation of blood sugars such as excess fructose, sucrose and maltose that the cells do not require due to excessive sugar consumption.

Dr. Samuel West's book *The Golden Seven Plus One* describes how cancer is caused by trapped blood sugars and proteins in the lymphatic system, storage vessels and ducts. Dr. West diagrams the cellular environment showing normal cells as close together in a dry state, and how excess fluids cause cells to become surrounded with excess fluids and enter a wet state. Excess fluids result from mineral imbalances due to processed foods. The wet state leads to cancer through fermentation of glucose between the cells. When fungal mycelia invade the cell, they cause sufficient injury to generate a current of injury response to heal the damage. The current of injury causes these cells to multiply.

Dr. Costantini, author of several books on the fungal cause of disease, sees fungi related to all cancers. Dr. Majid Ali's research also ties fungi directly to the cancer process. Fermentation, a fungal process, produces enzymes to block off oxygen from the fermenting material. Fungi create low-oxygen microspheres so that anaerobic glycolysis, or fermentation, can proceed without the interference of oxygen.

Fungal mycelia formation and fungal budding

In the *Journal of Integrative Medicine* (Winter, 1997), by Dr. Majid Ali, M.D., we find a significant reference to fungi and blood clotting. This quotation is important to the theme of this book because it supplies documentation explaining how and why the intracellular spaces become clogged with trapped blood proteins allowing for the spread of cancer.

In the following reference, Dr. Ali describes how fungal mycelia create microspheres of low-oxygen areas. The research explains another relationship between fungi and cancer. Fungi deprive cells of oxygen, and this leads to fermentation of glycogen. Dr. Ali describes his personal observation of fungal mycelia causing blood plasma (lymphatic fluids) to congeal as observed in live blood-cell analysis. The *Journal of Integrative Medicine* provides the following information (Page 46):

We observed *zones of plasma congealing surrounding fungal organisms.* We observed this phenomenon to occur within ten to sixty minutes in almost all instances in which we studied the morphology of fungal organisms continuously in freshly prepared unstained peripheral blood smears. We also observed fungal spores germinate within one to ten hours in most cases.

The zones of congealing-plasma surrounding fungal organisms increase in area, trap platelets and cellular debris, and grow into microclots, and finally into micro-plaques. Such findings suggest fungal organisms play a role in pathogenesis *(spread of disease).*

Dr. Ali's research supports Dr. Costantini's fungal research showing a direct connection between fungi and all cancers, through the mechanism of trapping blood proteins for fermentation and blocking off oxygen from the cells. Fungal enzymes produce zones of congealed blood proteins (micro-plaques), thereby creating a low-oxygen microsphere suitable for anaerobic life and replication.

Combining Dr. Ali's observations with Dr. Warburg's, we can now see how the fungal process of fermentation leads to the growth and spread of cancer.

The microspheres result in human cells and tissue becoming overwhelmed with microbes and contaminants. Blood proteins are trapped, oxygen is reduced, the production of ATP stops, the immune system is compromised, fermentation begins, glucose is not oxidized directly but is converted to chitin, and microbial proteins. The environment becomes supportive of microbial infections as carbon dioxide levels rise, and microbes are allowed to take over cellular metabolism and replication.

The interrelationship between fungi, bacteria, and cancer cells is now obvious. Fungi prepare the low-oxygen environment and provide nucleotides for replication. Bacteria provide DNA polymerase enzymes and coenzymes for replication and differentiation. Fermentation provides high-energy primers to initiate chemical action with stable DNA molecules, and fermentation allows glucose to be converted into microbial proteins and cell-wall components.

The final step in the process is amalgamation of chitin and other proteins into cell-wall membranes.

The blocking of oxygen and the accumulation of carbon dioxide, from intracellular spaces, creates the primordial condition necessary for anaerobic microbes to multiply and survive. In addition, the raised carbon dioxide levels cause the expression of dormant primitive genes to support rapid fermentation. The human cell is converted to a more primitive life form because bacteria are using the cell to produce vital nutrients for their needs.

I might add that Dr. Ali's research also supports the findings of the research of Dr. Philpott into Alzheimer's. Microbes produce "micro-plaques" and Alzheimer's brain tissue is characteristically plaque-filled. This supports the theory that microbes in the brain cause Alzheimer's disease. Because of the blood-brain barrier, drugs are not effective for curing Alzheimer's, but pulsed magnetic fields as described in Chapter 26 could do so very well. Alzheimer's is another disease in which freedom of choice in health care is required before we can treat patients effectively. Restricting advancement of alternative cures for cancer results in restricting cures for all microbial diseases, including the dreaded living death known as Alzheimer's.

I am going to digress for a moment. If you have a loved one with Alzheimer's, please stop and think about the implications of the medical monopoly on health care with a mindset limited to drug therapy. The suppression of cancer cures results in suppression of treatment for other diseases. It follows that freedom of choice in treating cancer is required before we can have effective non-drug treatment of Alzheimer's and other diseases. The medical monopoly on health care must be taken away from those who deny the public free access to alternative health care. Chapter 26 lists several effective cures that should be made available immediately to help Alzheimer victims.

One of the greatest medical errors is the rejection of treatments for disease based in the lymphatic system. How often have you had your lymphatic fluids checked? If you have swollen lymph nodes, you need lymphatic cleansing, not surgical removal of swollen nodes. How many medical treatments are there that actually support better health by cleansing the lymphatic system and lymph nodes? None.

The only lymphatic system treatment I know of was introduced by Dr. Gaston Naessens, and is known worldwide as 714X. The persecution of Dr. Naessens and the suppression of his cure for cancer and AIDS are painful reminders of the ongoing suppression of effective cancer cures. A second lymphatic system cleanse exists in a series of exercises that help pump the lymph through the body. This exercise program is listed in SOURCES under the heading of Multi-Versa

Let's review the lymphatic system to see how electro-magnetic pulses can be used to prevent and cure cancer and other diseases by destroying microorganisms and stopping fermentation.

Lymphatic system existed before arterial system

Fred Soyka in his book *The Ion Effect* describes how the lymphatic system was formed in living things before the blood system. When you think about it, every living thing has liquids in circulation or within the cell walls. Even cells have tiny tubes that allow for transfer of liquids within the cell.

Fred Soyka writes about the lymphatic system (Page 62):

Human lymph glands and ducts form a circulatory system that medical scientists believe to have existed in animal life forms before they evolved to the point where blood and a vein-and-artery circulatory system came into being. Precisely how important the lymphatic system is to animal life remains a mystery, although it is known that many kinds of cancer spread from one part of the body to another through the lymph glands and that these glands and ducts are part of the total circulatory system that carries body chemicals to the place where they are needed.

Replication of multi-celled living things obviously occurred before the development of a blood, heart, artery, and vein system. We can assume that the method used by the body to control replication was distributed through the lymphatic or nervous system as the body developed. The mystery of how cells communicate and how the mind/body connection directs replication and growth may someday be found to be a function of ionic energy and electrolytes in the lymphatic liquids. Enzymes control the function but we still do not know what controls the output of enzymes. The controlling mechanism of the replication process is still a mystery because we are looking in the wrong place. The autonomic nervous system relies on the proper function of the primitive ionic energy fields within the body.

Cleansing and maintaining the lymphatic system should be one of the major processes used to combat disease. In the next chapter, we will see how electromedicine is ideal for this purpose.

---

12. Control cancer with electromagnetic therapy

Let's focus now on how cancer can be controlled by applying magnets or electronic energy to enzymes, microbes, and cancer cells. Consider life as an electrical phenomenon and disease as an electrical energy deficiency or disruption.

Enzyme function and magnetism

Enzymes are paramagnetic due to the combination of oxygen, proteins, and minerals. A mineral oxide is simply a combination of a mineral with oxygen, such as iron oxide or magnesium oxide. In the CRM Books publication *BIOLOGY, An Appreciation of Life,* written by a group of 21 scientific contributors, we have a reference to life using energy from the earth (Page 49):

> Probably the central feature of living systems is to reproduce themselves. All living systems utilize the flow of energy through the universe to reproduce and to maintain life. A living system uses this energy to produce complex molecules and to maintain highly integrated and ordered structures.

These scientists describe life as an electromagnetic phenomenon dependent on the magnetism of the earth. Living things demonstrate the presence of measurable amounts of electrical energy and therefore must generate magnetic fields.

If we combine the concept that all biochemical actions are controlled by enzymes, and that all-living systems utilize the flow of energy through the universe, we can surmise that enzyme function is fueled by some form of magnetism.

The cell is an electromagnetic resonator

Author George Lakhovsky in his book *The Secret of Life* describes his concept that a cell is *"nothing but an electromagnetic resonator, capable of emitting and absorbing radiations of a very high frequency.*" Life of a cell is a vibrational frequency induced by vibrational frequencies in the lymphatic system. Dr. Hulda Clark has measured these frequencies using a device that measures frequency by resonance. Minerals as well as living and dead creatures have a resonant frequency.

Life in a single-celled life form, such as a bacterium, vibrates at a frequency of its own. In her books Dr. Clark has charts showing the "bioradiation of pathogens" which range from 77 Khz to 900 Khz?

Lakhovsky **tells us life in multi-celled creatures is the result of** "*harmony of multiple radiations which react upon one another.*" Ancient Hindu medicine recognizes the body as being energized through a number of 'chakras' or lines of energy running through the body. This is ionic energy flowing along cell-wall membranes.

Western medicine recognizes the existence of 'circadian rhythms' or daily patterns in activities that correspond with the time of day or night. The energy of life is related to the spin of the earth through the ether or energy of space. This is energy from ionic particles smaller than electrons and that found in nerves. Ghosts, assuming they exist, would be living things made of this ether-energy, and the life-force is made up of this ether-energy. The life-force gives structure and form to the body by polarizing ionic energy through crystals. Taken together, there is a large body of evidence that supports a concept that living things generate electrical energy and this energy flows from the earth and our environment. Life energy is generated by resonance, and crystalloid minerals serve as the mechanism to convert ionic energy to life energy.

What is resonance? Perhaps the easiest way to explain resonance is through the function of music. If you pluck a guitar string it will vibrate and produce a sound. The wooden box forming the guitar will resonate to the vibration and amplify the sound. In addition, the other strings will start to vibrate due to resonance.

It is possible that the DNA crystal-like structure forming our genes resonates to the thought waves from the mind, and emotions from the body, as well as the subconscious mind and life-force. Through resonance, genes are expressed and tRNA formed to provide the enzymes and proteins required by the body to function as a living thing. Perhaps the resonating strand of DNA attracts the molecules required to form the corresponding strand of RNA just like one guitar string makes another resonate. In other words, genes are crystals that resonate according to thoughts and emotions thereby connecting the physical reality of the body to the mental, emotional, and spiritual reality.

Dr. Hulda Clark's book *The Cure for All Diseases* (Pages 562-570), contains charts listing the vibrational frequencies of all common microbes and parasites. The huge majority of these microbes vibrate at a frequency between 77,000 Hz to 900,000Hz. Human cells vibrate at a frequency that starts about 1,562,000 Hz and rises to 9,457,000 Hz.

For comparison to broadcasting stations, the 107 AM radio stations operate from 535,000 Hz to 1,605,000 Hz, TV stations 1 to 6 vibrate from 54MHz to 108MHz, UHF TV stations 14-69 range from 470MHz to 890MHz and cellular phones at 806 MHz.

The large gaps between microbial frequencies and human frequencies (900,000 Hz to 1,562 000Hz) allows for selective killing of parasites by zapping them. Zappers work effectively in the range of 31,000 Hz, far below any human frequencies. The fact that broadcast frequencies overlap human frequencies, without harm, supports confidence in the safety of this device.

In order to understand and accept forms of cancer treatment, based on electrical energy of magnetic fields, we must consider the vital part played by the lymphatic system and body fluids. The portion of our body called the lymphatic system is the least protected from microbial life forms, as this area is technically outside of cellular walls and cellular defenses. By energizing our lymphatic fluid with electromagnetic impulses, we support the immune system in its most vulnerable area. Fungi and microbes in body fluids can be killed and their enzymes destroyed. This concept provides the scientific basis for cancer therapy without drugs. This is also the scientific reason to believe in the simple nine-volt device called a zapper, as developed by Dr. Hulda Clark.

Square wave vibrational frequency kills microbes

In order to explain how microbes can be killed electronically, I would like to draw a comparison that we are all familiar with through common knowledge.

We have all been taught to avoid having electrical devices near bathtubs. Supposedly, if a person is having a bath, and a radio or other 110-volt electrical device falls into the bath water, the person will be electrocuted. According to physics, electric currents follow the route of least resistance. Since the bathtub is metal, or has metal fittings, and the tub is connected to copper tubes leading to the ground, one must ask why doesn't the current flow harmlessly to the ground?

Since I have never witnessed such an accident, perhaps the statement it is not true. However, this is not a good time to ask: "Why should I believe you?" I am not prepared to prove it is false. Testing could be fatal! I am willing to believe it is true because it makes sense.

The answer, I believe, is that all of the water in the bathtub is momentarily charged with the voltage. Since the human body is more than 50 per cent liquid, the body is also charged with the voltage. Even if the person is sitting up in the tub, his or her whole body is equally charged, not just the portion under water.

The same principle takes effect when you touch an electric wire or zap yourself for microbes. When you receive an electrical frequency through the hands or wrist, the energy zaps all tissues in your body. Because human cells vibrate at a much higher frequency than pathogens, one can selectively zap single-celled parasites without damage or unwanted side effects. We can also kill them in the lymphatic system and in pools of trapped blood sugars where they cannot be reached by other means. We can even zap them in our brain tissue without harm. Zapping could be a great benefit to psychotic and Alzheimer's patients.

The fact that microbial parasites and human cells operate at different vibrational frequencies is the basis for electromedicine. This explains why microbes can be killed and microbial enzymes suppressed with a micro current harmless to human cells. An electric field contacting any part of the body is measurable at all parts of the body. A vibrational frequency designed to destroy microbes by connecting through the hands, wrists, or feet reaches all parts of the body in contact with the lymphatic system.

Several other devices are available to treat the lymphatic system. One of the most effective is a strong magnetic pulse and another is a strong magnetic field that goes around the body. Some doctors have even patented a system that works extremely well by removing blood from the body for electrocuting parasites, but this life-saving drug-free invention is being ignored and suppressed. *(See notes on Patent 5188738.)*. It is unforgivable that mainstream medicine has neglected cleansing the lymphatic system with electromagnetism as a treatment for disease.

If you do a patent search on the Internet you will actually find two numbers for this suppressed patent. Both were issued to Kaali Steven of Dobbs Ferry, N.Y. Patent 5139684 was issued in 1992, and revised patent 5188738 was issued in 1993. The major claim is *"the electrical treatment of bacteria, and/or virus, and/or parasites and/or fungus contained within blood and/or other body fluids..."* The patent was developed at the Albert Einstein College of Medicine in New York according to the Dec. 1992 issue of a magazine called *Longevity*. We will discuss this patent later in conjunction with the legal issues of making claims for electrocuting parasites. First, let's review the scientific rational for using magnetic and vibrational devices to help cure cancer.

Magnetism and its effects on the living system

A great deal of specialized knowledge is required to use magnets safely and effectively. Its also rather difficult to understand the basic concepts.

There is considerable confusion in the definition of terms because the North pole of the earth attracts the south pole of a magnet. However, convention identifies the pole of the magnet that points north as the North pole. This problem has led to the development of a scientific convention and an industrial convention for identifying magnets. If a bar magnet is suspended with freedom to rotate, the industrial convention identifies the pole pointing to the north as the North pole. The scientific convention prefers to identify the pole that points toward the north as the south pole or negative energy pole. The end of the magnet that points south becomes the north pole, or positive energy pole. *The scientific convention recognizes the negative pole as the healer and the positive pole as the adversary to good health but this is not all that simple.* Positive polarity also has many beneficial functions and a balanced polarity also has many useful functions.

Back in 1974, authors Albert Roy Davis and Walter C. Rawls, Jr. published a book called *Magnetism and its Effects on the Living System.* This book collects research from around the world in the field of biomagnetics (biology and magnets). With this knowledge, they proved that they could enhance healing of injured cells and improve health of test animals by applying the South-seeking pole. Alternatively, if desired, they could cause microbes and worms to suffer reduced activity and replication by applying the North-seeking pole at a very low level. The low level was damaging to microbial life forms but did not show any adverse side effects to human cells.

Another problem faced by both conventions is based on how the earth's magnetic field is drawn. It was previously thought that the magnetic energy traveled through space in a circular motion exiting from the tip of the North pole, and entering near the tip of the South pole. According to Davis and Rawls, this concept is not correct.

In a bar magnet there is a narrow area at the center known as the Bloch Wall where no magnetic lines of force are evident. Researchers now believe that the earth has a Bloch Wall at the equator as well. The earth is divided magnetically at the equator into two distinct energy flow patterns. In the Northern Hemisphere, energy exits the earth near the equator and enters the earth at the North pole. In the Southern Hemisphere, energy exits the earth at the South Pole and enters the earth at the equator. Magnetic energies appear to be making a figure 8 pattern passing through the center of the earth. Alternately, there are two independent energy fields, one flowing from the equator into the North pole region, and the other flowing from the South

Pole into the equator region. In this case, magnetic energies flow through the earth as well as through the atmosphere and ionosphere.

By adding the spin of the earth through these lines of force, nature creates two giant generators. Living things use this energy, and life functions can be modified by increasing or decreasing the magnetic fields appropriately.

Just as the spin of the earth creates a flow of air from west to east, known as the west winds, the spin of the earth creates a flow of magnetic lines of force through the atoms and molecules of matter. This is the force that spins diatomic molecules, such as water, producing the Brownian motion of colloids in suspension; the force that creates and drives electrons; and the force that gives energy to enzymes and all living things. In addition, this force can be captured as free energy with crystals. The DNA molecules are crystals that capture this free energy and convert it to life energy. Increasing the magnetic field increases the speed of bioactive reactions in living things. The current of injury produced by the body causes DNA to separate because the ionic hydrogen bonds of DNA molecules can be cancelled out by a negative magnetic field produced by the body. Indeed, this is the only force capable of initiating DNA separation so the replication, through chemical action, can take place. That is why the defective gene theory as the cause of out-of-control replication, or cancer, is totally invalid.

In the book, *Cancer, The Magnetic/Oxygen Answer* by William H. Philpott, M.D., we find a clear explanation for the effect of magnetism on DNA and the concept of positive and negative magnetic fields (Page 1)

> The static magnetic field from a permanent magnet is an energy field by virtue of the movement of electrons in the field. A negative field spins electrons counterclockwise while a positive magnetic field spins electrons clockwise. A magnetometer is a scientific instrument used to identify poles of a permanent static field D.C. magnet. A magnetometer is also equally used to identify the positive and negative poles of an electric current by identifying the positive and negative magnetic fields produced by the electric current. It has been recommended hat the electric pole definition of positive and negative be used rather than the traditional north-seeking and south-seeking magnetic polarities. Since the human electromagnetism functions as an electric circuit of the central-peripheral nervous system and a static magnet fields in DNA, it is especially useful to use the electric polarity definition of positive [+] for electric and [+qM] for magnetic and [-] for electric and [-qM] for magnetic when applying magnetic fields to humans which thus avoids a necessary translation of polarity terms....

This energy can also be used to help cure cancer or speed healing. In the book *Discovery of Magnetic Health*, by George Washins we read (Page 196):

> For over 18 years, Davis and Rawls experimented with the effects of magnetic fields on the development of tumors and cancers. This mainly involved the transplanting of cancerous tumors into healthy rats, rabbits, mice, and other animals. Results showed that when the north (scientific negative) pole was applied, the pathological conditions improved and development of tumors and cancers slowed down or were stopped in over 90 percent of the cases, depending on the stage of the disease and age and physical condition of the animal. When the south (scientific positive) was applied, the invariable result was an aggravation of the pathological condition and a more rapid development of the tumors.

> Concerning injuries, in every case where internal repair is occurring, whether animal, or human, an increase in negative bioelectric potential takes place on the external surface of the affected region. Upon recovery, the negative potential drops and returns to normal.

There are numerous sources of information supporting the need for greater use of electromedicine. The following quotation from Davis and Rawls, *Magnetism and its Effect on Living Things*, helps explain why low voltage currents from zappers are so effective for improving health (Page 90):

THE AMINO ACIDS AND
RESULTANT PROTEIN DEVELOPMENT

> Taking a sample of any of the many types of amino acids — the basic building block of the protein structure—and exposing them to the S pole energies of a biomagnet, can and will inspire a higher degree of energy and development resulting in a higher valued substance. These facts were discovered in the research towards the arrest of cancers by dual and separate magnetic pole field effects.

> Everything that can be done with the positive S pole energies of a magnet to inspire strength and biological development can, to a large degree, be reversed with the N pole energies. This was discovered after hundreds of exposures of these energies to the living systems, organs, or segments, as each responded in the same manner.

The facts, as they now present themselves, are that when we use the N pole negative energies we do not stop the production or development of life systems, instead we simply arrest their actions or developments without the use of toxins or poisons to obtain this effect. This provides us with a better approach to disease arrest, as in the case of cancer treatment.

The important point in the above reference, from a scientific point of view, is that an energy field arrests the action of bacterial and fungal life systems. That is exactly what a zapper does. The zapper produces a small but effective positive offset square wave. The positive field arrests the enzymes produced by fungi and parasites. The zapper eliminates microbial polymerase growth hormone to arrest the growth of cancer cells. It also kills the microbes. This is the scientific basis for magnets and biomagnet devices in healthcare.

It is also possible that some local areas of the planet, such as where your home or subdivision is built, has a higher than average negative or positive field. Regions of high cancer incidence can be explained as geophysical anomalies in the magnetic fields of the planet.

Because of the extensive difference in the frequencies of human cells and microbes, we can safely zap or magnetically degrade microbes and their enzymes without danger to human cells. The special positive offset square wave of a zapper designed by Dr. Clark interferes with the normal alternating current through magnetic resonance of microbial cells and enzymes, rendering them ineffective. This is why we are now seeing more and more cancer patients recover from cancer based on Dr. Clark's cleansing protocol. The zapper is scientifically sound and proven safe and effective. Unfortunately, we may never see it supported by the existing cancer service industry because of the suppression of non-drug therapies.

In the human body, the lymphatic system is an electromagnetic vibrational fluid that gives the body a unified vibrational field. The trace minerals called electrolytes in the extracellular liquids are vital for the functions of vibration and cellular communication. Similarly, the electrolytes inside the protoplasm of cells resonate to the vibrational frequency of the lymphatic fluids. The secret of life lies in the vibrational frequency of the cells and the electrical conductivity of the lymphatic system and cell membranes. Essential trace minerals, essential amino acids, and essential fatty acids are essential for this very reason. However, oxygen is the key to understanding why these nutrients are essential. Oxygen requires an alkaline environment in order to function. An acid environment, produced by fungi and bacteria, or faulty nutrition, results in oxygen depletion. Lack of oxygen results in loss of aerobic metabolism and cellular energy. Fermentation of excess sugar in the lymphatic system leads to loss of oxygen in the cells.

Philpott goes on to say (Page 2).

It has been observed that the negative field is alkalinizing which supports the presence of oxygen and the positive magnetic field is acidifying which produces an oxygen deficit. In fact, all acidic states produce an oxygen deficit.

Philpott's book is must reading for anyone interested in this subject. He goes on to explain how Alzheimer's disease and diabetes (both types) are microbial diseases. He also states that infections cause autoimmune reactions. He writes (Page 6).

Infections are acidifying, produce numerous acid toxins, evoke immunologic reactions, and precipitates autoimmune reactions, Infections may be bacterial, viral, fungal or intestinal parasites. Focal infections are important sources of rheumatoid diseases.

Philpott supports the statement that growth and spread of cancer follows from fermentation of blood sugars trapped in storage vessels and ducts. Fermentation increases acidity, and decreases oxygen levels in adjacent cells. He also supports the concept that increasing oxygen levels in the body cures cancer by oxidizing the available acids. Alkaline minerals such as calcium are also essential for curing cancer for this very reason.

Hulda Clark's design for a hand-held zapper destroys microbes not only by electrocuting them but also by disturbing their metabolic enzymes. The voltage is that from one-half of a nine-volt battery. The current level is too weak to damage human cells.

We tested oxygen levels in the body before and after using a zapper. Invariably, the oxygen levels shot up from three to five percent with just a few minutes of zapping. The increased energy field supports an increase in oxygen. We also theorize that red blood cells that sometimes clump together in rolls are caused to separate by zapping. With more red blood cells free to absorb oxygen from the lungs, more oxygen can be absorbed and transported throughout the body.

A similar system to Clark's zapper can be found in retired physicist Bob Beck's wrist-band zapper. This device destroys parasites in the blood stream as blood flows past the wrists, but uses a higher voltage. Bones in the wrist force blood to flow near the surface where the zapping process can proceed without removing blood from the body. Simply attaching bands around the wrists allows for zapping. Any point in our body where we can feel our pulse provides a suitable location to electrocute microorganisms in flowing arterial blood. Beck's invention is a modifications of the suppressed U.S. medical patent number 5,188,738 which takes blood out of the body, electrocutes the microbes, and returns the blood to the veins. Using either method, cancer and AIDS can be cured and all viruses in the blood destroyed. No side effects are experienced and no drugs are consumed.

That's the problem. No drugs are consumed. Zappers give individuals the power to look after their own health and control microbial infections using nine-volt batteries instead of medical intervention and drugs. The cost of health care can be reduced to the cost of recharging batteries or of replacing them from time to time.

The whole problem of contaminated blood from blood donors could be solved if donated blood were purified electronically before storage. More significant is the fact that blood donors are getting hard to find due to the qualification program. If patent 5,188,738 were used for sterilizing blood as it is collected, all donated blood would be safe to use. All microbial life forms and stages in blood can be destroyed before storage, or later in storage.

Reducing infection without antibiotics

I had an experience that convinces me that microbial infection caught in the early stages can be killed electronically, at home, without antibiotics. At a New Year's Eve dinner, a piece of lobster shell (or something in the food) cut into my lower right jaw just below the tooth line. (I don't know how this happened as I normally don't chew the shells.) Infection occurred during the night and by morning, my jaw was too swollen for me to eat toast. I immediately applied a zapper (as designed by Dr. Hulda Clark) to the jaw, on and off for about three hours. By noon, the swelling was down and the pain had ceased. By evening, I was able to eat normally with only a slight reminder of the swelling. Next day there was no sign of the infection.

Similarly, a friend broke a tooth on a Friday afternoon and was in considerable pain that evening. He applied the zapper against the broken tooth area and the pain disappeared. Pain, in this case, was probably caused by a lack of electrical energy due to the break in the tooth. In any case, he enjoyed a pain-free weekend thanks to the zapper.

In my opinion, every home should have a zapper in the first aid kit, and every emergency waiting room should have zappers available for people to use as they wait for medical treatment. Schools should have zappers available for student use to prevent infections from minor injuries..

In some cases, zappers appear to be effective against viral infections, colds and the flu, but not in all cases. Catching them early appears to be important. Others report tremendous benefits over mental illness and chronic fatigue, but others do not experience the same benefits. Perhaps, more research is needed in finding the correct frequency or length of program to overcome established infections. We could be doing so much more to treat injuries, reduce pain, and save on medical costs than we are doing now. Starting to treat disease electronically through the arterial and lymphatic system should be the major focus of a new vision in health care.

Incidentally, you can build your own zapper from parts available at Radio Shack by following the diagrams in Dr. Clark's books. However, it is much better to purchase one ready made with extra features and a printed circuit. Look for ads in alternative health magazines.

Homeopathic remedies are based on vibrational energies

Homeopathic medicine contains vibrational energy and supports health by providing the vibrational frequency required by certain cells and organs. Mainstream medicine scoffs at homeopathic medicine because it cannot measure any chemicals in it. The fact that animals benefit from homeopathic medicine shows that homeopathy is not simply the power of suggestion at work.

Homeopathy is based on a concept that like begets like. A resonating solution ingested into the body will cause other liquids to resonate accordingly. You don't have to measure chemicals in a homeopathic remedy because the value is in a vibrational frequency that stimulates the body. If you just consider for a moment that all life functions are controlled by enzymes, and enzymes consist of paramagnetic vibrational fields, you have a simple explanation for the reason why homeopathic remedies work. Like begets like. A frequency in one substance creates the same frequency in another substance. Trace minerals in homeopathic form can be very effective. Vibrational medicine can work to destroy microbial enzymes or to support and increase the production and strength of human enzymes. We control health by controlling enzymes. We can control unwanted enzymes by disrupting their vibrational frequency. We increase good enzymes by applying the negative field of a magnet or consuming appropriate supplements.

Energy testing for diagnosis of disease conditions is possible

Most alternative health care specialists rely on measuring subtle vibrational energy levels in their patients. Some use electro-dermal screening devices, others use muscle testing, and so on. If a food supplement is desired by the body, there is a positive response to it by the body, and conversely, if the item is toxic to the body there will be a strong negative response to it. Electro-dermal devices test the energy levels in the skin or epidermis. There is no doubt that subtle changes in vibrational frequencies can be made through changes in our environment and nutrition.

Mainstream medicine scoffs at energy testing describing it as unscientific. One of the charges placed against Dr. Krop of Toronto by the Ontario Medical Association stems from the use of equipment for energy testing. The fact that it works for the immediate benefit of the patient without any possible injury to the patient has no bearing on the issue. The enforcement of accepted medical procedure on all doctors keeps mainstream medicine in the dark ages and wastes billions of tax dollars through lack of advancement in medicine.

In contrast to our country's restricted medical view, some countries are now opening their doors to electro-medicine. Look at the following newspaper heading from the Sarasota ECO report (Dec. 97), describing a cancer treatment now available in the Dominican Republic.

> **Cancer cells can be precisely targeted and destroyed by physicians using pulsed magnetic fields at this innovative cancer center in the Dominican Republic.**

What is probably the most valuable but suppressed cancer cure available in the world today utilizes the electrical difference of cancer cells to identify them, and a similar frequency to destroy them. This method uses totally safe and non-invasive magnetic frequency. This is available in Dominican Republic (operated by American medical doctors Armstrong and Reynolds since 1996) at the Center for Cell Specific Cancer Therapy in Santa Domingo.

If all Canadian cancer hospitals had a pulsed magnetic field generator to destroy cancer cells, we could save billions on conventional therapy. No chemotherapy drugs would be needed, no radiation, and few, if any operations.

Why is progress held back and innovation rejected? Who makes these decisions? Is it a committee or an individual? In every organization, if you go far enough, you reach the top person. How can he or she be held accountable for not adopting effective cancer cures? How can suppression of cancer cures be stopped?

13. Summary of the cancer process

Let's summarize the conditions required for microbes to initiate cancer and for cancer to spread in our bodies. Some of the material in this summary will be discussed more fully in the chapters that follow. This summary will help you connect the previous chapters with new information about conditions leading to the spread of cancer.

The scientific basis for cancer lies within the primitive genetic structure of human cells. Scientists believe mammals descended from earlier life forms because about 45 per cent of the mammalian genetic structure can be found in earlier life forms. That is why we have interchangeable microscopic parts and why DNA polymerase enzymes from bacteria will assist replication of human DNA in epithelial cells. All human tumor-producing cancers occur in epithelial cells and membranes because these cells are the only ones with cell-wall traits shared by microbial single-celled life forms.

Microbial cell wall material is referred to as chitin. Human finger nails and cuticles are forms of chitin. It is very likely that human cells have dormant DNA to produce chitin. These may become expressed in cancer cells through the process of dedifferentiation.

Mammalian cells have the unique capacity to produce energy by metabolism of food nutrients using oxygen, if available, or by fermentation of food nutrients if oxygen is not available. The dual capacity has been inherited and is perfectly normal.

Descendants of ancient living things that do not have the genetic capacity for the oxidative process survive as parasites in living things that do have this capability. These parasites have evolved the capacity to produce enzymes to exclude oxygen from their immediate environment and to create low-oxygen microspheres. They have also evolved the capacity to disrupt the citric acid cycle and to prevent the oxidation of food nutrients they desire for metabolism.

Larger parasites that infect humankind such as flukes and worms are also hosts to these anaerobic microbes. Two significant events occur when large parasites damage epithelial tissue between areas where blood flows near storage vessels or ducts. Fermentation starts if blood flows into a storage vessel or duct where it is trapped. Injury caused by parasites, host to fungi and bacteria, result in infectious tissue at the location of the injury. Trapped blood starts to ferment and supports fungal growth that leads to cancer.

In addition, the body's natural defense mechanism to heal an injury goes into action. A current of injury develops around the damaged tissue and cells start to replicate in order to repair the damage. The fermenting blood glucose provides necessary pentose phosphate and other growth factors to support replication of the stable DNA molecules.

Cancer spreads by modifying the environment of adjacent cells. Infection spreads after the cellular environment of adjacent cells is modified to support the fungal process of fermentation. Cancer initiates after cell-wall injury occurs due to parasitic and microbial infection and the body's attempt to repair the injury.

Proteins produced by fermentation disrupt the citric acid cycle, reducing production of ATP. Cells lose the energy vital to defend themselves against microbes and cells become infected. Infection leads to microbes taking over metabolic processes within the cell and control of replication. Consequently, cancer spreads to other cells and areas.

The lymphatic system provides the nourishment for fungal/yeast fermentation and an easy method to invade surrounding human cells. Mycelia develop and grow into and along the lymphatic system and invade membrane epithelial tissue as toxins create an ever-expanding oxygen-free microsphere. The result is a cancer tumor.

Keeping the lymphatic fluids clear of trapped blood proteins through exercise and nutrition is one of the primary cures for cancer. Keeping the body free of large parasites and flukes is obviously the most critical issue. Taking immediate care of injuries that do not heal is a close second. To prevent cancer we must prevent infection of internal blood clots and trapped blood sugars.

If the true cause of cancer were being taught to the public by our health protection branch, we could have a healthier and more productive society. We could improve quality of life, increase productivity, and GNP, and could reduce taxes. Among other things, tax revenues could be used for building universities and developing skilled youth to maintain a competitive edge in the world economy.

I think this is worth fighting for. What about you?

14. Cure cancer by eliminating toxic ammonia

I mentioned in the introduction that I began my search for the cause of cancer after watching my brother die from this horrible disease. When I last saw him alive he was connected to an oxygen tank, weighed less than 70 pounds, and was no more than skin and bones. What happened to all the protein that had formerly made up about one 100 additional pounds of tissue? How is living flesh metabolized during the cancer process?

Cancer tumors consume blood proteins, release ammonia

In Guyton's *Textbook of Medical Physiology* (Page 864), we can find the following reference to cancer cells consuming protein:

> For instance, if any particular tissue loses proteins, it can synthesize new proteins from the amino acids of the blood; in turn, these are replenished by degradation of protein from other cells of the body. These effects are particularly noticeable in relation to protein synthesis in cancer cells. **Cancer cells are prolific users of amino acids, and simultaneously, the proteins of other tissues become markedly depleted.**

The text doesn't say why cancer cells are prolific users of amino acids. They just are, and this reference explains why cancer victims lose protein tissue throughout the body although their cancer is highly localized.

How is the process of amino acid catabolism controlled by microbes?

In order to understand how non-invasive cancer cells consume protein, I reviewed several medical textbooks looking for answers to two questions.

1. How is the more powerful oxidative process shut down in favor of the weaker fermentation process so that cancer can spread?

2. How do cancer cells switch from metabolizing glycogen, a sugar, to metabolizing protein?

What I found in this research suggests there is a simple way to cure cancer with two amino acids that protect the cells from ammonia toxicity. Ammonia production explains how microbes shut down the citric acid cycle and production of ATP.

In *Harper's Review of Biochemistry* (Page 273), we learn that ammonia can deplete or reverse an essential enzyme required in the citric acid cycle.

Ammonia is toxic to the central nervous system by mechanisms that are not fully understood but likely involve the reversal of the glutamate dehydrogenase pathway and the consequent depletion of a-ketoglutarate, a necessary intermediate in the citric acid cycle.

This enzyme is a carrier or substrate for hydrogen. Ammonia depletes supplies of the essential enzyme a-ketoglutarate because ammonia (NH3) can supply large quantities of hydrogen. The citric acid cycle cannot proceed without this enzyme.

The second significant reference points out that metabolism of protein in the citric acid or Krebs cycle requires removal of nitrogen from the protein molecule, producing more ammonia and a carbohydrate base. This reference can be found in *Human Physiology*, by E. B. Mason (Page 444):

Amino acids can lose their nitrogen-containing amino groups and be converted to a-keto acids that can enter the Krebs cycle with the resultant production of ammonia.

The important point in this reference is that the process of protein metabolism produces more ammonia creating a chain reaction.

In *Harper's Review of Biochemistry*, Chapter 21, (Page 275), *Catabolism of Amino Acid Nitrogen* we learn that ammonia is catalyzed by the active and important enzyme *l-glutamate dehydrogenase*.

The amino groups of most amino acids ultimately are transferred to α-ketoglutarate by transamination, forming l-glutamate. Release of this nitrogen as ammonia is catalyzed by l-glutamate dehydrogenase, an enzyme of high activity widely distributed in mammalian tissue.

Transamination is a process in which amino acid molecules are switched with carbohydrate molecules in a process for breaking down proteins.

Here is the information I was looking for, because it explains how ammonia disrupts the metabolic process for normal human cells to utilize proteins. The essential enzyme *l-glutamate dehydrogenase* is depleted by ammonia toxicity

Ammonia produced by microbes stops the oxidative process and allows microbes to take over control of metabolism of amino acids. The resultant metabolism produces more ammonia for the spread of cancer. Fermentation of proteins, with the progressive breakdown of carbohydrates in protein, accounts for the spread of anaerobic life forms.

In the early stages of cancer growth, if cells are replicating due to natural growth, as in children, or due to the repair of injury as in adults, ammonia toxicity from fermentation of trapped blood sugars and proteins allows for microbes to take control of cellular metabolism in adjacent cells. After stopping the citric acid cycle, even if oxygen is available, the metabolic process is shut down by the '*the reversal of the glutamate dehydrogenase pathway and the consequent depletion of a-ketoglutarate.*'

Confirmation of the above process can be found in Dr. Guyton's *Textbook of Medical Physiology.* In describing the citric acid cycle, he writes (Page 843. Italics added):

As noted in several points in this discussion, hydrogen atoms are released during different chemical reactions – 4 hydrogen atoms during glycolysis, 4 during the formation of acetyl Co-A from pyruvic acid, and 16 in the citric acid cycle; this makes a total of 24 hydrogen atoms. However, the hydrogen atoms are not simply turned loose in the intracellular fluid. Instead, they are released in packets of two, *and in each instance the release is catalyzed by a specific protein enzyme called a dehydrogenase.* Twenty of the 24 hydrogen atoms immediately combine with nicotinamide adenine dinucleotide (NAD+), a derivative of the vitamin niacin. ...

This reaction will not occur without the initial intermediation of the dehydrogenase nor without the availability of (NAD+) to act as a hydrogen carrier. Both the free hydrogen bound with NAD+ subsequently enter into the oxidative chemical reactions that form tremendous quantities of ATP, as will be discussed later.

Saying that the citric acid cycle cannot function without the dehydrogenase and saying that ammonia eliminates dehydrogenase

confirms that ammonia toxicity shuts down the citric acid cycle. The fermentation of glycogen follows from ammonia toxicity in cells. Ammonia toxicity and the resultant fermentation leads to cancer and supports the spread of cancer.

I have not found any books or articles associating ammonia directly with the cause or spread of cancer. In my search for information, I checked my medical textbooks. I could not find anything on 'ammonia toxicity' in the indexes. I also checked the product safety data information available on the Internet. Ammonia is listed, but the only information on ammonia as a cause of cancer is that ammonia has never been tested as a carcinogen. Is this part of the *misinformation* package by the cancer establishment or has it just been overlooked?

Ammonia toxicity should be classified as the leading secondary cause of cancer because it stops production of ATP, shuts down the immune system, and allows microbes to proliferate freely. Ammonia toxicity is actually the cause of several so-called autoimmune diseases related to nerves. It is also significant that parasites and cancer tumors produce ammonia. Let's take a closer look at the effects of ammonia toxicity in the body.

Structure of ammonia is closely similar to water

Ammonia is a common gas (formula NH_3) with one nitrogen atom combined with three hydrogen atoms. Ammonia dissolves readily in water to form ammonium (NH_4).

In *Harper's Review of Biochemistry*, Chapter 2, *WATER*, we find a comparison of the water molecule to ammonia. The two are very similar being described as irregular tetrahedrons (*pyramid shaped*) with dipole features (positive and negative charges with opposite polarity separated by a distance).

Isaac Asimov gives a simple explanation of the dipole nature of water in *Asimov's New Guide to Science* (Page 519):

Hence, the oxygen atom, by virtue of its excessive portion of electrons, has a slight excess of negative charge. By the same token, the hydrogen atom, suffering from an electron deficiency, has a slight excess of positive charge. A molecule containing an oxygen-hydrogen pair, such as water or ethyl alcohol, possesses a small concentration of negative charge in one part of the molecule and a small concentration of positive charge in another. It possesses two poles of charge, so to speak, and is called a polar molecule.

This structure explains why water is the universal solvent and is an active participant in many biochemical reactions, and why water often determines the properties of those reactions. The magnetic dipole feature, positive (south seeking) at one point and negative (north seeking) at the other provides for its chemical and biological versatility. Water can combine with either acid or alkaline substances because it has a positive and negative pole. Like a magnet, one pole or the other will be attracted to any chemical with polarity or an unstable molecule.

Ammonia has the same physical structure and chemical versatility as water but is more reactive. In ammonia gas (CH_3), one of the carbon-to-hydrogen bonds is an unstable double bond and the molecule will accept another hydrogen atom to become the more stable liquid ammonium (CH_4). It is this unstable molecule in ammonia that enables ammonia to take hydrogen from living nerve tissue and disrupt enzyme function.

That's why ammonium is used in so many household cleansers and formulations and why it is so toxic to humans. Ammonia cannot be allowed to accumulate in living tissue because it disrupts enzymes and attacks nerves by displacing water. Ammonia virtually destroys life, although it is a byproduct of life. Fish excrete ammonia through their gills. If ammonia levels rise too high in fish-tank water, fish die from ammonia poisoning. Bubbling air (oxygen) or ozone through the water reduces ammonia levels.

People with cancer symptoms often show symptoms of ammonia poisoning, such as being easily confused and lethargic. The concept that excess ammonia leads to reduced production of ATP has also been established as a cause for mental fatigue. In an Internet report on *Metabolism, Protein and Nitrogen Homeostasis*, we find the following data:

> One common metabolite of nitrogen that is formed from many nitrogen-containing compounds, and is used as a source of nitrogen for biosynthesis, is ammonia. High levels of ammonia, however, are quite toxic. The brain appears to be the organ that is sensitive to high levels of ammonia.
>
> In the presence of high levels of ammonia, the equilibrium for the glutamate dehydrogenase reaction lies in favor of glutamate, which will then lead to the formation of glutamine. **Both of these reactions diminish the level of the Krebs' cycle intermediates and *oxaloacetate* is not regenerated. The brain becomes deprived of its source of ATP, leading to symptoms of ammonia toxicity.**

A further complication is that both glutamine and asparate, which can be readily formed from glutamate, have neurotransmitter functions.

Oxaloacetate is another essential enzyme in the citric acid cycle. In the brain, the energy production cycle is shut down by ammonia disrupting another enzyme critical for producing energy in brain tissue. Mental fatigue can be the result of ammonia toxicity. In addition, as we shall see later, ammonia appears to have an important part in the process of brain dysfunction known as Alzheimer's.

Without the essential regeneration of the oxaloacetate enzyme in the brain, the citric acid cycle and production of ATP is stopped. Obviously, the same principle applies to other cells as the citric acid cycle is shared by all cells. The resulting lack of ATP explains why the immune system fails to defend against further invasion and replication of microbes. Ammonia toxicity can cause numerous diseases.

Ammonia is produced naturally in the body by cells during the metabolism of protein, but this ammonia is safely catalyzed into other products. Ammonia is also produced in the kidneys to counter high acidic levels in the blood and urine. This form of ammonia is considered as "physiological ammonia" and is considered useful to the body. Excess ammonia produced by other means is toxic to the body.

The immune system function within a cell is limited to its ability to assemble defensive enzymes. ATP is the first requirement. In addition, minerals are required for the production of enzymes. Selenium, for example, is required for production of Glutathione peroxidase that serves as an antibiotic to destroy invaders.

Without adequate ATP and minerals to assemble defensive enzymes and chemically break down the viral DNA, microbes, and related microbial enzymes, human cells cannot defeat microbial infection. Without adequate ATP, the cell's immune system simply shuts down. A cell without ATP is like a motor without gas! Human cells cannot produce the enzymes required to destroy microbial enzymes produced by cellular parasites. Microbes are free to carry on with their life processes, including rapid replication and mutation of normal human cells during the replication process.

Dr. Clark advises her cancer patients to consume a minimum of 4,000 calories of food nutrients per day in order to supply the nutrition required to build new cells and repair old ones, as well as to help destroy microbes and microbial enzymes. These nutrients must also be consumed from a select group of easy-to-digest, malonic acid-free products. Fresh and raw vegetables, boiled dairy products, and other plant-derived foods are listed in her books. In her latest book, *The Cure for All Advanced Cancers*, she outlines a 21-day metabolic feast that includes over 50 valuable cancer-curing nutrients. Several of these are directly related to eliminating ammonia toxicity. Others serve to increase oxidation and respiration at the cellular level.

Numerous authors advise cancer patients to take enzymes that increase oxidation and respiration of cells, because all cancer cells are lacking in respiration capacity. By increasing respiration, you slow the spread of cancer. Ozone, hydrogen peroxide (35% food grade), and numerous oxygen supplements are recommended in alternative therapy books. Trace minerals and digestive enzymes for food metabolism should also be used.

As a cost saving move, many hospitals have now switched over to fast-food providers to feed their patients, or meals are prepared at privately owned commercial facilities, frozen, and delivered to hospitals hundreds of miles away. Meals are simply reheated for serving. Money is saved by reducing kitchen staff. However, fresh and raw enzyme-filled nutrients are destroyed in the process.

Considering the billions of dollars we spend on health care, saving money on hospital meals is not wise. Hospital patients need better-than-average food intake with mineral supplements. Hospital patients should have a mineral analysis and be fed as well as possible according to their mineral and vitamin deficiencies. Why is this vital and cost-saving method neglected? Who benefits by the process? It is certainly not the patient. In the end, it costs more, not less, because the functional cause of illness is not addressed.

Immune system dysfunction is a metabolic disorder

Let's look at common knowledge about how the immune system functions or fails to function. Have you ever read books or have you been taught that the immune system requires ATP and the ability to produce defensive **enzymes to destroy infections inside cells?** I don't recall learning the names of any defensive enzymes.

Lloyd Motz's book *The Universe, Its Beginning and End, Chapter 10, The Origin and Nature of Life* discusses the immune system function to fight viral infection within the cell as based on enzymes and ATP. I am repeating this reference in order to discuss the issue of immune system function (Page 257):

At this point, the intruding DNA of the virus is attacked by the natural immunological defenses of the cell, which in most cases destroy the foreign DNA. But if these cell defenses are not strong enough to devour the injected DNA molecules, these molecules, using their own genetic code, induce the cell to manufacture new viruses from its own nucleotides and amino acids, and within 10 minutes of the intrusion, new empty protein virus coats are formed inside the cell.

"If these cell defenses are not strong enough" is a vital point that has been missed by books on the immune system written for the public. These books tell us about defensive cells but very little is said about defensive enzymes as suggested by Motz in the above quotation. By putting more emphasis on the study of the enzyme portion of the immune system within a cell, we could focus on supporting the immune system better. These enzymes are mineral dependent, and this dependency connects the cancer process to mineral deficiencies.

A good example of this problem is found in the book *The Immune System Handbook* by Charlene A Day. In a chart labeled *Cells of the Immune System,* we learn a great deal about immune-system cells. These cells are produced within bone marrow and distributed through the arterial and lymphatic system as cells, not enzymes. In a second chapter, we learn about the bad guys being all the known viral, microbial and parasitic life forms that the body identifies as non-self and destroys. All these cells have names, but there is no mention of the critical enzymes produced in cells to defend them from invading enzymes. The information is well presented and easy to understand, but it lacks detail about enzymes.

Diseases such as cancer should be considered as continuous biochemical reactions controlled by microbial enzymes. Cancer is cured through the immune system by interrupting the function and production of microbial enzymes causing out-of-control replication and mutation of cells.

It follows that preventing and curing cancer requires elimination of ammonia toxicity in order to revive the citric acid-cycle and production of ATP. Control of ammonia is accomplished through control of the urea cycle that is required to convert ammonia to urea. Cleansing the kidneys and liver are significant steps in the control of ammonia. Again, it all depends on the availability of minerals and enzymes.

The importance of a balanced diet with adequate proteins and minerals cannot be overlooked. In *Harper's Review of Biochemistry* we learn (Page 265):

There are, for practical purposes, 20 amino acids present in mammalian proteins. If, during protein synthesis, a single one of these amino acids is missing, protein synthesis ceases. Since continual synthesis and degradation of proteins, (protein turnover) is characteristic of all forms of life, the availability of α-amino acids in for example, humans must reflect their distribution in human proteins. If not, protein synthesis becomes nutrient-restricted.

In Canada, all of these vital amino acid food supplements are restricted from sale to the public. Canadians may import them for personal use (which indicates their relative safety) but not for resale. In the cancer process, two vital amino acids, arginine and ornithine, if restricted, lead to an incapacity to convert ammonia to urea. In Canada, regulations enforced by the Health Protection Branch actually promote cancer.

Metabolic disorders of the urea cycle lead to cancer

In *Harper's Review of Biochemistry* (Pages 279-281), we learn about the significance of urea synthesis.

A moderately active man consuming about 300 grams of carbohydrate, 100 grams of fat, and 100 grams of protein must excrete about 16.5 grams of nitrogen daily. Ninety-five per cent is eliminated by the kidneys and the remaining 5% in the feces. The major pathway of nitrogen excretion in humans is urea synthesized in the liver, released into the blood, and cleared by the kidney.

...Note that urea formation is a cyclic process. The ornithine used in reaction 2 is regenerated in reaction 5. There is thus no net loss or gain of ornithine, citruilline, argininoscuccinte, or arginine during urea synthesis; however, ammonium ion, CO_2, ATP and aspartate are consumed.

Note that aspartate is consumed. How can it be replaced through supplements since amino supplements are illegal?

The text explains there are five enzyme-controlled steps in the cycle used by the body to remove excess ammonia. All five steps can be disrupted by a nutritional deficiency of enzymes, or by a deficiency of the amino acids ornithine and arginine or aspartate. Since aspartate is consumed, the loss of this amino acid results in loss of capacity to eliminate ammonia. The text goes on with even more vital information:

Metabolic disorders associated with deficiency of the five enzymes of hepatic urea syntheses are known. The rate-limiting reactions of urea synthesis appear to be catalyzed by carbamoyl phosphate synthase, *(reaction 1)*, Ornithine transcarbamoylase, *(reaction2)*, and arginase *(reaction 5)*.

Since the urea cycle converts ammonia to the non-toxic compound urea, all disorders of urea synthesis cause ammonia intoxication.

This intoxication is more severe when the metabolic block occurs in reactions 1 or 2, since some covalent linking of ammonia to carbon has already occurred if citrulline can be synthesized. Clinical symptoms common to all urea cycle disorders include vomiting in infancy, avoidance of high-protein foods, intermittent ataxia (incoordination and clumsiness), irritability, lethargy, and mental retardation.

The large intestine is a source of considerable quantities of ammonia, presumably as a product of the putrefactive activity of nitrogenous substrates (i.e. red meat) by the intestinal bacteria. This ammonia is absorbed into portal circulation, but under normal conditions, it is rapidly removed from the blood by the liver. In liver disease, this function of the liver may be impaired, in which case the concentration of ammonia in the peripheral blood will rise to toxic levels. It is believed that ammonia toxification may play a role in the genesis of hepatic coma in some patients.

The liver consists of 'hepatic cellular plates' hence the name of diseases related to the liver are characterized as "hepatic" conditions. An 'hepatic coma' is caused by ammonia toxicity produced by intestinal bacteria from dietary protein, and from urea present in liquids secreted into the intestinal tract. This ammonia absorbed directly into the portal vein and portal venous blood flows into the hepatic vein that carries blood to the liver. Ammonia toxicity can lead directly to a hepatic coma or loss of consciousness due to toxins in the blood.

Hepatic comas and cancer are associated with impairment of the liver because a toxic liver cannot break down ammonia fast enough to prevent ammonia toxicity. Cancer is also associated with impaired kidney function. In *Harper's Review of Biology*, we read how kidney disease excretes excessive amounts of arginine and ornithine essential for converting ammonia to urea. On page 304 we read:

Sulfur-containing Amino Acids.

Cystinuria: in this inherited metabolic disease, urinary excretion of cystine is 20-30 times normal. Execration of lysine, arginine, and ornithine is also markedly increased. Cystinuria is considered due to a renal transport defect.

Although cystinuria is considered an inherited metabolic disease, it is also possible that microbial toxins cause the renal problem. Kidney failure can result in toxic overloads of homocysteine as well as depletion of essential amino acids such as lysine, arginine and ornithine. Homocysteine, as we shall see later, is the major cause of heart failure.

When I studied the work of Rene Caisse and the treatment of cancer patients, I learned that Caisse also used several herbs for a kidney stimulant. Without knowing why, we made up this formula to go along with our essiac.

Similarly, Dr. Clark recommends the use of a six week kidney cleanse as part of the cure for cancer. Obviously, if our kidneys are not functioning properly, we are not likely going to cure cancer.

Ammonia toxicity from parasites and tumors

It is generally believed that the body can eliminate ammonia before it reaches a toxic level. However, this is not true if the body is faced with a diet deficient in minerals and essential amino acids. Ammonia toxicity is also increased by high protein diets.

In *Harper's Review of Biochemistry* (Page 276), we have documentation that an impaired liver fails to detoxify ammonia:

With severely impaired hepatic (liver) function or development of collateral communications between the portal and system veins, portal blood may bypass the liver. Ammonia may thus rise to toxic levels in the systemic blood.

Surgically produced shunting procedures are also conducive to ammonia intoxication, particularly after ingestion of protein or after gastrointestinal hemorrhage, which provides *blood proteins to colonic bacteria*.

When you think about it, blood proteins are a potent source of ammonia if fermentation occurs anywhere in the body. In addition, parasitic larvae in the blood stream are a significant source of ammonia toxicity. That's why cancer can start from internal bleeding into ducts and storage vessels, or in cartilage and bone fractures.

Ammonia toxicity from parasitic infection has been recorded in sheep. A report in the *"Online Journal of Veterinary Research"* clearly explodes any myth that the body can handle large volumes of ammonia produced by microbes or cancer tumors in the body. The article is entitled *"Immunosuppression by unionized ammonia in sheep infested by Lucilia cuprina larvae."* In research done on sheep infested with *Lucilia cuprina larvae*, tests show the concentration of ammonia increased many times higher than normal and the levels of zinc and immune system cells decreased significantly. The capacity of the liver to remove ammonia in sheep infected with larvae could not detoxify the ammonia fast enough to stop it from accumulating and causing illness.

Please recall that Dr. Fibiger created cancer in laboratory mice by feeding them cockroaches infected with parasitic larvae from horses. One should note that three immediate cancer concerns arise from the presence of larvae in the blood stream.

1. excessive ammonia

2. depletion of zinc

3. a weakened immune system.

Zinc is one of the essential trace minerals for defensive enzymes. When parasites succeed in leaving the arterial system, they may cause internal bleeding into storage vessels or ducts, and injury to the tissue.

When one does a live blood-cell analysis, one can observe these squirming little parasites swimming in the blood serum. The frequency of observed parasites, yeast and fungus indicates the levels of parasites in the body. When one scans a tiny portion of one drop of blood and sees even one parasite, there are billions in the body. It is not uncommon to see hundreds of parasites in a single drop of blood. A herbal parasite cleanse combined with zapping can eliminate these parasites in a matter of days. Why isn't this process accepted into mainstream medicine?

Farmers recognize the significance of ammonia toxicity in animals, and some purchase products to add to the drinking water of their stock to reduce the effects of ammonia. On the Internet, under H & S Corporation, you can purchase YS-50 "Ammonia and Odor control for Poultry and Animal Use."

Similarly, people who raise fish for pleasure or as a business are instructed how to maintain low ammonia levels in the water. Fish excrete ammonia through the gills. If ammonia levels rise too high, fish die of ammonia toxicity. (See *Ammonia Toxicity* by Randy or Deb Carey at carey/spacestar.net)

Humans, on the other hand, are encouraged to use ammonia-based cleansing products and personal care products. Why are we not fully informed about the dangers of ammonia such as immune system dysfunction and cancer? On the Internet under "Let's Stop Poisoning Our Children," we can find a strong warning about the dangers of household cleansers:

LONG-TERM HEALTH HAZARDS
OF HOUSEHOLD PRODUCTS

Most poisonings happen slowly, over a long period of time, by daily exposure to toxins in the air, and toxic chemicals that come into contact with the skin. Household products are among the most toxic substances that we encounter daily. In one study conducted over a fifteen-year period, women who worked at home had a 54% higher death rate from cancer than women who had jobs away from home. The study concluded that the increased death rate in women was due to the daily exposure to hazardous chemicals found in ordinary household products.

Tobacco companies add ammonia to cigarette tobacco to enhance the flavor. According to the Blue Cross and Blue Shield consumer fraud lawsuit against tobacco companies, "internal documents say ammonia changes the chemistry of smoke, increasing the nicotine to smokers." Is ammonia one of the major reasons why smokers get cancer of the lungs? I believe it is. With all this evidence that ammonia may be related to lung cancer, why hasn't this product been tested as a carcinogen?

In the textbook *Fundamentals of Clinical Chemistry*, *4th* *edition*, by Tietz, we find several pages describing ammonia metabolism, the toxicity of ammonia, and how ammonia levels are measured in the body.

In order to obtain reliable results from measurements for ammonia, the following advice is given (Page 557):

Smoking: by the patient or the phlebotomist *(person who draws blood)* is a source of ammonia contamination in the specimen. The patient must not smoke after midnight before the morning when the fasting blood specimen is to be drawn.

If ammonia contamination of the blood sample can occur from the phlebotomist or by a single cigarette taken several hours earlier, consider how much ammonia contamination we get from second-hand smoke, and how much ammonia a pack-a-day smoker takes into his or her system. Consider the plight of infants strapped in a car seat, with the car filled with smoke. Since women are generally smaller than men are and their lung capacity is also smaller, consider the extra damage that occurs in women smokers. Lung cancer in older women now causes more premature deaths than does breast cancer. Ammonia toxicity is probably the most significant reason for lung cancer in smokers and family members who are exposed to second-hand smoke. Ammonia toxicity shuts down the oxidative process of lung tissue and ammonia accumulates in the lymphatic system.

Also according to *Fundamentals of Clinical Chemistry*, the second most important consideration for accuracy of measurements in testing for blood levels of ammonia relate to the atmosphere:

Laboratory atmosphere is a source of ammonia contamination for the specimen and for the assay method. To minimize contamination of specimens and glassware by ammonia in laboratory atmosphere, the blood collection and subsequent analysis should ideally be done in a special laboratory.

Obviously, ammonia is a very toxic substance and we absorb it from cigarette smoke, the atmosphere, cleaning products, and personal care products. Childhood cancer can be related to ammonia toxicity in the room atmosphere. Has anyone ever bothered to check?

If we look into Judi Vance's book, **Beauty to Die For, the Cosmetic Consequence** (Page 132), we find more about the dangers of ammonia. Ammonia is listed as "carcinogenic, mutagenic, toxic or causes adverse reactions." *Mutagenic* means capable of mutating genetic structures.

Vance goes on to expose the following ammonia compounds used in beauty products and personal care products. *(These few examples have been selected from a long list.)*

1) Ammonium chloride, used in permanent wave solutions.

1) Ammonium cocoylisethionate, used as a surfactant and cleaning agent.

2) Ammonium laureth sulfate, used in hair products and bubble baths. Laureth means it contains ether, a substance that is considered carcinogenic and toxic.

3) Ammonium lauryle sulfate, used mainly in shampoo.

4) Ammonium nitrate, which is a well-known carcinogen.

5) Ammonium thioglycolate, used in permanent wave solutions.

The skin and scalp, with an abundance of hair follicles, can absorb chemicals from our personal care products. Is the development and increase in Alzheimer's directly related to people absorbing ammonia and toxins into their scalp and brain from shampoo, hair coloring, hair rinses and permanents? I haven't seen any documentation, but people who work in hair salons claim hair stylists have a higher-than-average frequency of cancer.

Vance tells us that the large majority of people who experience chronic fatigue are women. Could disruption of the production of ATP in the brain, and hence the mental fatigue, be a direct result of ammonia toxicity, which can be eliminated by changing personal care products?

It would seem wise for cancer patients to avoid all contact with ammonia and second-hand smoke. People with cancer who continue to smoke probably have a subconscious death wish.

Let's look now at how ammonia causes cancer to spread.

How cancer spreads and how to stop it from spreading

In another Internet report, we learn that cancer tumors in the brain excrete ammonia and disrupt the nervous system. This report by William T. Chance, Ph. D., tells us cancer tumors secrete ammonia.

The presence of a growing tumor induces profound behavioral and metabolic alterations in the host, including loss of appetite. These neuro-chemical aberrations appear to be secondary to brain detoxification of **ammonia, which is secreted by the tumor.**

I understand this to mean that the 'brain detoxification of ammonia' is through a process that is under human control. The ammonia is secreted by the cancer tumor is very significant. I was surprised to learn that tumors secrete ammonia. I have never seen this expressed elsewhere.

Mainstream medicine knows that both ammonia and growth hormones are secreted by cancer tumors. That's all that is needed to cause cancer to spread from a cancer tumor to adjacent cells.

In addition, ammonium in the blood stream is released in the lungs as ammonia, enabling cancer to spread to the lungs and other parts of the body. Cancer can also spread to the liver by cancer cells in the blood stream, but oxygen levels must be reduced in order to have anaerobic cancer cells survive. Microbes replicating in tumors create conditions that pollute adjacent cells and cause the spread of cancer. Excess microbial growth hormone and ammonia are not accidental. They are produced by microbes to cause replication of human cells.

We stop cancer from spreading by eliminating toxic ammonia so that the citric acid cycle in adjacent cells is not interrupted. If cells can continue to oxidize nutrients, fermentation cannot occur and the immune system defenses remain strong. Eliminating excess ammonia is a function of the amino acids arginine and aspartate which are required to convert ammonia to urea.

Arginine required to eliminate ammonia as urea

Let's look now at the mechanisms used by the body to eliminate ammonia. The amino acid arginine combines with ammonia to produce urea.

In the text *Foundation of Biology*, by W. D. McElroy and various authors, there is significant chapter entitled *Genes and Enzymes*. Arginine is used as the example to illustrate how cells, through production of enzymes, control the synthesis of arginine in the body. In the first step, carbon dioxide and ammonia are combined to produce glutamic acid. The last three steps of the process result in the conversion of glutamic acid to ornithine; ornithine to citrulline; and citrulline to arginine. *If any of these processes are blocked by lack of an essential enzyme, arginine cannot be produced.*

In the book, *Life Extension* (Page 289), by Durk Pearson and Sandy Shaw, there are numerous references to the importance of arginine supplements. Three-gram and four-gram servings were taken on a daily basis without harm. Servings of L-Dopa, L-ornithine, and L-arginine up to 5 grams daily caused significant release of growth hormones making "a normal 65-year-old's growth-hormone levels resemble those of a young adult or even a teenager." Obviously, the direct consumption of amino acids can have a beneficial effect on health and vitality.

Shortly after *Life Extension* became a best seller in Canada and the USA, the FDA and HPB combined efforts to ban amino acids from the public. The U.S. FDA failed and amino acids are not restricted for sale in USA. However, Canada's "Health" Protection Branch succeeded in regulating these Natural Health Products off the market. There is no valid scientific reason for doing so. We don't hear about any adverse reactions and deaths in occurring in countries where amino acids are still not regulated. In Canada, if anyone makes a drug related claim for a product, the product automatically becomes a drug, by definition of drugs, and therefore, must be controlled as a drug.

Excess sugar consumption leads to ammonia toxicity

When Dr. Fibiger of Denmark first initiated cancer in the laboratory back in 1913, he used mice and cockroaches from a sugar warehouse. This was the only place he could find wild mice with cancer.

In Fibiger's research, eggs from parasitic worms were hatched inside cockroaches, matured into larvae and were eaten by mice. Mice developed stomach cancer from the larvae that may have burrowed into tissue forming the intestinal tract. Their growth would lead to further injury and cause cancer. Since parasitic larvae are growing rapidly, they would also produce large quantities of DNA polymerase.

Cells that lack minerals essential for defensive enzymes cannot destroy invading microbes. Healthy, wild mice, not living on sugar, do not experience cancer due to a stronger immune system. Their bodies do not become mineral deficient due to an excess of other minerals. Wholesome natural plant foods metabolize faster and provide a balanced source of digestible fats and bioactive minerals. The resulting higher oxidative energy and the capacity to destroy microbial enzymes in the cells prevents microbial infection and cancer.

Why did cancer occur only in mineral deficient mice?

High sugar diets with subsequent loss of minerals interfere with the production of enzymes required to assemble arginine. Arginine is required

to convert ammonia to urea for elimination from the body. Arginine is also a major source of an enzyme used in the citric acid cycle. Without arginine, the body suffers ammonia toxicity and depletion of essential enzymes required for maintaining production of ATP.

Sugar depletes our mineral base, destroys essential enzymes, and increases fermentation. Ammonia produced by fermentation reaches toxic levels and disrupts the citric acid cycle. The modern era of disease and the cancer epidemic are a result of commercial processing and marketing of toxic-food items and processed products with long shelf life. Sugar based foods filled with glucose are one of the major problems. Refined fats are another.

Sugar and processed food cause of cancer epidemic

In her book, *Lick the Sugar Habit*, Nancy Appleton tells her readers about the dangers of sugar hidden in our processed foods. Most of us are unaware of how much sugar we consume through processed foods. She writes (Page 9. Italics added):

Glucose, as high in calories as refined sugar, is in effect a predigested food that undergoes no processing at all in the stomach or intestines. Yet there is no law requiring that glucose be listed with other ingredients on the label of any package! **The food industry uses glucose as a cheap filler; since it is not as sweet as sugar and therefore unrecognizable, many people consume large quantities of glucose without realizing it.** If you eat packaged foods such as cereal, bakery goods, sauces, and processed meats, chances are you are getting more sugar than you bargained for—maybe 130 pounds more.

The 130 pounds refers to the average amount of sugar that was being produced annually, per person, in the USA. That's over 10 pounds per month per person, even though many people take very little. Is it any wonder we have a cancer epidemic?

15. Use amino acids to help cure cancer

In this chapter, we will review cases of cancer being cured by increased use of amino acids. Anyone who wants to prevent and cure cancer, and stop it from spreading, must first deal with the problem of ammonia toxicity. Amino acids provide the means by which to eliminate excess ammonia.

In the medical textbook *Harper's Review of Biochemistry* (Page 277), we find medical interest in amino acids to fight cancer because cancer tumors consume essential amino acids.

Asparaginase and glutaminase have both been investigated as antitumor agents, since certain tumors exhibit abnormally high requirements for glutamine and asparagine.

The above quotation from Harper's is significant because it describes another reason why the body lacks arginine and thereby fails to eliminate ammonia. Tumors consume glutamine and asparagine. This explains why the citric-acid cycle is deprived of glutamine essential for enzymes needed to maintain the citric acid cycle. It also explains why the body is depleted of essential asparagine to convert ammonia to urea.

Mainstream medicine has investigated these amino acids as antitumor agents. The fact that they have made a toxic chemotherapy drug called Asparaginase indicates their research was promising.

In *Everyone's Guide to Cancer Therapy* (Page 664), we learn that Asparaginase is one of the chemotherapy drugs used for acute lymphoblastic leukemia and lymphomas. The possible side effects include fever, allergic reaction, neurological problems (seizures, reduced level of consciousness, drowsiness), stroke, liver malfunction, weakness, increased blood sugar, pancreatitis, kidney failure, loss of appetite, nausea, vomiting, abdominal discomfort, sore mouth, and malabsorption. Other than that, there are no undesired side effects!

It would be interesting to know how they discover these side effects. Is it all trial and error with human guinea pigs? How can a natural product have so many toxic side effects? What do they do to it? Why not just use arginine?

It appears that the profit motive, and commercial success of a cancer treatment, is dependent on modifying the product so that it can be patented and controlled. The fact that it works in its natural state does not qualify it for use in treating cancer.

Virtually complete inhibition of cancer with amino acids

In Ralph W. Moss's book *Cancer Therapy, The Independent Consumers Guide*, we find this reference to another effective cure for cancer.

According to Moss, the cure includes the amino acid arginine with acetimide (Page 285). The following information should be classified as incredible but true.

*Arginine also helps detoxify the liver, assists in the release of growth hormones, maintains a healthy immune system, and **detoxifies poisonous ammonia**.*

Feeding a carcinogen to rats caused liver cancer in 50 per cent of the animals after 12 to 15 months.

Giving arginine along with the chemical acetimide led to virtually complete inhibition of the carcinogenic process.

Assuming you had cancer, what would you give for anything that promised *virtually complete inhibition of the carcinogenic process?* Is there any reason to believe the above quotation has any merit? How can such a valuable cancer cure be overlooked by mainstream orthodox medicine as well as the majority of alternative health care specialists?

Perhaps these claims for arginine and acetimide are not true. Why should I believe you? Let's take a closer look.

Arginine and acetimide to cure cancer

While attending a health conference in Los Angeles, I listened to one of the speaker's review the court case of the FDA versus Jimmy Keller. Mr. Keller *(not a doctor)* ran a cancer clinic in Mexico and reportedly had a success rate over 80% with all types of cancer patients. Many of his patients were late-stage desperate cancer victims. The speaker related how one afternoon, two station wagons, one with armed men in brown uniforms drove up to the clinic door. The group in brown uniforms, who appeared to be Mexican customs officials, picked Jimmy Keller up, loaded him into the first station wagon, and drove him to the U.S./Mexican border. At this point, the other group took him off to prison in United States.

According to the speaker, the Cancer Establishment gets angry when medical doctors move to Mexico and set up a clinic to cure cancer. However, they get damn mad when ordinary people do it. Jimmy Keller first learned of tumorex when his cancer was treated by an injection into his tumor and his cancer was cured. After that, he set up a clinic in Mexico to help others.

After being illegally abducted from Mexico, he was tried and sentenced to a U.S. federal prison for 'wire fraud.' One of the charges against him was that he used an unapproved *arginine* preparation called Tumorex. Conditions for his release from prison two years later were that he must not treat people for cancer or talk in public. The speech was given by a friend so as not to break the conditions for his release from prison.

The Jimmy Keller story is truly fascinating. In 1991, The Times Mirror Company of Los Angeles printed a story on Keller. You can read this story on the Internet, under Faith, Hope, and Fraud. Just search under Tumorex.

From the transcript of the court case FDA vs Jimmy Keller we learn: that tumorex was a live-cell polypeptide **smuggled out of West Germany. In fact, it was mainly water and L-Arginine, a common, everyday amino acid.**

The effect of Tumorex injected into a tumor was very dramatic. In the report called *Faith, Hope, and Fraud* about his work, we read (Page 5):

> The instant he gave an injection, people would start feeling heat in their tumors (a thermometer placed on the tumor, Keller said, showed a temperature rise of one to two degrees). There was a pulling, tingling, grabbing sensation. One patient said it felt like a thousand little fingers pulling at her tumors. People with brain tumors heard popping and cracking sounds as if fireworks were going off in their heads. Tumorex didn't always work with everyone, but when it did, Keller said, the results could be spectacular. Within hours, patients reported, tumors began to soften and shrink, and within days, they began to disappear. "On open tumors," Keller said, "you could actually see bubbles."

Isn't that fascinating? How can arginine stop cancer? What is the function of acetimide?

In **Harper's Review of Biochemistry** (Page 66), the text discusses the function of high-energy phosphates as the currency of the cell. Phosphates are stored in arginine.

Another group of compounds, act as storage forms of high-energy phosphates. These include creatine phosphate (phosphagen) occurring in vertebrate muscle and brain, and arginine phosphate, in invertebrate muscle.

Under physiological conditions, phosphagens permit ATP concentrations to be maintained in muscle while ATP is rapidly being utilized as a source of energy for muscular contraction.

Arginine phosphate is a storage form of ATP. It appears that arginine is capable of donating ATP energy directly into the cancer process. ATP could renew the immune system function and disturb the progressive break down of glucose. The production of high-energy phosphate molecules would cease, more ATP would be produced, and cancer replication would stop.

In *Harper's Review of Biochemistry Chapter 22, Catabolism of the Carbon Skeleton of Amino Acids* (Page 284), we have a significant series of diagrams that detail how amino acids are broken down or catabolized. In this diagram, five essential enzymes in the citric acid cycle are shown. These include Citrate, α-Ketoglutarate, Succinyl-CoA, Fumarate, and Oxaloacetate.

Oxaloacetate is required for delivery of oxygen, and is dependent on the amino acid aspartate. Similarly, the essential enzyme α-Ketoglutarate is dependent on the availability of arginine.

In metabolism of the amino acid arginine, nitrogen is first removed from the arginine molecule. Nitrogen combines with ammonia to produce urea and thereby reduces ammonia toxicity. The citric acid cycle and production of ATP for human energy can be revived as soon as the toxic levels of ammonia are reduced. That is where arginine comes in as a cure for cancer.

Arginine cures cancer in a two-step process.

In the first step, nitrogen is removed, combined with ammonia and allows the citric acid cycle to start. In the second step, the balance of the arginine molecule is quickly and easily converted into the essential enzyme αketoglutarate. The text reads as follows:

Note that an early step, frequently the first reaction in amino acid catabolism, involves removal of the αnitrogen… Once removed, the nitrogen enters the general metabolic pool. Depending upon demand, it may then be reutilized for anabolic processes or, if in excess, converted to urea and excreted. The remaining nitrogen-free carbon skeleton is converted to αketoglutarate.

Here's the biological reason why arginine is effective in treating cancer. Nitrogen reduces ammonia toxicity and the remaining portion of the arginine molecule converts to the vital enzyme αketoglutarate to revive the citric acid cycle.

Ammonia toxicity stops the citric acid cycle and arginine revives it. Nitrogen from arginine eliminates excess ammonia and the remaining amino acid skeleton converts to the vital enzyme αketoglutarate. These two steps renew the citric acid process converting lactic acid, a by-product from fermentation, to ATP. Cancer growth stops because the higher energy and temperature levels resulting from oxidation, and lack of fermentation, return the cellular environment to normal. Virtual elimination of the cancer process is possible with this vital amino acid.

After nitrogen is removed, the remaining skeleton from arginine has numerous hydroxyl appendages and would function as an anti-oxidant. Perhaps bubbles on the surface of a tumor and the sensations described above within the tumor arise from the anti-oxidant activity. In addition, a tumor would contain high levels of lactic acid. As soon as the citric acid cycle is restarted, cells within the tumor would produce ATP from the lactic acid reserves. The cancer process will be reversed very quickly.

Here is the chemical pathway taken directly from *Harper's Review of Biochemistry*, a medical university textbook that indirectly outlines the chemistry explaining how the amino acid arginine stops cancer. You can stop cancer if you combine arginine (in sufficient quantity) with an antifungal agent to stop fermentation. By stopping fermentation, you stop production of additional ammonia so that the cancer process can be stopped.

Eliminating ammonia toxicity with nitrogen and providing the essential enzyme αketoglutarate will revive the citric acid cycle. Human cells will gain vital ATP energy, cancer cells and microbes will lose nucleotides for growth. We can SWITCH metabolism back to the aerobic process and stop fermentation.

When Levine and Suzuki described the polymerase chain reaction in a book called *The Secret of Life,* they explained how the normal bacterial DNA polymerase enzyme would not stand up to heating and cooling cycles required for continuous replication. DNA polymerase from hot-spring bacteria was selected instead. If bacterial polymerase does not stand up to frequent heating and cooling cycles in a test tube, it probably does not stand up within a highly oxidative cell. With the renewed production of ATP, microbial DNA polymerase would break down and the mutation of replicating cells would cease. Perhaps the extra heat destroys other vital microbial enzymes and co-enzymes as well leading to immediate death of these microbes.

Some observations indicate that people who exercise and perspire vigorously do not experience cancer. Increased body temperature, perspiration, and exercise lead to cleansing of pollutants and microbial enzymes and reduced fermentation of trapped blood sugars and proteins.

Numerous cancer cures involve fasting. If we eliminate fungal food, fungal processes must stop. Periods of fasting from all carbon-rich foods such as sugars and starches leads to reduced fungal and yeast infection because these microbes depend on carbon for energy.

In summary, medical textbooks show tumor cells consume arginine. A chemotherapy drug called Asparaginase uses arginine as a base but has horrendous side effects. Research shows arginine blocks tumors in mice and rats, and arginine was used by Jimmy Keller in his cancer treatment. It was so effective he was abducted from Mexico and put in U.S. prison because of his success. I doubt if the FDA would have gone to this trouble if it didn't work. The popularity of the treatment led to Keller's abduction and closure of his clinic. Testimonials available on the Internet attest to its effectiveness. Various authors report research indicating it stops tumor growth. The fact that arginine is not endorsed as a cancer treatment is a good example of a suppressed cancer cure.

The fact that Canadians are deprived of this valuable amino acid supplement by regulations is cause for a class-action suit against those who are responsible for these regulations.

Let's take a look at the contribution of acetimide to the cancer cure.

Acetimide helps stop fungal growth

Acetamide (C_2H_5NO) is formed by removing a molecule of water from a compound of ammonia and acetic acid, producing a white crystalline solid used for organic synthesis. None of the components, which are carbon, hydrogen, oxygen, and nitrogen, are toxic to human cells and the compound tests safely with rats. Acetic acid is vinegar.

There is only one reference that I can find to explain how acetimide could help cure cancer. Acetimide is antifungal and would stop fermentation of blood sugars and blood proteins. As you know, Dr. Costantini claims all drugs or other nutrients that cure any human disease have only one thing in common. They are all antifungal or antimycotoxic. This text was referred to in Chapter 3.

Here's what you will find on the Internet if you search under *acetimide*. Acetimide is used to make Cymoxanil, an antifungal spray for fruit and vegetables.

Cymoxanil was first introduced in 1977. It is an acetimide compound used as both a curative and preventative foliar fungicide. *In Europe it is being sold for use on grapes, potatoes, tomatoes, hops, sugarbeets and other vegetable crops.* Cymoxanil is currently not registered in the U.S.A.

Cymoxanil's mode of action is as a local systemic. It penetrates rapidly and when inside the plant, it cannot be washed off by rain (*a systemic enters the system*). It controls diseases (fungal types) during the incubation period and prevents the appearance of damage on the crop.

There's the one-two punch for cancer.

1. Arginine eliminates ammonia and restarts the citric acid cycle.
2. Acetimide eliminates fermentation and all the related oxygen-free microspheres, ammonia toxicity and fungal chitin used to mutate cell-wall membranes.

I started this research simply to see if there was any validity in claims by Ralph Moss that: **Giving arginine along with the chemical acetimide led to virtually complete inhibition of the carcinogenic process.** As the references show, there is more reason to believe these claims than there is to doubt them.

Is acetimide safe to take internally? Rats used for testing purposes as mentioned in the preceding reference from Dr. Moss were not harmed by it. The West German fungal spray for fruit and vegetables "penetrates rapidly and when inside the plant cannot be washed off." It is being used for a large variety of crops that are consumed fresh. Obviously, ingestion of this residual spray is safe for human consumption.

If you want the complete Jimmy Keller story from "Cathy" who was in the clinic at the time of the raid and abduction, check out the Internet by searching under TCMherbal Forum, or just Jimmy Keller and FDA. Cathy reports how she was almost healed of her life-threatening condition while at the clinic. Someone else, who does not wish to be identified, relates how Cathy died a few years later from the chemotherapy cancer treatments she was forced to endure due to the loss of Keller's protocol. The article on Faith Hope and Fraud list numerous testimonials of people who were permanently healed of tumors by this method.

Parasite cleansing is essential for a permanent cancer cure

In the book *The Amino Revolution* Dr. Robert Erdmann, PH.D, we learn that arginine reduces the size of tumors (Page 132):

> In tests on mice, scientists have found that arginine supplementation inhibits the growth of cancer tumors and often reduces their size.

In Dr. Clark's book, *The Cure for All Cancers*, arginine is recommended as very important for cancer patients to reduce ammonia toxicity in conjunction with a parasite cleanse. Dr. Clark writes (Page 15):.

These are the only essential herbs you will need to cure your cancer *(Black Walnut, Wormwood and Cloves)*. They will last through the first 18 days of the parasite program *(based on quantities in the bottles from sources she recommends)*.

Two additional items, ornithine and arginine, improve this recipe. Parasites produce a great deal of ammonia as their waste product. Ammonia is their equivalent to urine and is set free in our bodies by parasites in large amounts. Ammonia is very toxic, especially to the brain.

If you kill off all of the parasites using the above-mentioned herbs, or others like them, you will eliminate most of the sources for ammonia. However, it is still in the air you breathe and in many household and personal care products. Taking extra arginine is still good advice. Dr. Clark gives important advice about eliminating parasites:

Do not try to substitute drugs for herbs to kill parasites. Drug parasiticides can be extremely toxic, even in small doses needed. Nor do they kill all the stages.

In review, by stopping the citric acid cycle with ammonia, microbes and cancer cells obtain the nutrients they require for growth. Dr. Warburg was right when he claimed the prime cause of cancer is the switch from oxidative metabolism to fermentation of glucose. The essential step in the process of cancer is the switching of energy production from aerobic to anaerobic glycolysis. Switching over provides microbes with control of temperature cycles for replication, provides the energy source and nutrients for growth of cancer cells and the production of ammonia. In due time, injury to the cell wall will turn on the current of injury and initiate replication, mutation and cancer.

Dr. Costantini tells us that the success of chemotherapy drugs comes from reducing the capacity of microbial enzymes to stop the oxidative process or in killing the fungi.

This is probably why Dr. Hulda Clark's parasite cleanse was selected by Chinese cancer specialists for use in China and why arginine/ornithine supplements increase the effectiveness of a parasite cleanse. Dr. Clark has put together a complete package. Her books should be in every home as a reference for better health and treatment for disease. A simple *Cancer Curing Program* based on detoxification and nutrition should be compulsory at every cancer clinic in the world. Maybe some day it will be.

Mr. Keller's Tumorex and research into curing cancer has been totally wasted by the cancer industry. Ornithine and Arginine in bulk form are banned in Canada. Ammonia, on the other hand, has never been researched (outside of this book) as a carcinogen. No regulations apply against its use in the home or for personal care products such as shampoos or as an additive in cigarette tobacco.

Avoiding ammonia toxicity through lifestyle changes

It is your personal responsibility to eliminate sources of ammonia from your environment. No one can do this for you. This information about ammonia could be a valuable and effective step for prevention and/or treatment of active cancer and neurological diseases.

By eliminating as many sources of ammonia as possible from your external and internal environments, you can avoid polluting your body. Less ammonia will result in more energy and a stronger immune system.

By ensuring your diet provides an adequate amount of amino acids (arginine or its precursors) to combine with ammonia and reduce it to urea, you can help break the ammonia/fermentation cycle. If you feel drowsy after a heavy protein meal, your brain is probably suffering ammonia toxicity. Ammonia toxicity is directly associated with Alzheimer's and nerve damage, so you might well consider taking trace mineral supplements before your meals, digestive enzymes with your meals, and not eating too much protein (meat) at one time.

Ammonia also results from fermentation of glucose and proteins through a fungal process. By reducing levels of fungi and parasites in our body, we can reduce the rate of fermentation and thereby reduce production of ammonia. Zapping microbes is an excellent way to reduce ammonia production and avoid mental fatigue. (Zapping will be discussed more fully in Chapter 16).

In order to prevent fermentation of blood proteins, we must keep our lymphatic system clear of trapped blood proteins, through exercise and nutrition. Rebounding on a home rebounder (a miniature trampoline) is one of the most efficient methods we have for pumping and cleansing the lymphatic system. A few minutes daily spent lying head down on a slant-board is also helpful. Special lymphatic system exercises and lymphatic massage as described in the Multiversa Health Strategy are also very beneficial.

These exercises direct the discharge of lymph fluids into the colon. The exercises serve to cleanse lymph nodes in all parts of the body. (See bibliography under Coville for source.)

The fermentation and production of ammonia also occur in our small and large colon due to putrefaction of meat. Proper combining of food to avoid putrefaction, and maintenance of a healthy intestinal flora, will help reduce production of ammonia.

By destroying anaerobic bacteria and fungi, we eliminate the low-oxygen microspheres they produce. By maintaining adequate oxygen levels, we maintain the production of ATP and keep the immune system strong enough to overcome microbial infections.

By periodic cleansing of the lymphatic system and removing blocked blood proteins, we help reduce fermentation. A diet of easily digested foods, combined with fasting and exercise, will help to cleanse the cells of waste. To fast, for health purposes, doesn't mean to stop eating. Rather, it means to drink lots of water, eat lightly, and to eat only fresh and raw vegetables and fruit so that the body can produce energy for cleansing.

Author Harvey Diamond's recent books *You Can Prevent Breast Cancer*, as well as *Fit-For-Life 3* contain valuable information describing brief but frequent one-day and two-day fasts to allow the body to cleanse the lymphatic system of trapped blood proteins and cellular debris. Harvey Diamond also stressed the need to add enzymes to every meal containing cooked foods. Without these enzymes, the body must produce enzymes for digestion. Sprinkling food enzymes on every meal made of cooked and processed foods is great advice for older people.

Increased oxygen intake is also important during a fast. Fresh vegetables contain about 45% oxygen and support health in many ways. Fresh vegetables are our chief natural source of arginine. Processed and canned vegetables, on the other hand, have no oxygen or arginine content. Perhaps this explains why so many cancer cures are based on a strict, fresh vegetarian diet.

714X reduces ammonia toxicity of lymphatic system

Christopher Bird's book, *The Persecution and Trial of Gaston Naessens*, with the subtitle *The True Story of the Efforts to Suppress Alternative Treatment for Cancer, AIDS, and other Immunologically Based Diseases*, is a classic on suppression of effective cancer cures. Gaston Naessens has created a worldwide following. Thousands claim to have used his formula 714X to cure both cancer and AIDS.

Naessens has produced two commercially available videos that show slides of live blood in which we can see red blood cells with parasites inside them, and watch as the parasites multiply, rupture the cell wall, and spill out thousands of small but living particles into the blood plasma. These mature into larger tube-shaped organisms filled with *granular structures* (grain-like) that also burst into the blood plasma. After bursting, the outer shell remains as granular debris in the blood stream.

These videos are also important for the cancer issue. The reduced blood flow caused by partially blocked arteries contributes to cancer by reducing delivery of oxygen to the cells. Similarly, swollen lymph nodes in the lymphatic system reduce capacity to remove intracellular wastes from the intracellular spaces. In addition, hardening of the arteries may lead to rupture of plaque and consequent internal bleeding.

Granular debris causes hardening of the arteries.

According to Dr. Costantini, who specializes in granuloma diseases, the reason we have hardening of the arteries, but not the veins, is because of the way blood flows, pulsating in arteries, smooth flowing in veins. With pulsating blood, granular microbial products and debris compress to form hardening of the arteries. Veins, on the other hand, which do not have a similar pulsating flow of blood, do not harden, although veins contain the same level of granuloma debris as the arteries. Cholesterol coating which forms a plaque of granuloma debris is a defense mechanism to smooth over the granuloma. Cholesterol helps maintain flexibility, and *maintain lower blood pressure* in order to circulate blood.

Dr. Costantini supports the concept that cholesterol is a defense mechanism of the body. He writes in Fungalbionics on the Internet:

Cholesterol binding reduces injurious effects of toxins

Benson et all (1989) found that the microbial-derived toxic metabolite (antibiotic) mycosubtilin has a strong lytic action *(destruction of cells)* upon fungi and erythrocytes. . . . The protective benefits of cholesterol binding of the toxic microbial metabolite thus preventing disruption of the cellular membrane provides evidence of a heretofore unrecognized purpose for the presence of cholesterol in the cellular membranes of all living cells; antitoxicity.

In time, this defensive mechanism fails by blocking the arteries with layers of granuloma debris coated over with layers of cholesterol. The artery loses elasticity and blood flow is restricted, blood pressure increases, until the system fails when the plague ruptures. It all starts with parasitic debris from microbes living and dying in the blood stream.

Bacteria and fungi live relatively short lives compared to humans. They also have cell wall membranes made up of sugars known as *mannans*, *glucans*, *chitin*, and *glycoproteins*. Microorganisms with rigid molecules in the cell-wall membrane that live in our blood steam must also die in our blood stream. Over time, these billions of dead bodies cause granuloma diseases and hardening of the arteries. Studies show that people with high build up of dental plaque also have high frequency of heart attacks, and people who are given antibiotics have reduced frequency of heart attacks. The explanation of blood circulation health problems appear to be microbial overload and nutritional deficiencies.

On the Internet at www.gordonresearch.com we find an 8 page article on the true cause of heart attacks. The article reads as follows:

Medicine's understanding of what causes heart attacks is being rewritten. Vulnerable plaque, something that cardiologists can't see, is responsible for 85% of heart attacks. Dr. Steven Nissen of the Cleveland Clinic then adds "The rupture of a plaque will be the cause of death of about half of all of us in the United States.

There are numerous cases of people in their teens and early twenties dying of hardening of the arteries and heart attacks, similar to that of older people. Back in the late 1960's Dr. Kilmer McCully discovered that high levels of homocysteine in the blood accounted for these early-in-life heart attacks. He fed rabbits high protein diets, similar in the protein levels of humans, and the animals developed heart diseases. Dr. McCully proved that heart disease could be caused by excessive buildup of the amino acid homocysteine. When we see healthy young men collapse and die on the basketball court or other sporting event, we are probably watching a heart attack brought on by a high protein diet and lack of trace minerals.

The article goes on to say:

One would think that discovering what could be the cause of the biggest health problem in North America would garner McCully some praise. For his efforts, McCully was effectively fired from Harvard. He subsequently went to the VA Hospital in Providence, Rhode Island, and continued his studies. He is still there.

In 1988, he published a study showing that men with homocysteine levels only 12% higher than average have a 3.4 time greater risk of having a heart attack.

Isn't that incredible! Risk of heart attacks is increase over 3 times by a 12% rise in homocysteine. Homocysteine is an amino acid. A partial explanation describing how homocysteine leads to heart attacks is described by

Paul Frankel, Ph.D. and Terri Mitchell on the Internet at www.lef.org/magazaine. He writes:

> Homocystinuria is a condition of enzyme deficiency that allows homocysteine to accumulate. homocysteine is a by-product of methionine metabolism, which becomes toxic if allowed to accumulate.

The Internet article goes on to describe how the cause of heart disease is in the blood. Nutritional factors can make a difference to supply the enzymes needed by the body to eliminate the problem. The two major supplements are folic acid of 400 mcg. to 2 mg. per day, plus vitamin B6 and vitamin B12. In the book *Prescription for Natural Healing*, by Dr. James Balach, we read under the heading for Vitamin B6:

> Vitamin B6 plays a role in cancer immunity and aids in the prevention of arteriosclerosis. It inhibits the formation of a toxic chemical called homocysteine, which attacks the heart muscles and allows the deposition of cholesterol around the heart muscle.

Have you ever seen homocysteine listed as a possible cause of heart attacks in literature from the heart and stroke industry? I know I haven't. Why isn't it at least mentioned as a potential cause?

Homocysteine is derived from Methionine found in meats, legumes, soy, nuts, dairy, eggs, fish, garlic, onions, nuts seeds and some grains. These are excellent food items, but must be taken in moderation. A diet consisting of 40% carbohydrates, 30% protein, and 30% fats will ensure that too much protein is no being consumed. Periodic cleansing of fungus and bacteria will help reduce incidence of heart attack through granuloma accumulation.

Blood circulation diseases caused by microbes

Medical reporter Carolyn Abraham reported in the Canadian newspaper *Globe and Mail* (Feb 26, 1999) that researchers at the Princess Margaret hospital in Toronto have identified a link between heart disease and Chlamydia, a bacterial infection. Nearly everyone gets this infection, because it is most often spread like a cold by coughing and sneezing.

The recent medical observation that people on antibiotics have fewer heart problems makes sense. Antibiotics reduce microbial levels in the blood and thereby reduce dead cells and granuloma.

Dr. Costantini believes microbial toxins in the body can account for all degenerative diseases. This means that all of our degenerative diseases will respond to anti-fungal treatments and various forms of electronic medicine as well as herbs, homeopathics, and metabolic therapy using amino acids. Cleansing the body of toxins and microbial debris is a positive step toward better health. Cleansing the lymphatic system, liver, colon, and kidneys results in increased cleansing capacity for the cells in these organs. We take time to cleanse the fluid filters in our cars. Why not take time to cleanse the fluid filters in our body?

The only lymphatic system cleanser available that I know of at this time is Gaston Naessen's formula 714X. Let's review how this formula can cure cancer and other infectious diseases.

714X contains nitrogen and trace minerals

In technical information on 714X, we find that the compound does not contain any protein or immunoglobulins, so it is not a vaccine. Rather it contains 18 trace minerals, and nitrogen. It is a health product to enhance the immune system and energize the cells. The formula is injected directly into the lymphatic system nodes. Injection results in reduced fermentation in the lymphatic liquids and reduced production of ammonia.

The formula 714X works on three levels. Primarily it liquefies the lymph so that the body can get rid of trapped blood proteins. Enlarged lymph glands are normally removed by an operation, leaving the body without this very essential defense mechanism. 714X liquefies the lymph and solves the problem while saving the lymph nodes.

Also, 714X provides nitrogen for cellular repair. Nitrogen is an important component of proteins and enzymes needed by the body for repair and operation. In addition, nitrogen is an important component of urea, which is needed by the body to eliminate ammonia.

After Naessens' more than 20 years of successful healing with 714X and without one unexpected negative side effect, mainstream medicine still refuses to incorporate 714X into standard treatment. If you are interested in seeing these amazing videos of parasites in red blood cells and blood plasma, you can purchase copies. See SOURCES appendix for details. After watching these videos, if you have an opportunity to have your blood tested by a darkfield microscope specialist, you can interpret what you observe with considerable accuracy and detail. You will know the condition of your health without anyone holding back the truth or getting you to over react and purchase products you don't need. In addition, if you change your lifestyle and try some alternative health therapies, you can go back for a second reading and see the results. You can safely take control of your health.

16. Use oxygen and ozone to help cure cancer

The purpose of this chapter is to expose misinformation about the free-radical theory of disease. Oxygen, hydrogen peroxide, and ozone are effective cancer cures that are being suppressed as dangerous free radicals. There is no truth in the concept that oxygen, in any form, is a dangerous free radical because the body has developed enzymes to protect against oxygen. The Western world has bought a false theory—a theory that has benefited only mainstream medicine.

Free radicals are said to be an atom or molecule that is highly reactive because it has at least one unpaired electron. Because unpaired electrons join so readily with other compounds, free radicals can attack cells and cause a lot of damage in the body. That may be true for some atoms other than oxygen. Oxygen is safely catalyzed in all human cells.

Back in 1954, Dr. Denham Harman, Professor of Medicine and Biochemistry at the University of Nebraska, published a paper implicating free radicals as a major cause of degenerative diseases. Since then, practically all educators have accepted the theory and enlarged upon it to include oxygen and all oxygen-related compounds. Let's review three of these typical modern-day expressions of the oxygen, free radical problem.

Author Jean Carpenter, in her 1995 book *Stop Aging Now,* describes how respiration creates oxygen free radicals. She writes about the dangers of breathing normal air. She is not even talking about the pollutants in the air. She is talking about oxygen (Page 12):

THE DANGER IS IN THE AIR

Oxygen is what it is all about… free radicals, including the pervasive *superoxides created by respiration*, careen out of control through the body, attacking cells, turning their fats rancid, rusting their proteins, piercing their membranes and corrupting their genetic code until the cells become dysfunctional and sometimes give up and die.

Similarly, author Stephen Masely, M.D. in his 1996 publication, *The 28-day Antioxidant Diet Program* (Pages 4 to 9), writes (Emphasis added):

When our bodies burn fuel with oxygen (a process called oxidation), we produce free radicals –toxic products that, in excess, can cause illness, accelerate aging, and lead to death. . . genetic DNA material can be damaged, making your cells more susceptible to aging and cancer. . . A normal cell takes 100,000 "hits" from free radicals every day. That's one hit per second!

Similarly, Dr. Hari Sharma, author of *Freedom from Disease,* established a clear connection between chronic inflammation, oxygen free radicals and cancer. He writes (Page 89):

The initiation phase of cancer is often caused by chronic inflammation, a fact that has been known for many years but has only recently been explained. In chronic inflammation, white blood cells are constantly releasing showers of free radicals. The neutrophils and macrophages spew superoxide and hydrogen peroxide in all directions, and both can enter nearby cells and travel to the cell nucleus to damage genetic material. Hydroxy radicals and hypochlorous acid released in intracellular spaces have the effect. . .

Please note that the "the initiation phase of cancer is often caused by chronic inflammation" and that the white blood cells spew hydrogen peroxide, which is used to fight infection. If the body produces hydrogen peroxide to fight infection, would drinking a light solution of hydrogen peroxide or ozonated water help support the immune system? Yes.

The cause, cure and cover-up of cancer is clearly demonstrated by the above reference. Chronic inflammation is the cause of cancer, hydrogen peroxide is nature's cure, and medical interpretation blaming hydrogen peroxide as the cause of cancer illustrates the cover-up. The initiation of cancer is caused by a chronic inflammation due to injury and parasites. Hydrogen peroxide is produced by the body to fight inflammation. Supplementing our body with hydrogen peroxide, (or ozone and other oxygen-compounds) helps cure cancer. How could it be otherwise?

It is highly improbable that someone who has dedicated his or her life to cancer research hasn't figured this out. All the information needed to understand the cause of cancer is in the public domain. It only took me five or six years to connect it for myself, after I committed myself to solving the problem. Real progress only came after I started questioning and rejecting the false dogma of modern medicine.

I have watched a video of a woman who was given less than a week to live due to cancer. She is speaking to a group in order to support the use of hydrogen peroxide for treating cancer. She claims to have cured her cancer by bathing in peroxide, using peroxide for colonics and douches, rinsing her mouth and drinking it. She realized she had nothing to lose by trying it. When I first watched the video, I mentally rejected it as preposterous. Now I believe she was telling the truth. Peroxide tastes horrible. It may make you vomit, due to rapid oxidation of microbes in the stomach. Vomiting is uncomfortable, but not harmful. It may give you diarrhea, but so do some other bowel cleansing processes. The oxygen in dilute hydrogen peroxide will not harm you. It certainly won't mutate your DNA as suggested in the above quotations. It will destroy microbial infection and stop the mutation of new cells. If it does that, it can cure cancer.

Getting back to the breathing of oxygen, Sharma goes on to establish the normal source of free radicals as a by-product of metabolism (Page 27):

> . . . Oxygen is used to burn glucose molecules that act as the
> body's fuel In the energy freeing operation, oxy radicals are thrown
> off as destructive by-products.

After considerable research, I now believe the whole concept about oxygen, free radicals is false information knowingly used for financial gain. There is not a shred of scientific evidence that oxygen is a dangerous free radical. Oxygen we breathe is not dangerous, respiration does not produce dangerous oxygen free radicals and metabolism does not produce them.

None of the metabolic activities produces dangerous free radicals of oxygen. Proof of this is found in medical university textbooks and other research. I doubt that anyone can graduate from medical university without knowing that the dangerous oxygen free radical concept is a lie.

Let's look at the following references in defense of oxygen.

Metabolism does not create reactive oxygen radicals

The outstanding author and scientist Isaac Asimov has a chapter on *The Biological Sciences* in his book **Asimov's New Guide to Science**. Here he describes how oxidation requires oxygen, (rather than gives off oxygen free radicals) and describes the potential energy difference between oxidation and fermentation. He writes (Page 580):

> The mammalian body cannot convert lactic acid to ethyl alcohol
> (as yeast can); instead, by another route of metabolism, the body
> bypasses ethyl alcohol and breaks down lactic acid all the way to
> carbon dioxide (CO_2) and water. In so doing, **it consumes oxygen**

and produces a great deal more energy than is produced by the non-oxygen conversion of glucose to lactic acid.

Normal metabolism consumes oxygen. Asimov refers to free radicals only once in his text, and that is free radicals produced by radiation. Normal life processes such as respiration and metabolism do not create oxygen free radicals.

The textbook used by most of the world's medical students explains why metabolism does not produce dangerous radicals. Enzymes do not allow single hydrogen ions to combine with oxygen to produce highly unstable and reactive molecules. Dr. Guyton, in the **Textbook of Medical Physiology,** in describing the citric acid cycle, writes (Page 843. My italics added):

> . . . hydrogen atoms are released during different chemical reactions – 4 hydrogen atoms during glycolysis, 4 during the formation of acetyl Co-A from pyruvic acid, and 16 in the citric acid cycle; this makes a total of 24 hydrogen atoms. However, the hydrogen atoms are not simply turned loose in the intracellular fluid. **Instead, they are** *released in packets of two,* and in each instance **the release is catalyzed by a specific protein enzyme called a** *dehydrogenase.* Twenty of the 24 hydrogen atoms immediately combine with nicotinamide adenine dinucleotide (NAD+), a derivative of the vitamin niacin . . .

The remaining four hydrogen atoms combine with oxygen in pairs, resulting in H_2O or water. Water is not a dangerous free radical.

There is a direct connection between hydrogen and oxygen free radicals because it is believed that if a single hydrogen atom bonds with oxygen, the compound will be lacking one additional electron and becomes highly reactive. This is called a hydroxyl (OH) radical with a single unpaired reactive molecule. The fact that enzymes deliver hydrogen atoms in pairs eliminates this problem.

Similarly, hydrogen peroxide (H_2O_2) does not produce dangerous free radicals. One of the two atoms of oxygen in peroxide attacks the anaerobic life form, which cannot produce defensive enzymes, and the remaining molecule is water. That is why blisters swell up with liquid. Perhaps the mechanism enabling cysts and ulcers to initiate cancer is that inflammations and swelling produce blisters in the cell wall, blisters lead to cell wall damage and initiation of the current of injury. Supplementing the body with peroxide or other oxygen supplements would support the immune system defenses.

Hydrogen peroxide does not attack fat or lipid molecules in skin tissue, because enzymes do not allow this to happen. The fact that oxygen attacks fat stored in containers has nothing to do with fat in human tissue. Fats and oils in storage containers lose the protective enzyme reserves and oxidation takes place. Fats in cells renew and maintain a safe supply of protective enzymes to combine oxygen atoms into harmless oxygen molecules.

The quantum theory states that chemical actions do not occur continuously, but in steps, as all stable molecules, such as DNA, require a minimum quantum of energy before chemical reactions can take place. A single hydrogen ion or oxygen atom does not have the quantum of energy necessary to initiate molecular changes in DNA. If numerous reactive hydrogen or oxygen atoms come together, they react with one-another instantly, and become stable diatomic atoms or compounds.

Information in Professor Guyton's textbook for medical students discusses the citric acid cycle and never mentions dangerous free radicals because hydrogen atoms are always handled in pairs. They are not simply turned loose nor are they combined with oxygen to form hydroxyl (OH) radicals.

Dr. Sharma's book goes on to list diseases now linked to oxy radicals and ROS (*Radical Oxygen Species*) (Page 24):

cancer	heart disease	strokes
emphysema diabetes	arteriosclerosis	ulcers
Atherosclerosis cataracts	Crohn's disease	diabetes
rheumatoid arthritis	Raynaud's disease	senility

We are being led to believe that human degenerative diseases, including cancer, are caused by reactive oxygen radicals. Since we can't stop breathing, we have a serious problem. We cannot control our health. We must rely on specialists who will tell us what to do, for a fee, of course. Since this problem has just been discovered, funds will be needed to research the problem.

Dr Sharma gives a list of the "BIOCHEMICAL BAD BOYS" (Page 45), carefully listing the ROS (Radical Oxygen Species) These are specifically:

1. *superoxide*

2. *hydroxy radical*

3. *lipid peroxy radical*

4. *singlet oxygen*

5. *hydrogen peroxide*

6. *hypochlorous acid.*

On page 78, we learn that oxygen free radicals damage cell membranes. If this is true, there would be a cell-wall injury, a current of injury, and cancer could result. Let's take a closer look.

DAMAGE TO CELL MEMBRANES

Free radical attack on cell membranes can be especially damaging. Attack on a single membrane molecule touches off a destructive chain reaction. The damage spreads down the membrane, and eventually results in a class of free radicals that move out to attack every vulnerable molecule in the cell.

The truth is that oxygen does not cause any diseases. Lack of oxygen does. Lack of oxygen leads to lack of energy and immune system dysfunction. The fundamental reason why oxygen could be considered a dangerous free radical is without scientific basis. Dr. Sharma gives the scientific explanation for the reactivity of oxygen based on a *quirk in the quantum theory* (Page 47. My emphasis added):

WHY OXYGEN STARTS IT ALL

It is not a pretty line-up. And the common denominator is oxygen. But why? Compared with every other compound in a living system (except for some of its own oxy radical off-spring), oxygen has the greatest need for electrons. What are the properties of oxygen that give it such a ravenous electron hunger?

The answer lies in a quantum mechanical quirk in oxygen's structure. An oxygen atom has six electrons in its outer shell, a shell that can adopt eight electrons total. One might expect that these six electrons would pair up two by two, leaving one empty orbital. If this were the case, the oxygen atom would still have a reasonably strong desire to pick up an additional pair of electrons to fill the last orbital in its outer shell. All atoms would rather have their outer shell full.

But oxygen is not a common case. Only four of its outer shell electrons pair off two by two. The last two electrons can't get together. *They are both spin up. They repel each other and must occupy separate orbitals, alone and unpaired.*

Oxygen thus has two unpaired electrons and its drive for additional electrons is thus uncommonly great. In a sense, in fact, oxygen is a free radical twice over.

Please note the first statement used to explain the danger of oxygen molecules: "*The answer lies in a quantum mechanical quirk*". There are no quirks or exceptions to the quantum theory mentioned in scientific books such as *Asimov's New Guide to Science*. In my opinion, any medical theory that requires a *quirk in the quantum theory* is immediately suspect of error. It is far more likely that we have an error in the concept of the quantum theory. It is even more likely that this misinformation is propaganda.

Let's look now at references that prove the oxygen molecule is a stable atom and is not a dangerous free radical twice over.

In Lloyd Motz's description of the oxygen molecule, we have a uniquely different concept from that expressed by Dr. Sharma in the reference above. The unique features of an atom are determined by the electrons and how they orbit the nucleus. Every electron has four quantum numbers by which to identify its orbit. In oxygen molecules, the directional spin of the electrons is key to understanding the stability of the oxygen atom and why it is not a dangerous free radical. The following quote is from the book *The Universe, Its Beginning and End* (Page 230):

> Consider now a homopolar (shared electron orbit) bond. The normal states of such gases as hydrogen, nitrogen, and oxygen are not the atomic states H, N, and O, but the molecular states H_2, N_2, and O_2. To see why this is so, observe two hydrogen atoms brought close together. Whether they repel each other or attract each other and thus combine to form a molecule, depends entirely on the two electrons that are spinning. If the two electrons are both spinning clockwise, or both spinning counter clockwise, the two atoms repel each other and the H_2 molecule is not formed; but if one is spinning clockwise and the other counterclockwise, the atoms attract each other and are then bound together to form the H_2 molecule. The way the atoms attract each other is a purely quantum mechanical phenomenon; the two electrons being indistinguishable, behave as though they were exchanging places at a certain frequency, and this exchange binds the two atoms together. It is as though the two protons were juggling the electrons between them and were held together by this juggling act; the two protons share the two indistinguishable electrons. It is important to note that because of quantization, in both the ionic bond and covalent bond only definite stable molecular patterns can occur, and this insures molecular stability. A molecule cannot change its structure gradually but only in discrete steps that require discrete amounts of energy. Ordinary thermal motion does not have enough energy for this.

Let's review this very important statement: *because of quantization, in both the ionic bond and covalent bond only definite stable molecular patterns can occur, and this insures molecular stability.*

We are being told that atoms of hydrogen, nitrogen, and oxygen form *stable molecules* of these substances. We understand that the electrons must be spinning in opposite directions and that the molecules are stable. In contrast, Dr. Sharma bases the dangerous reactivity of the oxygen molecule on the concept that the two electrons are spinning in the same direction. Let me repeat this important statement: *They are both spin up. They repel each other and must occupy separate orbitals, alone and unpaired.*

If both electrons were spin up, the diatomic oxygen molecule could not form. *Oxygen is a diatomic molecule; therefore Sharma is wrong.* **In chemistry, the very definition of a free radical is a chemical species that contains an unpaired electron. In order to establish oxygen as a dangerous free radical, it is essential that an atom of oxygen be identified as having one or two unpaired electrons. The whole concept is false and illustrates medical misinformation.**

In contrast to Sharma, Motz explains that these electrons do not occupy separate orbitals. The electrons exchange places at a certain rhythmic frequency. The two nuclei are the same size and the two orbits identical in diameter or distance from their respective nucleus. In individual atoms, the two electrons have the same quantum number because all atoms of oxygen are identical. As a diatomic molecule with two atoms, the electrons spin in opposite directions and share the same orbital. They do not occupy separate orbits alone and unpaired.

In chemistry there is a term called the Pauli Exclusion Principle which states that no two electrons in the same atom can have the same values for all four of their quantum number. Spins are only positive (+1/2) or negative (-1/2). There are no spin up or spin down electrons. The preposterous medical theory promoting oxygen as a dangerous free radical is without scientific basis.

The oxygen atoms do not repel each other, otherwise, the molecule could not be formed and we could not have diatomic molecules of oxygen. This is not the case in the real world. In forming a diatomic molecule of oxygen, energy is needed to reverse the spin of one electron. It takes a minimum quantity of energy to form a diatomic oxygen molecule. It takes an equal minimum quantity of energy to separate the diatomic molecule into two atoms of oxygen. That is why the oxygen molecule is stable and cannot be considered as a dangerous free radical.

Let's look at a second opinion that explains why oxygen is not a dangerous free radical, and why oxygen does not destroy tissue in human cells.

Dr. Majid Ali has written several books and numerous articles on the fungal cause of disease as well as the importance of oxygen to maintain health.

An explanation for the biochemical safety of oxygen can be found in the *Journal of Oxidative Medicine* (Page 18):

Diatomic oxygen (consisting of two atoms) in ambient air is considered a radical because it contains two unpaired electrons. This structural characteristic of oxygen, according to thermodynamics, should allow oxygen to cause immediate combustion of all organic molecules that are exposed to it. Why does that not happen? *The explanation is that two unpaired electrons of diatomic oxygen in two different orbitals have the same spin quantum number.* If oxygen were to directly oxidize organic molecules, it would have to accept two electrons from a donor with spins that are opposite to its own two unpaired electrons so as to be properly accommodated into vacant spaces in oxygen's two orbitals containing unpaired electrons. This, of course, cannot be achieved by electrons in covalent bonds, *which spin in opposite directions.*

Such spin restriction explains oxygen's poor reactivity even though it is a good oxidizer. This explains why organic molecules do not spontaneously undergo combustion in oxygen.

This also explains why glucose in oxygen, like ATP in water, is kinetically stable even though it is thermodynamically unstable. For oxygen to be reduced, it requires a *paramagnetic catalyst* such as heme iron or a copper chelate, which scrabble, so to speak, the electron spin in the donor.

Please note that both Lloyd Motz and Dr. Ali say that electrons in diatomic oxygen spin in opposite directions, and oxygen is safe. In contrast, Dr. Sharma says the two electrons spin in the same direction and oxygen is a dangerous free radical. Only one of these two divergent views can be correct. It is obvious that oxygen is a stable molecule because we need enzymes to make hydrogen combine with oxygen.

Dr. Ali writes (same source as above): For oxygen to be reduced, it requires a *paramagnetic catalyst* such as heme iron or a copper chelate, which scrabble, so to speak, the electron spin in the donor."

Paramagnetic enzymes modify the electric spin of the donor so that it will combine with oxygen. Paramagnets are crystals that take on a temporary magnetic charge, possibly due to an ionic field.

Based on the research of Ali and Motz, and observations of the real world, there is no reason to believe that oxygen is a dangerous free radical. I find this as unbelievable as you probably do. Why are we being told that oxygen is a dangerous free radical and we must take anti-oxidants to prevent damage from oxygen free radicals?

I now suspect that the oxygen free radical theory is a ploy designed to frighten people away from using ozone and oxygen therapies. The theory keeps us occupied chasing better health down the wrong road. It also serves to help explain the cause of so many modern diseases and the frequency of them. Moreover, the theory provides a free ticket to focus cancer research on something other than defective genes and viruses as the cause of cancer.

Let me take you on an imaginary trip into a government sponsored research center. I have spent several years in a research center when I worked at the National Research Center in Ottawa. I know what it is like to go from one research project to another. Although I never sat in on a project discussion, I imagine it would go something like this.

Imagine a group of white-lab-coated cancer researchers sitting around the lounge having coffee and brainstorming about initiating another long-term research projects in order to keep their jobs. In this case they have already spent millions on researching defective genes and virus and need something new. Researching fungi as a cause of cancer is not allowed. Then someone gets a bright idea. "Let's research oxygen," he says. "Let's say oxygen destroys tissue, causes defective genes, and may cause cancer." "Yaaa," says another, "that would work. Let's call oxygen a dangerous free radicals and confuse the issue by grouping oxygen with the real free radicals like fluoride, and ammonia." And a third person adds, "Let's research antioxidants to block the damage of oxygen free radicals and then research the benefits of antioxidants to prevent cancer."

Someone should write a script for a movie depicting how the western world has been taken in by the false theory of dangerous oxygen free radicals. The script should spend considerable time depicting the research grants wasted on this issue. That's the fundamental benefit. There have been numerous research grants provided to research the oxygen free radical concept.

In *Freedom from Disease,* we read about research projects now designed to test the anti-oxidant theory. Research is needed into the mechanism by which free radicals cause aging and disease, research is needed for antioxidant drugs, research is needed to determine what antioxidants to take, in what combinations, and in what doses.

Here's a typical example. Dr. Sharma writes (Page 35):

> These questions are now mainstream science, as illustrated by
> a recent $17-million research grant from the National Institute of

Health. The grant funds a five-year study of 40,000 women to test the long-term effects of vitamin E and beta-carotene on heart disease and cancer.

What a waste of research dollars!

How could they possibly identify a positive connection between health related conditions based on use of vitamin E and beta-carotene? These food items are in fresh fruits and vegetables, nuts, grains, and multi-vitamin supplements. How could they identify how many other antioxidants were in the diets of these 40,000 women? How could they adjust for the effect of different life-styles, disease, and general nutrition?

The National Institute of Health authorities and employees who benefit from research grants such as this must laugh their way to the bank. That five-year study must be over by now. What were the results? Have they ever been published? Does it really matter?

The textbook *Harper's Review of Biochemistry* (1983 edition), does not support the oxygen free radical theory. The entire concept of "oxygen free radical" is not in the index. The word "anti-oxidant" is listed in the index only once, and this is concerning rancidity of oil during storage in containers. One cannot compare enzyme-controlled chemical reactions in living things to chemical reaction in storage containers because living things produce enzymes to catalyze oxygen whereas containers do not. However, the rancidity of oil in containers is often quoted as proof of the free-radical danger of oxygen.

What about all the other bad boys listed by Sharma in his text: superoxide, hydroxy radical, lipid peroxy radical, singlet oxygen, hydrogen peroxide, and hypochlorous acid?

In *Harper's Review of Biochemistry*, hypochlorous acid is not even in the index. The other terms appear in reference to the concept of superoxide metabolism. The theoretical toxicity of oxygen is discussed and dismissed because no evidence of superoxide toxicity has been found. The text reads as follows (Page 129):

Superoxide metabolism

Oxygen is a potentially toxic substance, the toxicity of which has hitherto been attributed to the formation of hydrogen peroxide. Recently, however, the ease with which oxygen can be reduced in tissues to the superoxide anion free radical and the occurrence of superoxide dismutase in aerobic organisms (*although not in obligate anaerobes*) has suggested that the toxicity of oxygen is due to its conversion to superoxide (Friedovich, 1975).

However, no direct evidence of superoxide toxicity has yet been obtained.

Isn't that unbelievable? "No direct evidence of superoxide toxicity has yet been obtained." That theoretical concept is the only basis for the danger in oxygen free radicals, the hydroxyl radicals, peroxide and ozone.

In case you are just skimming or otherwise missed the point:

> As of 1983, when the dangerous oxygen free radical concept was being highly promoted, *no direct evidence of superoxide toxicity had yet been discovered.* The dangerous oxygen free radical did not exist then, and it does not exist now.

Millions of dollars have been spent on antioxidants and millions of people are protecting themselves from a danger that does not exist. Like misinformation on cholesterol, defective genes, and autoimmune diseases, the dangers of oxygen free radicals is *misinformation* purposefully promoted for financial gain by an abusive medical establishment. How else can one explain the conflict between information in texts used in medical schools to educate medical students, and the obvious misinformation directed towards the public?

Harper's Review of Biochemistry explains how virtually all chemical reactions in living things are safely controlled by enzymes (Page 129):

The function of superoxide dismutase seems to be that of protecting aerobic organisms against the potential deleterious effects of superoxide. . .The distribution of the dismutase is widespread, being present in all major aerobic tissues. Although exposure of animals to an atmosphere of 100% oxygen causes an adaptive increase of the enzyme, particularly in the lungs, prolonged exposure leads to lung damage and death. Antioxidants such as Vitamin E act as scavengers of free radicals and reduce the toxicity of oxygen.

The text says that injury from oxygen, lung damage and death does not occur until exposure to 100% oxygen for a prolonged period of time is experienced. The air we breathe is only 20% oxygen, and millions of animals breathe it without injury. Enzymes protect living tissue from oxygen.

Inside a living body, oxygen free radicals are produced during peroxide formation **but these are safely scavenged by vitamins, heme compounds and enzymes.** This 600-page text on biochemistry has only one statement to say about dangerous free radicals. Here is what is written (Page 197):

Rancidity of oil during storage

Rancidity is a chemical change that results in unpleasant odors and taste in fat. The oxygen of the air attacks the double bond fatty acids to form a peroxide linkage. Lead and copper catalyzes rancidity; exclusion of oxygen or addition of an antioxidant delays the process. Free radicals are produced, leading to a chain reaction, during peroxide formation, and these can damage living tissue *unless antioxidants, e.g., tocopherols (vitamin E), are present to scavenge the free radicals.* **Peroxidation is also catalyzed in vivo by heme compounds and by the enzyme lipoxygenase found in platelets.**

Free radicals are not produced in living systems if enzymes are available to scavenge free radicals. Within living things the "unless antioxidants are present" takes effect. We may be short on Vitamin E, but we always have a variety of enzymes that are capable of using oxygen.

I cannot find any valid research to support the theory that oxygen in the air we breathe can be dangerous to our health, or that oxygen is dangerous to living tissue inside our body.

The textbook *Basic and Clinical Immunology* describes hydrogen peroxide only as a valuable antibiotic (Page 219):

Hydrogen peroxide (H_2O_2) has direct antimicrobial activity. In addition, it may act in concert with ascorbic acid and certain metal ions to kill ingested microorganisms by nonenzymatic means. Some microorganisms are more susceptible to H_2O_2 than others, depending on their ability to catalase or peroxidase.

The microorganisms that are more susceptible to peroxide are the anaerobic life forms that cause inflammation and cancer. The good bacteria in our body are aerobic bacteria and produce defensive enzymes to help destroy their enemy—the anaerobic bacteria and fungi.

It is most amazing that there are hundreds of references to oxygen as a benefit to health in texts on biology and immunology. This is in direct conflict with the popular press listing the dangers of oxygen, ozone, peroxide, and the hydroxyl radical (OH).

Textbooks describe antioxidants as substances that inhibit or block destructive oxidation reactions. Examples are vitamin C and E, the minerals selenium and germanium, the enzymes catalase and superoxide dismutase, (SOD) coenzyme Q10 and some amino acids.

As far as I can discover in my series of medical textbooks, there are no destructive oxidation reactions to human flesh and tissue. All oxygen related chemical actions are enzyme controlled. Oxygen, in any natural form, is not a dangerous free radical. Oxygen is nature's most effective antibiotic against anaerobic microbes and cancer cells precisely because oxygen reacts with their enzymes and tissues. Anaerobic microbes have no defense against oxygen or antioxidants because they cannot produce the enzymes required. The true benefit of taking the antioxidants listed above is to destroy microbial life forms and reduce parasites in the body. The antioxidants listed above might be better called antibiotics.

Antioxidants are chemically referred to as *phenols*. Antioxidants function because they have a phenolic appendage (OH) or a reactive oxygen atom ready to accept another electron.

Polyphenols are molecules with more than one phenolic appendage. Polyphenols have many hydroxyl groups (-OH) surrounding the core. It is because of the hydroxyl groups that the polyphenols are some of the best antioxidants, and therefore antibiotics, available. The hydroxyl groups in vitamin C and vitamin E are responsible for their antioxidant and antibiotic activity. The antioxidant activity can be used to protect us from dangerous free radicals in toxins and mycotoxins as well as toxic metals such as lead and mercury. That is why the cure for cancer should include large doses of Vitamin C, selenium, and other antioxidants, but this has nothing to do with protecting us from oxygen and oxygen free radicals.

Ozone and hydrogen peroxide provide safe cancer treatments

For an expression of the typical medical mindset on peroxide, let's refer to Dr. Hari Sharma, MD, in *Freedom From Disease* (Page 46):

> Hydrogen peroxide. Hydrogen peroxide is an ROS *(Reactive Oxygen Species)* which can persist indefinitely. It is also highly mobile; it can penetrate a cell membrane from the outside to do damage within. It can touch off peroxy chain reactions in the cell membrane and will slowly degrade many biological molecules. At low concentrations, it is not deadly to a cell, but by reacting with superoxide or metal ions, it gives birth to the lethal hydroxy radical.

Dr. Sharma is not alone in expressing these views. Ask any doctor if it is safe to consume peroxide and most will tell you it is not safe. These views conflict with opposing statements based on scientific research.

Here are opposing points of view expressing the safety of oxygen therapies and hydrogen peroxide.

In medical researcher Ed. McCabe's book, *Oxygen Therapies,* we find this following reference (Page 82). The original source is IBOM Newsletter, Vol. 1, No. 2. April 1987.

Hydrogen peroxide is not only important to the body's normal function but it's oxidizing ability can be used to oxidize weak protozoa and yeast, inhibit viruses, oxidize fatty deposits on the arterial walls, increase oxygen tension between cells, stimulate oxidative enzymes, return elasticity to the arterial walls, dilate coronary vessels, and regulate membrane transport.

Please note the statement: *return elasticity to the arterial walls.* Cancer is initiated when the arterial walls allow internal bleeding into ducts and vessels. The consequent fermentation of trapped blood leads to mycelia growth, invasion of adjoining cells, and cancer. Consumption of hydrogenated fats and oils produce cells that are also hydrogenated. Hydrogenation is a process of adding more hydrogen atoms to the fats and oils to increase their shelf life. Peroxide gives you an abundance of oxygen in your blood to help return the elasticity of the arterial walls to prevent cancer, strokes, and hardening of the arteries. I know people who drink a few drops of hydrogen peroxide in a glass of water every day and never catch a cold. In our home, we also use it regularly without any medical problems.

The book, *Oxygen Therapies* is a collection of references to research showing the safety and value of oxygen as a treatment for disease. There are thousands of researched articles attesting to the capacity of oxygen to cure diseases. The person who is most responsible for publicizing the benefits of hydrogen peroxide as a low-cost source of oxygen is Father Richard Willhelm, based on the research of Dr. Edward Rosenow, of the Mayo Clinic. Rosenow was successful in curing many psychiatric patients with hydrogen peroxide. The peroxide destroyed virus, fungi, and bacteria in the brain and body and eliminated the mycotoxins that were making these people psychotic. Oxygen is used by the brain in large amounts and oxygen passes through the blood/brain barriers.

Before the advent of antibiotics, hydrogen peroxide was the primary means by which doctors treated infections. I have one book with recommendations for the use of peroxide from more than 300 doctors. In the medical text *"The Therapeutical Applications of Hydrozone and Glycozone,* by Charles Marchand published in 1904, we have this significant reference (Page 232):

Peroxide of hydrogen is one of the most useful agents which we have in the treatment of diseases of the nose, throat and ear; its germicidal antiseptic properties and its capacity for destroying pus and decaying organic matter, without injurious effect on healthy tissue, renders it almost indispensable in many cases.

Peroxide of Hydrogen is not toxic, in fact it is safe for internal medication, and the amount which may be taken without injurious effect, is well illustrated by a case, in which patient took six, four ounce bottles of peroxide in one night. He was not injured but actually believed he had been benefited.

Robert Stroud (The Birdman of Alcatraz) who was confined to solitary confinement for over 50 years, used hydrogen peroxide to treat birds in his jail cell. I know several people who have taken this extremely low-cost antibiotic for years, without harmful side effects. It is ideal for swimming pools, well water and cisterns. It keeps water fresh and clear and helps avoid the real damage and danger of chlorine and microorganisms. It is ideal for cleansing your skin of microbes during a bath or shower. No home should be without it.

Unfortunately, the 3% drugstore type now has stabilizers and additives that make it unsuitable for internal use. When people condemn hydrogen peroxide for internal use, they may be condemning the additives. The body makes hydrogen peroxide. It cannot be all that bad. Peroxide and ozone are effective for increasing oxygen levels in the body without damage to normal cells. Hydrogen peroxide taken internally is very effective for curing cancer.

The following quotation comes from Ed McCabe's book *Oxygen therapies* (Page 102) (I have added bullets to highlight the major points.)

One study exposed lung breast and uterine cancer cells, along side normal cells, to ozone over an 8-day period.

- at .3ppm the cancer growth was inhibited 40%.

- at 5ppm yielded a 60% inhibition

- at 8ppm yielded a 90% inhibition and at this level the normal cells showed the first signs of change, lowering activity by 50%.

In *Oxygen Therapies* (Page 82), we find reference to similar results using oxygen with cancer cells in vitro. In laboratory work, high oxygen levels are referred to as high *tensions*. J.B. Kizer, Biochemist/Physicist, Gungnir Research, Portsmouth, Ohio, writes as follows:

Since Warburg's discovery, *(that cancer cells are anaerobic)* this difference in respiration has remained the most fundamental (and some say, only) physiological difference consistently found between normal and cancer cells. Using cell culture studies, I decided to examine the differential response of normal and cancer cells to changes in oxygen environment.

The results that I found were rather remarkable. I found that...high O₂ tensions were lethal to cancer tissue whereas, in general, normal tissues were not harmed by high oxygen tensions.

German doctors have applied ozone therapy millions of times with no toxic side effects. The issue is well presented in a 1993 commercial video called *Ozone and the Politics of Medicine.* (See the SOURCES index for information.) Ozone is safe when used as directed. The research by Dr. Majid Ali regarding the nature of diatomic molecules explains why oxygen in its various forms is not toxic to human cells. In my opinion, we should not be afraid to use oxygen supplements, hydrogen peroxide, and ozone therapy. Indeed, we should fight for the right to have them used by professional caregivers and recommended by mainstream medicine. Millions of lives could be saved and millions of tax dollars made available for other health-care benefits and education. The frightful concept that we may not have any suitable antibiotics because microbes outsmart the antibiotic is false. We will always have oxygen because anaerobic microbes cannot produce enzymes to outsmart oxygen molecules.

Warburg discovered that oxidative enzymes contain iron

In the textbook *Foundations of Biology,* we find reference to this significant discovery by Dr. Otto Warburg (Page 249):

He (Dr. Warburg) was intrigued by the ability of iron-containing compounds to catalyze the oxidation of many different organic substances by using molecular oxygen. Warburg suspected that the iron contained in these compounds was responsible for the catalytic activity. He reasoned that an iron-containing substance is needed in the cell if oxygen is to be activated and used. A search led to the discovery of several iron-containing compounds, the function of which is to carry electrons to molecular oxygen. The compounds are called CYTOCHROMES.

It turned out that a second coenzyme was needed to transport electrons (plus the proton H+) from reduced DPN to molecular oxygen –FLAVON, a derivative of the vitamin riboflavin. It soon became clear that when hydrogen atoms (electrons plus protons H+)

were removed from various substances they were transported by DPN flavin, and iron-containing cytochromes to molecular oxygen with a resulting production of H_2O.

It was this discovery that earned Warburg his Nobel Prize in 1931. He was also nominated for a second Nobel Prize years later for his discovery of a hydrogen transfer enzyme called nicotinamide. Through his research, Warburg has identified the essential metabolic difference between normal human cells and cancer cells. He argued that enzyme production and the switch in metabolism was the cause of cancer, but to no avail. This valuable research has been ignored and suppressed.

How often have you heard or read about Otto Warburg or his research into cancer in mainstream medicine publications? Have you ever even heard of him?

Warburg also explained why fermentation always occurs after the citric acid cycle is interrupted. Both processes share a common enzyme, the nicotinamide. Therefore, this enzyme is always present to take over and switch cellular metabolism to the fermentation process.

Lung cancer leads to death from lack of oxygen transfer enzyme

Dr. Enderlein has established how lactic acid binds with iron to produce "lactic acid ferric oxydul" ($Fe[C_3H_5O_3]-3H_2O$) with catastrophic consequences of the entire respiratory system." Without available free iron for the enzymes needed to transport oxygen from the lungs, human cells cannot function. Cancer patients die even though all their organs can function. As lactic acid builds up, oxygenation decreases, and more lactic acid is produced. Once this chain reaction starts, death through oxygen suffocation follows. (See EXPLORE, Vol. 9, 1999, Page 23.)

In conclusion to this chapter, Health Canada, established to protect public health, has actually banned a low-cost, non-toxic, readily available product capable of inhibiting cancer tumor growth by 60 to 90% and destroying cancer. The banning of ozone therapy in Canada for cancer treatment should be considered a crime against humanity. A class-action suit should be initiated over this issue in order to make ozone therapy available to Canadians. The money we save on taxes for health care would be far greater than the cost of the court action.

17. Eliminate parasites and pollutants to help cure cancer

The purpose of this chapter is to discuss methods for killing fungi and parasites in the body and to discuss the scientific basis for electromagnetic therapy. This issue leads to the legality of manufacturing and selling electromagnetic devices for treating cancer as well as for treating all other microbial diseases. From a legal point of view, having parasites is not considered a disease. Everyone has some fungus in their system. Therefore, it follows that providing a method to eliminate parasites is not a medical issue. No disease is involved.

Based on the theory that cancer starts when microbial growth factors cause normal cells to mutate the proteins in the cancer cell wall, it is obvious that one of the most significant steps to curing cancer is to eliminate fungi and parasites from the body. Since mainstream medicine does not offer any parasite cleansing programs, we have a few problems. Occasionally, we hear about cancer being cured by fungal antibiotics, but this is not very frequent and no effort is made to research the phenomenon. How can we be sure a device or method is safe?

Dr. Costantini states that all cures for human degenerative diseases have only two things in common. They are antifungal or antimycotoxic. It follows that all degenerative diseases can be treated by electromagnetic frequencies which are antifungal or antimycotoxic. Antimycotoxic frequencies disturb the crystalloid structures of bioactive toxins produced by fungi. Cleansing the body of fungal parasites eliminates the source of mycotoxins and helps cure most degenerative diseases.

How does one do a parasite cleanse?

My best answer for that is to purchase and read books by Dr. Clark.

She is the only alternative therapy cancer specialist that I know who has put together a complete program to cleanse your body of toxins, pollutants, and parasites. Her program is described in her books. Her latest book, *Cure for ALL Advanced Cancers* includes a long list of supplements to take. Unfortunately for Canadians, some of these items are banned for sale in

Canada. Importing DHEA, a hormone made from Mexican wild yams, a food product, results in penalties applicable to drug trafficking. Amino acids such as arginine and ornithine are banned for sale in Canada. Ozone therapies are also banned in Canada and you may have difficulty finding an ozone generator. The real problem is political and economic.

Another question is whether to do a parasite cleanse with a zapper, or without. A parasite cleanse can be accomplished by mildly saturating the body for about three weeks with antifungal and antiparasitic herbs, or a parasite cleanse can be accomplished more effectively with fewer herbs and a zapper.

Another problem arises from the politics of medicine. As you will see by the end of this book, Canada's Health Protection Branch suppresses products and devices that would weaken the empire of the existing health care service business. Canada is not unique. History shows a definite program to suppress effective low-cost cancer cures worldwide, other than in Mexico and some island countries.

In Canada, Rene Caisse's medical files were burned to destroy evidence of cancer cures. Gaston Naessens was persecuted for developing a new insight into treating cancer. Even today, effective cancer treatments suppressed in the U.S. are also suppressed in Canada, such as Ozone therapy, Rife technology, CanCell, and Cell Specific Therapy. It is not likely that a zapper capable of destroying virus, fungi, and bacteria in the body will be welcomed into mainstream medicine.

Products and devices that empower people to take control of their own health infringe upon the medical monopoly to provide health care services. Just as the tribal 'medicine-man' guarded his exalted position in society, modern medicine-men do the same through medical associations closely similar in function to labor unions. Both types of associations have their place in society, but both can serve to exploit the public to benefit the workers. No other union has ever had the power taken by the medical authorities to control treatment of disease, eliminate competition, and exploit tax revenues.

One must recognize that a zapper is not a cure for any disease. It is a tool to kill fungi and parasites. It helps the body heal itself to cure diseases caused by infection. The zapper is an electromagnetic tool that generates a functional frequency, just as a microwave oven generates a functional frequency. As you read this page, your body is being zapped, so to speak, with the functional frequency of all your local radio and TV stations. The frequency of a zapper is below that of radio stations, and the current received is less than half of the nine-volt battery. Many people check the strength of a 9 volt battery by placing their tongue on the battery posts. Just as radio waves are considered harmless, zapping with a device producing a similar wave is not potentially harmful. The stability of molecules as described by the quantum theory demands a large quantum of energy to damage DNA molecules and functional proteins.

The key to understanding the function and safety of a zapper, is that the low frequency from a zapper affects only the parasitic life forms of a similar low frequency. Anaerobic parasites that cause human diseases function in a low-range of frequencies. It is not the voltage from the nine-volt battery that kills. It is the off-beat pulsating positive polarity and corresponding magnetic pulses that disturbs microbial paramagnetic enzymes and their function. The jamming of a radio station is closely similar in concept as the zapper jams the bioradiation of parasites.

Resonance in crystalloid structures can be compared to someone pushing a child on a swing. A small push at the right time keeps the swing in motion. An equally small off-beat push disturbs the motion. Much the same type of thing happens to fungi or parasites from the off-beat magnetic frequency of a zapper.

The scientific basis for electromagnetic therapy is very simple. DNA is a crystalloid structure that resonates according to the life form controlling it. RNA is a crystalloid structure transcribed from the DNA crystalloid form and resonates at the same frequency. Functional proteins and enzymes translated from RNA duplicate the crystalloid form and resonate at the same frequency. Proteins are molecules with a specific frequency. Life is a combination of resonant frequencies. DNA is a template for construction of these crystalloid forms we call enzymes and proteins.

The zapper produces a positive offset square wave that disturbs the magnetic resonance of parasitic life forms and the enzymes they produce. Similarly, permanent magnets are able to polarize atoms in the nucleotides and cause a change in polarity. If you place an iron rod beside a permanent magnet for a few hours, the iron rod will pick up a magnetic charge and become a magnet with north and south polarity. The same type of thing happens to molecules in the body that contain iron. Red blood cells sometimes stick together in stacks with limited capacity to transport oxygen. By applying a magnetic field to your body, these stacks separate, enabling you to transfer more oxygen. Zapping does the same thing and measurements using sophisticated oxygen-level measuring devices show an immediate increase in oxygen levels after zapping.

Hundreds of people have tried magnetic therapy and find it beneficial. When and if the monopoly on health care is broken, health care will come out of the dark ages. Free market forces and human ingenuity will produce electromagnetic devices to save lives and millions of tax dollars. But this will not happen until the people organize and make it happen.

The legality of electromagnetic devices to kill parasites

Is it legal to manufacture and distribute an electromagnetic device such as a zapper to help kill parasites?

As far as I can make out it is not illegal to make or import them. It is illegal to make unsubstantiated claims unless the claims are scientifically verifiable and have been proven to authorities. Due to the monopoly on healthcare, *scientifically verifiable* needs defining. Who makes the decisions: scientists or restrictive medical authorities? The following information states the position of the HPB quite clearly.

Please note, due to the length of the quotation, I have not indented the margins. The reference can be found on the Internet under Health Canada. For emphasis of significant points, I have used italics.

ELECTROMAGNETIC DEVICES INTRODUCTION

"Electromagnetic devices sold for home use are often represented as cure-alls and miracle cures. *Some promoters make claims that are not scientifically verifiable and are therefore illegal and deceptive.* The Health Protection Branch has received numerous complaints from people who purchased electromagnetic devices and found them to be ineffective.

These devices usually consist of an electrical control unit or generator, and come with attachments such as local applicators or pads, and cylinders and rings that can be placed around the body or limbs. They can sell for up to five thousands dollars ($5000.00).

Tactics used to promote the sale of these electromagnetic devices include newspaper and magazine ads, word of mouth advertising, and private and public meetings where users of the device, often distributors themselves, present moving and effective testimonials. The promoters often try to imply that the medical profession is trying to prevent access by the public to this therapy while giving the erroneous impression that their claims for the devices are scientifically valid.

CONSUMER, BE AWARE

Consumers should be suspicious of electromagnetic devices that are advertised as an effective treatment for almost every type of ailment, including chronic pain and serious diseases. As well, these products may be misrepresented, and wrongfully promoted, as useful for a wide range of conditions, for example:

- improving blood circulation;

- relaxing the nervous system;

- producing anti-inflammatory effects;

- stimulating cell repair and regeneration;

- not only alleviating symptoms but also influencing the profound causes of illness;

- helping the human body maintain and improve health by reinforcing the body's natural defense and healing mechanisms;

- helping in the process of detoxification, activating the elimination of toxins;

- treating anxiety, arthritis, arthrosis, arteriosclerosis, asthma, back, knee and shoulder pain, burn-out, bursitis, chronic fatigue, depression, diabetes, eczema, hypertension, hypotension, inflammation, insomnia, kidney stones, migraines, phobias, psoriasis, ulcers, etc.

These types of claims are false and misleading! **The effectiveness of electromagnetic fields has only been demonstrated in the promotion of bone regrowth in non-healing bone fractures,** with a specialized electromagnetic device, and following a controlled scientific protocol for this purpose. Non-healing bone fracture is not a common condition and is usually treated under medical supervision. The fact that there is *one recognized medical use for this type of device* under very specific conditions does not make this type of therapy effective for any other type of ailment.

The majority of these devices *do not pose a direct health hazard* to the user. Nevertheless, they can pose an indirect hazard if they cause a patient to delay seeking proper medical treatment for a serious condition. In any case, there is always an economic loss to the user. Additionally, consumers are often upset when the expected results are not obtained and they realize that they have been deceived.

ROLE OF THE HEALTH PROTECTION BRANCH

All medical devices sold in Canada must comply with the Medical Devices Regulations of the Food and Drugs Act. Although the Health Protection

Branch does not routinely test devices for safety and effectiveness, manufacturers are required to do so.

While the Branch has the authority to investigate medical devices problems and to stop the sale of devices when necessary, the Branch concentrates its efforts and resources to serious problems, where there is potential for injury. Problems of a less serious nature, such as deceptive claims, are usually addressed through educational efforts such as this ISSUES document.

WHAT YOU, THE CONSUMER, CAN DO

Consult your family physician or other health care professional if you have a medical problem and are considering buying a device of this type. This will ensure that your problems are treated promptly and properly, and not allowed to deteriorate to an untreatable state. By obtaining professional medical advice you may also save a considerable amount of money and avoid the potential disappointment of being misled.

Be skeptical of electromagnetic devices that claim to treat a wide variety and range of ailments with cures that are quick, painless, simple and miraculous. Ask for all the promotional material for the product. Read the information carefully. Remember that the only medically recognized application of electromagnetic devices is for the promotion of bone regrowth in non-healing bone fractures, and only if the device is specially designed for this purpose and used under specific conditions. (These devices are not usually advertised to the general public.) Any other claim is false and misleading. Beware of personal testimonials. *In most cases, testimonials have not been supported by scientific or medical evidence, and should not be accepted as proof that a product is effective.* Also, be suspicious of claims that the therapy or the product is commonly used in other countries. Other countries may have less stringent regulatory requirements and may not require that claims be supported by data.

Remember that statements such as "Duly registered/Notified with Health Canada" are no indication that the product is endorsed or approved by the Department, but might be used to mislead the consumer into believing that they are. These statements simply means that the manufacturer has informed Health Canada that a device is being offered for sale in Canada, which manufacturers are required to do by law. Notification is not approval by Health Canada.

Do not hesitate to report any complaints and concerns about electromagnetic devices or other suspect medical devices to your local Health Protection Branch Regional Office. You can also report problems with medical devices to the toll-free Medical Devices Hotline at 1-800-267-9675.

In short, be suspicious of aggressive, miracle cure advertising promoting expensive products, and most importantly, remember that if it sounds too good to be true, it probably is!

January 12, 1995

Electromagnetic Devices is one of a series of Issues produced by the Health Protection Branch of Health Canada for the public, media, and special interest groups. For additional copies of Issues contact: Health Canada"

End of report.

Discussion of false and misleading claims

There is one main point that should be carefully noted.

These types of claims are false and misleading! The effectiveness of electromagnetic fields has only been demonstrated in the promotion of bone regrowth in non-healing bone fractures, with a specialized electromagnetic device, and following a controlled scientific protocol for this purpose

It seems to me that the statement that these *claims are false and misleading*, is itself a false and misleading statement. The benefits of electromagnetic therapy outside of bone healing have been scientifically established through the medical patent for electrocuting microbes in blood. In addition, claims to increase healing with electromagnetic stimulation have been established for both bones and tissue. Why would claims for rapid healing of cells other than bone not be accepted? What is so special about bone cell growth since it follows tissue growth?

The research of Robert Becker illustrates that electromagnetic frequencies increase growth. Cancer starts with an injury to epithelial cells. New growth is required to repair the injury, and new growth can be enhanced by electromagnetic devices. Increasing electrical stimulation of epithelial cells will lead to faster replication and healing, just as it increases bone growth.

In my opinion, magnetic healing for tissue cells is just not being recognized by a suppressive medical society. In the book, *365 Surprising Scientific Facts, Breakthroughs, and Discoveries,* by Sharon B. McGrayne, she discusses the significance of accidents in leading to important discoveries. On Page 5, we learn that that the study of "the effect of electric fields on cell division" led to the discovery of "cisplatin, the first heavy metal anticancer drug." After discovering electric fields increased rate of cell division, they developed toxic heavy metal drugs to retard the rate of cell division. As a result, new cells to repair an injury cannot be formed and the real cause of cancer is not corrected.

Heavy metals are toxic. Drugs are costly. Why not just use a harmless electromagnetic energy field to increase cell division and allow the body to heal the injury? The drug cisplatin is just another instance of pharmaceutical companies designing the wrong drugs to solve a problem that could be solved much more effectively and cheaper with electrotherapy.

The following reference from the Internet relates to the suppressed cancer cure using blood electrification to eliminate microorganisms in blood. This method had proven itself effective for curing AIDS and other viral diseases but it is not available in Canada or the U.S. It also establishes credibility in the effectiveness of vibrational devices to kill virus, fungi, and bacteria.

Would proof that a patent was issued for devices such as this qualify as scientific verification for the principle of zapping blood to kill microorganisms in the body? If so, would it be legal to make claims that such a device is effective for killing parasites based on the claims in the patent? Let's review the abstract of this amazing patent that could save Canadian taxpayers millions of dollars, reduce pain and suffering, and save Canadian Medicare from a two-tier system.

Blood electrification. Patent 5,139,684, granted Aug 18 1992 (filed Nov 16, 1990)

Electrically conductive method and systems for treatment of blood and other body fluids and/or synthetic fluids with electric forces

Inventors: Dr. Steven Kaali and Peter Schwolsky

Abstract:

A new process and system for treatment of blood and/or other body fluids and/or synthetic fluids from a donor to a recipient or storage receptacle or in a recycling system using novel electrically conductive treatment vessels for treating blood and/or other body fluids and/or synthetic fluids with electric field forces of appropriate electric field strength to provide electric current flow through the blood or other body fluids at a magnitude that is biologically compatible but is sufficient to render the bacteria, virus, and/or fungus ineffective to infect normally healthy cells while maintaining the biological usefulness of the blood or other fluids. For this purpose the low voltage electric potentials applied to the treatment vessel should be of the order of from about 0.2 to 12 volts and should produce current flow densities in the blood or other fluids of from one microampere per square millimeter of electrode area exposed to the fluid being treated to about two milliamperes per square millimeter. Treatment time within this range of parameters may range for a period of time from about one minute to about 12 minutes.

U.S. References Cited: 15 patents: #'s 5049252, 3994799, 4473449, 5133932, 2490730, 3692648, 3753886, 3878564, 3965008, 4616640, 4770167, 4932421, 5058065, 5133932, 592735, 672231

Foreign References Cited: 1 patent: # SU 995848

Other References Cited:

Journal of the Clinical Investigation published by the American Society for Clinical Investigations, Inc, vol. 65, Feb 1980, pp. 38of:

Photodynamic Inactivation of Herpes Simplex Viruses- Lowell E Schnipper
Journal of Clinical Microbiology, vol. 17, No 2, Feb 1983:

Photodynamic Inactivation of Pseudorabier Virus with Methylene Blue Dye, Light and Electricity- Janine A Badyisk

Proceedings of the Society for Experimental Biology & Medicine, vol. 1, 1979, pp. 204-209: Inactivation of Herpes Simplex Virus with Methylene Blue, Light and Electricity- Mitchell R Swartz
To view a picture of the original patent click here, click 'View Images', and then click BACK twice to return here.

To see this patent description of experiments testing electric currents ability to disable HIV click here.

End of report.

The patent was issued in 1992 and immediately put into mothballs by mainstream medicine in all Western countries. Although the original patent specified removal of the blood, thereby restricting it to being a professional service, word leaked out that zapping blood internally was just as effective. There is no advantage to removing the blood providing care is taken to oxidize dead fungi and bacteria. Be careful to avoid overloading the body's cleansing system. The process empowers a person to take control of his or her own health and eliminates the need for medical fees, prescription fees, and drugs. Imagine how this could benefit the economy, reduce medical expenses, and reduce hospital corridor overload, if it were made available by mainstream medicine. In my opinion, hospital overload is a ploy to increase government funding for health care because alternative therapies are suppressed.

The zapping process is being described at alternative health fairs across Canada and USA as well as other publications not controlled by mainstream medicine. In 1991, press releases on the invention appeared in magazines such as Science News (March 30, Page 207), and newspapers such as The Houston Post, Wed. March 20, 1991. Thousands of people are now using a zapper for parasite cleansing. In my opinion, based on several years of use, electromagnetic devices to treat infection are safe and effective. These devices will help prevent cancer by eliminating fungi and bacteria. Mainstream medicine should be promoting them. They help treat infection and infection causes cancer. There is a lot more to curing cancer than eliminating parasites, but cancer cannot be cured without first doing so.

Let's review the following diseases or conditions that may benefit from electromagnetic therapy as *considered false and misleading by the Health Protection Branch*. Can any of these diseases be considered as viral or fungal? Can any of these be considered as a problem relating to epithelial layers in the body? If so, could they benefit from the proper electromagnetic therapy? The answer to all questions is "yes."

- arthritis, arteriosclerosis, asthma, back, knee and shoulder pain, bursitis, chronic fatigue, depression, diabetes, eczema, hypertension, hypotension, inflammation, insomnia, kidney stones, migraines, phobias, psoriasis, ulcers, etc.

Please note that the warning does not mention use for or against treating HIV infected blood, AIDS or other viral diseases. There is substantial medical proof in the medical patent 5,139,684 that zapping kills the HIV virus. Why wouldn't it kill other viruses? After reading this warning, would you have any reason to try one of these devices? All I see is a warning to be aware of unproven claims. By not mentioning these proven uses that led to a medical patent, they reader is led away from using them for proven uses as well. This is another example of deceptive misinformation produced by Canada's Health Protection Branch.

Diabetes deserves special mention, as there are about 2 million Canadians now taking regular insulin shots. Just as cancer cells do not knit with adjacent cells due to microbial contamination during replication, it is very probable that microbial proteins mutate insulin so that it fails to function. Insulin is required to transport proteins across cell-wall membranes, and mutated insulin cannot do so. As mentioned earlier, healthy cells require the transport mechanism of both insulin and growth hormones. One of the cancer markers is called 'insulin-like' growth factor. Is mutated insulin enzyme capable of transporting proteins and carbohydrates to feed cancer tumor cells due to cell wall mutations?

Receptors in the cell wall of cancer cells are different from receptors in the cell wall of normal cells, giving cancer cells a nutritional advantage from mutated insulin. If microbes have mutated both the cell-wall receptors and insulin—a glucose and protein carrier—the recognition of IGF (insulin-like growth factor) becomes obvious.

According to *Harper's Review of Biochemistry* (Page 511), insulin contains 21 amino acids in the A chain and 30 in the B chain, connected by 31 connecting peptides, so any mutation produced by substitution of human amino acids by microbial amino acids could account for the lack of normal function. Dr. Clark finds that people who follow a parasite cleanse program can reduce insulin dependency significantly within a few weeks. There is probably a microbial mutation in insulin that reduces the capacity of insulin to support metabolism of proteins and sugars by normal cells but increases it in cancer cells.

Dr. Johanna Budwig made the following point in a lecture she gave in 1959. The statement can be found in the book, *Flax oil as a true aid against arthritis, heart infarction, cancer and other diseases,* by (Page 12):

> The basic problem with diabetes is really impairment of the fats metabolism system and not that of the conversion of sugar. The sugar assimilation problem is secondary.

I have not found that statement repeated in any of the medical textbooks. Imagine what a bonus our health care system would have if 2 million diabetics could be relieved from taking daily insulin shots? Imagine too, what a bonus it would be to those with diabetes.

Effectively killing fungi and bacteria with an electromagnetic frequency in the safe voltage range of .02 volts has been scientifically established by research into patent 5,139,684. In my opinion, Health Canada is making statements that are false and misleading by refusing to recognize the microbial cause of cancer and suppressing electromagnetic therapy as a treatment for infection.

In the book *Discovery of Magnetic Health*, 1998 New Edition, by George Washnis, we can read more than 300 pages of testimonial material on the health benefits of magnetic therapies. Washnis says (Page 89):

> ... the individual's freedom of choice remains a cornerstone of the American system. . . the system does not allow the doctor and his patient the choice of treatments, even when that treatment is safe and reliable.

Considering the financial consequences to the health-care business of electromagnetic healthcare, it is profitable to permit electromagnetic stimulation of bones that do not heal, because these professional devices will increase business and profits. However, it is not profitable to permit use of hand-held electromagnet devices to eliminate fungal and parasitic infections that cause the majority of human diseases. A low-cost house-hold electromagnet stimulation device to cure disease is a threat to the healthcare industry. It is, however, quite a bonus to the electronics industry such as Radio Shack where you can buy the components to build your own zapper according to the design disclosed in books by Dr. Hulda Clark. Generally speaking, if you can locate a source for factory made quality and additional features, it is well worth while. The price of quality made zappers ranges from 90 to 300 dollars depending on features.

It is a well-known fact that numerous effective herbs have been suppressed from the Canadian marketplace. Herbs are simply plants with a recognized functional frequency in the proteins produced by them. When we consume food or herbs, the crystalloid molecules in the plants produced by them to fight viral and fungal infection, is ingested, and used by the body. Herbs are plants that produce molecules with a functional frequency to resist virus, fungi, and bacteria. It is perfectly logical that the different life-stages of bacteria and fungi, replicating in our body, must be attacked by corresponding different frequencies because each life stage has a unique frequency. If you do not attack all life-stages simultaneously, you must maintain an application program that allows eggs to hatch and early-life stages to mature into organisms with a bioradiation frequency that can be zapped.

A combination of three or four herbs will have a synergistic effect, not available from a single herb or drug. The concept of killing all life-stages of fungi and bacteria simultaneously to eliminate the cycle of life is perfectly scientific. The combination of electromagnetic frequencies and herbal remedies is scientifically sound. Maintaining a three-week cleanse is scientifically sound. It is far more scientific than taking a single toxic drug capable of killing only one life stage.

To do a parasite cleanse, you must kill all life-stages. Using herbs and electromagnetic energy makes perfect sense.

The weak voltage and vibrational frequency produced by a zapper does not enter all parts of the body, such as the contents of the colon, eyeballs, or testicles. The highly polarized membrane surrounding these organs, or their location in the body, does not allow the weak zapper energy to enter. Present research indicates that a zapper combined with herbs produces the most effective results. Destroying parasites in tissue does not have any lasting effect if the contents of the colon or an infected root-canal provides a continuous supply of more microbes. When an electromagnet device does not appear to be effective, the problem could be that of continuous reinfection. The whole field is relatively new and it is difficult to make headway when the government health department stands in the way of progress. If dedicated mainstream medical doctors were allowed to research and pursue this course openly, health-care costs would plummet beyond our greatest expectations.

18. Avoid hydrogenated oils to help prevent cancer

The Cancer Research Institute of Paris, equipped with the largest state-of-the art electron microscope in existence has found that the only substance that characterized the cancerous cells, as opposed to the normal cells, was isolated fat. It was the single distinguishing feature of cancerous cells in contrast to healthy ones.

The above statement can be found in the book, *Flax oil as a true aid against arthritis, heart infarction, cancer, and other diseases,* by Dr. Johanna Budwig (Page 4).

What is the significance of isolated fat being found in cancer cells but not in normal cells?

The process of catabolism and anabolism takes a considerable amount of ATP or energy. This would be missing in a cell functioning on fermentation, and fat molecules could not be broken down if they are hydrogenated already. Consequently, fat molecules would not be assimilated. Fungus and bacteria would have a distinct energy advantage to supply the cell-wall proteins and enzymes that mutate the cell wall.

It could also be that hydrogenated fats were not suitable for use as the lipid portion of the cell-wall membrane. It could be excess fat. Perhaps the cell prepared sufficient fat molecules to complete mitosis and build two new cell-wall membranes, but proteins were inserted instead. The amount of excess fat would be equal to the amount of microbial protein incorporated into the cell-wall membrane by microbial enzymes.

The focus of the above research illustrates that researchers have not been investigating the cell-wall membrane for abnormalities. They have not checked the plasma quality of the cell, because, in researching the contents of the cell, they had to destroy the cell-wall membrane.

The point of the reference is that the cause of cancer is not inside the cell or the DNA. The cause of cancer is in the cell-wall membrane and its plasma qualities. The replacement of normal unsaturated fat by hydrogenated fats will change the phospho-lipid traits of the cell wall. This probably allows for microbial invasion and infection.

Dr. Budwig is not alone in viewing a connection between saturated fats such as margarine and the cause of cancer. The President of the Nobel Prize Committee in Stockholm had already concluded that fat plays an important part in all human diseases. He is quoted as saying: "when living tissue rejects some fats, the body isolates them—and this is the crux—and deposits them in places where fats are not normally found". Bauer, whose book, *The Problem with Cancer,* has made him world famous, wrote in his 1966 edition "everything points to fats playing an enormous role in this problem."

Budwig goes on to say (Page 7), that the significant difference between the two fats is that saturated "fatty acid chains with their weak, unsaturated connections, form protein associations very easily. The fatty acids become water soluble through this association with protein." The saturated fatty acids cannot form associations with protein, cannot dissolve in water or cytoplasm, and remain as so much useless junk occupying the cell or cellular environment. A cell functioning on the fermentation process cannot ferment the fat, nor can it assemble enough energy in the form of ATP to break down the fat.

She writes (Page 9): "The solid fats which are not water soluble and cannot associate with proteins are no longer capable of circulating through the fine capillary networks. The blood thickens and circulation problems arise. . .The solidified, inert bulk fats act as further hindrances in the blood.

The most significant statement being made is that saturated fatty acids cannot be readily connected to protein to form the cell-wall protein-lipid molecules.

In the book *Fats and Oils* by Udo Erasmus (Page 272) we read:

Blood samples from people who have cancer, diabetes, and some kinds of liver disease (a frequent forerunner of cancer) consistently lack one of the essential fatty acids, the doubly unsaturated linoleic acid. These blood samples also consistently lack the substances of which linoleic acid is part: the phosphatides of the cell membranes; and a type of blood lipoprotein now identified as fatty acid-carrying albumin.

The lack of phosphatides helps to explain the polyploidy of cancer, the fact that cancer cells often have multiple sets of chromosomes. The genetic material divides, but the cell membranes can't be produced, due to the lack of the material from which they are made. Cell division remains incomplete.

The lack of the essential phosphatides is all that is required to create a cancer cell. That's the one essential type of molecule required to create a plasma barrier and an energy meridian to form a functional membrane. Without a strong barrier, cells become infected with fungus.

If cells replicate due to normal growth, and both microbial infection and the current of injury are absent, nutritional deficiencies of suitable cell-wall material would result in a cell being rejected for its membrane deficiencies. Perhaps some benign growths are caused this way. Lumps in the breast, for example, are formed from cells that replicate and are rejected due to chemical toxins such as estrogen, but the current of injury has not been turned on to cause rapid out-of-control replication. Subsequent injury (mammogram or probe) causes injury and cancer.

The other interesting point about the lack of any significant differences in the cell, other than fat, is that the metabolism of the cell may have switched, without any telltale sign in the DNA or other cell components. Defective genes are not required to switch metabolism as the process is environmental and within normal cell functions.

Here's where hormones such as estrogen or lipid molecules from chemicals or bacteria enter the cancer picture. In the absence of unsaturated fatty acids, the cell-wall membrane is assembled with whatever fat is available or whatever is most dominant in the cytoplasm. The cell wall is assembled, but the resonant frequency does not allow the new cell to knit with the normal cells. Cellular contaminants mutate the cell wall but only cause benign growths.

In support of the above concept that estrogen ends up in the cell-wall membrane, Budwig writes (Page 17):

> It has already been clearly established that carcinogens, or chemical substances which are known to cause cancer, attach themselves to the parts of the cell which reproduce the protein substance, and in the external lipoid membrane, which is where the highly unsaturated fats are localized.

According to Budwig, the highly saturated fats are localized in the lipoid membrane, and these fats lack the phosphatides necessary to form a phospholipid cell-wall membrane. All of this fits in perfectly with the cause of cancer rising from a mutated cell wall. In this case, the mutation is from toxins and contamination.

If a cell has toxins such as ammonia that stops the citric acid cycle, fermentation would continue to metabolize food nutrients. In addition, if these cells lack nutrients for a healthy plasma cell-wall membrane, these cells could continue to multiply and be continually rejected by the normal membrane cells. The cell walls would not contain chitin or microbial proteins, but they could contain DDT or estrogen molecules and lack the essential lipid layers and phosphatides necessary to knit with an existing membrane.

Since references to fungus and bacteria as carcinogens are not found in medical texts on cancer, I doubt if I could find any significant research establishing defective cell-wall membranes as the cause of cancer. Nevertheless, I continued to look for a significant distinguishing feature that would probably be identifiable in all cancer cells.

In the 1971 edition of *Textbook of Anatomy and Physiology*, I found a significant clue. The cell-wall membrane is described as being a double layer of *polarized lipid* molecules.

Polarization of the lipid layers was the answer. The cell membrane has two polarized layers of lipid-protein molecules although it is only about 75 Angstroms thick. In order to understand how such a thin membrane can function, it is necessary to view the bilateral layer as producing the effect of a 'magnetic-bottle' that allows it to function. This polarization of unsaturated lipids serves as the magnetic glue that forms the cell-wall membrane. Use of saturated fats in large sections of the cell wall fails to produce the magnetic-bottle effect. Consequently these cells do not attract to normal cells, and do not knit to repair an injury. In the future, researchers should look for the difference between normal cells and cancer cells by measuring the electrical conductivity of the cell wall.

In cancer cells, the protein portion of the lipid-protein molecules in the membrane consists of two different forms; one transcribed from human RNA, the other transcribed from microbial RNA. This would result in two different resonant frequencies from almost identical structures. Visual inspection of the lipid layer fails to identify the change in resonant frequency. To identify cancer cells, researchers should be measuring the resonant frequencies and comparing them to normal cells. Cancer tumors could be located by their resonant frequency.

These are the frequencies that Royal Rife discovered back in the 1930s and used to cure cancer patients, until his equipment was confiscated and his work was suppressed. With modern equipment, we should be able to identify cancer cell-wall membrane frequencies and possibly identify the cause of cancer, as being either microbial or contamination.

In my notes on the Rife frequency generator used to kill cancer cells using a modern hand held beam tube, we read:

Type of cancer	frequency (Khz)
Breast cancer	2008 –2128

Carcinoma	2127
Leukemia	2127
Sarcoma	2008

Several videocassettes are available that show bacteria swimming in a medium, which I think is blood plasma. As you view the video, you can see the cell-wall membrane disintegrate and the contents of the cell spill out. It is truly unbelievable that millions of people are being denied this amazing cancer cure. A three-day interval for treatment is required to allow the body to cleanse itself from the dead bacteria and contents of their cells. Imagine giving yourself a three minute painless electromagnetic energy wave every third day to destroy an existing tumor. Rife did this more than fifty years ago.

Although Royal Rife and Edgar Cayce were contemporary Americans, I cannot find any references that they knew each other. There are no references in Rife's work relating to the current of injury.

As I mentioned earlier, I have found only one reference to this theory describing how microbes cause cancer and that is from the readings of Edgar Cayce. Cayce said: "Cancer is that which lives upon the cellular force by the growth of itself...caused by breaking of tissue internally, which was not covered sufficiently by the leukocyte due to the low vitality in the system." A low vitality and leukocyte count could also account for pollutants entering the cell cytoplasm to mutate the cell membrane during normal mitosis.

Fat does not cause breast cancer

Fat is often implicated as being a cause of breast cancer. The fact that both male and female abdomens, hips and buttocks often have extensive fatty deposits but do not experience cancer frequently proves that fat deposits are not an immediate cause of cancer. Fat tissue does not contain sugar to cause fungal fermentation. Fat tissue does not replicate due to a field of injury because fat tissue does not contain a nucleus with DNA. Blood sugars and proteins are not deposited in the fat tissue as they are in the lymphatic system to nourish energy producing cells. If there is nothing to ferment, fermentation cannot take place and fungi cannot multiply.

Udo Erasmus in his book *Fats and Oils* (Page 101), tells us:

It has been shown that many kinds of cancers are associated with diets high in fats. It can also be shown that the increase in the occurrence of cancer parallels the increase in the consumption of fats of vegetable origin, and more closely with the increase in consumption of hydrogenated vegetable oils.

I believe the relationship between fat and cancer can be found in the mechanism of fermentation of excess food nutrients.

All cells have a phospho-lipid layer with proteins woven into the cell-wall membrane as receptors. This membrane is quite a remarkable achievement. It is capable of engulfing large protein molecules to bring them into the cell. It also allows nutrients into the cell for metabolism, allows waste products out, but keeps most of the contents of the cell from leaking out. The cell also gives form to the tissues. In addition to that, the cell converts glucose to energy and delivers excess energy to the body.

Fatty degeneration increases metabolic disorders

In order for the cell wall to take in large molecules of protein, the cell wall must flow around and engulf the molecule. When we consume hydrogenated oils and fats, such as deep-fried foods, margarine, or shortening, we load our body with a fat that does not provide the cell wall with the flexibility it needs. Consequently, large protein molecules in the lymphatic system cannot be assimilated into the cells. If these nutrients are not removed by the lymphatic system, they commence to ferment and produce ammonia.

Dr. Guyton teaches medical students how cells take in nutrients and discusses the consequences of the failure to do so. See *Textbook of Medical Physiology* (Pages 19 to 54) (Italics added.):

If a cell is to live and grow, it must obtain nutrients and other substances from the surrounding fluids. Substances can pass through a cell membrane in three separate ways:

(1) by diffusion through the pores in the membrane or through the membrane matrix itself.

(2) By active transport through the membrane, a mechanism in which enzyme systems and special carrier substances "carry" the substance through the membrane.

(3) By endocytosis (or pinocytosis), a mechanism by which the membrane actually engulfs particulate matter or extracellular fluid and its contents.

Dr. Guyton also states:

The real importance of pinocytosis to the body is that this is the only known means by which very large molecules, such as those of protein, can be transported to the interior of the cells.

Take a moment to apply the above information to the immune system and white blood cells that engulf invaders to render them harmless.

The outer wall of white blood cells must be able to engulf invaders in order to have a healthy immune system.

Have your cells become hydrogenated?

Dr. Cass Igram in his book *Eat Right to Live Long* has a major section on the dangers of hydrogenated oils. He writes (Page 35):

> Would you believe in the probability, you are 'partially hydrogenated?' Over the years, you have developed untold thousands of hardened (hydrogenated) cells. This is because these cells have inserted into their membranes trans-fatty-acids from a dose of margarine or from some French fries cooked in a deep fryer, etc.
>
> An example of this is what happens to white blood cells. These cells incorporate the hydrogenated fats you eat into their membranes. When this happens, the white cells become sluggish in function and their membranes actually become stiff! Such white blood cells are poor defenders against infection. This leaves the body wide open to all sorts of derangement of the immune system. Cancer or infections by yeast, bacteria and viruses can more easily take a foothold.
>
> Chemically altered and hydrogenated fats are no longer a food. They, in effect, become a poison, polluting the body's cells and organs. Once deposited within the tissues, these fats damage the cells and organs.

Consider reducing the amount of hydrogenated oils in your diet. You will have to avoid all deep fried-foods, baked goods cooked with shortening, margarine, baked goods containing lard, imitation ice cream, candy bars, chocolates, frozen or pre-packaged dinners, mayonnaise, and any products containing hydrogenated oils.

Udo Erasmus in his book on *Fats and Oils* describes the problems related to fatty degeneration complete with chemical terminology and diagrams. He describes how cell walls formed from hydrogenated oils do not have the same flexibility of as cell walls formed from normal oils. Then he writes the following summary of health-related damages from processed fats in Western society (Page 78):

> *Hydrogenation,* a process also introduced on a large scale in the 1930's for making margarine and shortenings as cheaper substitutes for butter and lard, respectively, has resulted in so many altered fat substances in our diet that just one of them, the *trans*-fatty acids,

make up twice as much food additives in our diet as all other food additives combined.

We ended up with fats and oils which are the nutritional equivalent of the refined sugars in carbohydrate nutrition: demineralized, de-vitaminized, fiber-less, empty calories which cannot be properly digested and metabolized, which rob the body of its stores of minerals and vitamins, which lead to deficiency states in these essential substances, and which lead to fatty degeneration in all of its many forms.

Based on the function of the cell wall to take in oxygen, mineral ions, and protein particles, as well as eliminate carbon dioxide and digestive residue, it is important to maintain a diet with essential fatty acids and oils that are non-hydrogenated. Developing a cancer free life-style includes learning about the dangers of margarine and hydrogenated oils. The low-cholesterol benefit of margarine is far outweighed by its saturated fat danger.

More mycotoxins in a high fat diet

Dr. Costantini's book *Fungalbionics*, provides an explanation for the apparent relationship between fat and cancer, as well as other diseases. Modern diets contain too much processed fat and oils, margarine, and deep-fried foods made from damaged crops (Page 70).

It is now commonly accepted that a high fat diet may increase the incidence of a number of cancers in humans. Not appreciated is the fact that plant-derived oils and margarine are made from the lowest quality stored grains and nuts (corn, peanuts, sunflower, etc.) **The "oil seeds" are characteristically colonized by very large numbers of toxicogenic fungi and may contain significant amounts of mycotoxins.**

Fat made from low-quality, damaged, fungi-infected plant material and oils will supply mycotoxins that lead to the destruction of enzymes and substrates. One might assume that high temperatures found in deep-frying will destroy the mycotoxins, but this is not the case. Poison mushrooms, for example, are still deadly after deep-frying because the heat does not destroy the mycotoxin. Mycotoxins survive food processing and cooking. As you see, there is more to curing cancer than just eliminating parasites. We must develop a cancer-free lifestyle.

19. Developing a cancer-free lifestyle

Knowing the true cause of cancer enables you to prevent cancer and treat it by removing the cause and mechanisms that support cancer. Only you can apply this knowledge to your life through modification of your lifestyle. This doesn't involve your doctor. Doctors specialize in treatment, not prevention. Prevention takes time, specialized knowledge, and costs money too. The benefits of good health and an active, full life are well worth the extra cost and effort.

Microbial enzymes disturb human-cell metabolism

Avoid thinking in terms of diseases, defective genes, microbes, and parasites. The correct term is simply *disease conditions*. Remember that enzymes control all biological chemical actions. There are only two sources for enzymes: human and microbial. Microbial enzymes, proteins, and lipids cause disease when they take the place of the corresponding human unit. Cancer is a process based on conditions in the body. We cure and prevent cancer by controlling the conditions that cause cancer.

Conditions allow for the fermentation of sugars, starches, and blood nutrients. Conditions allow for fungi and parasites to thrive, and conditions allow cells to be injured and replication required. You cannot focus on just one part of the problem.

Good health follows from maintaining conditions suitable for normal human cells to maintain aerobic metabolism. It all starts with ingestion, and assimilation of food nutrients at the cellular level. Remember Dr. Guyton's important points about cellular fluids (Page 3):

Intracellular fluids differ significantly from the extracellular fluids; particularly, it contains large amounts of potassium, magnesium, and phosphate ions instead of sodium and chloride ions found in the extracellular fluid. Special mechanisms for transporting ions through the cell membrane maintain these differences (Page 3)

Dr. Guyton goes on to say (Page 22):

In addition to membrane transport of sodium, energy from ATP is required for transport of potassium ions, chloride ions, urate ions, hydrogen ions, and still many other special substances. Membrane transport is so important to cellular function that some cells, the renal tubular cells for instance, use as much as 80% of the ATP formed in the cells for this purpose alone.

The importance of daily intake of essential fatty acids cannot be overstressed. The information required is far too much to do an adequate review in this book. Just as you should take the time to learn about minerals, you should also take time to learn about essential fatty acids and the dangers of hydrogenated oils.

Dr. Johanna Budwig (Seven time Nobel Prize nominee) explains why fats govern all aspects of the human body. In a nutshell, essential fatty acids are required for electrical energy and hormones. Books by Udo Erasmus and other researchers explain how processed oils destroy the ability of cell walls to maintain function. Margarine and processed oils are a major problem.

Our soils are depleted of minerals. Fertilizers containing only NPK (Nitrogen, Phosphorous, and Potassium) are deficient in 57 known minerals found in good soils. It is very difficult to obtain a diet adequate in minerals, even if we avoid processed and junk foods. Supplements are no longer an option. They are required. As Judi Vance writes in her book *Beauty to Die For, The Cosmetic Consequence*, "Health isn't a given, but it's yours for the taking." You take good health through what you eat, digest and assimilate.

Suggestions for a healthy metabolic lifestyle

The following note is presented so that you might educate yourself towards living a healthier lifestyle. I do not for a moment presume to have the background or training to advise you, or anyone, on specifics. You can learn a lot by going to health fairs and searching the Internet. Just be aware that there is a lot of misinformation being promoted by mainstream medicine and the processed food industry.

You are a unique person with a unique life-style, food preferences, and customs. Do not expect to find the perfect menu for your good health in someone's formula. Develop your own.

Become a professional health-care person for your body. Keep notes and references of your nutrition and emotions. Become aware of how you feel after what you have eaten and of what you do, such as exercise or physical work. Purchase a three-ring binder with at least 15 dividers. Take time every day to read and make notes about your food choices that day and why you made them. Good health is your most valuable asset in life. Take time to protect it.

Start your self-education process by creating a file on your lifestyle and how your present knowledge and beliefs affect your health. If you are not in good health, what are you doing that is wrong for you? Record what you do, eat, drink, and how you feel from doing what you do.

Give yourself a section in your notebook on oxygen, the most vital element in the body. Find out how many ways you can increase oxygen levels in your body. If you are ill, try an oxygen supplement. Ozonated water or water with a few drops of 35% food grade hydrogen peroxide is the least expensive and most effective method available to increase the oxygen in your system.

Give yourself another section on water. Some researchers claim distilled water is beneficial, others claim it is not. Through the above method, I discovered bottled distilled water to be the worst water for my health and energy levels. Distilled bottled water is polluted with chemicals from the container. It is also dead or lacking in vital trace minerals. Measure your distilled water with a pH tape. It will be acidic rather than neutral. The more you drink, the more acidic you become. Reverse-osmosis water is marginally better. Fresh tap water filtered through a solid carbon block or ceramic filter is ideal. Check it out and study the literature. Read the book, *Reverse Aging*, by Sang Whang for this most vital information on the magnetic charges in water. Water is an essential mineral. Drinking soft drinks or processed juices in place of water deprives your body of its most essential minerals and adds more sugar and toxins.

Remember that water is paramagnetic and is capable of serving as a catalyst for numerous chemical reactions in your body. Dr. William Phillpott, as well as numerous other researchers, report that ordinary water charged with the south-seeking pole of a magnet will greatly increase the value of water you drink. The addition of trace minerals helps water carry a negative charge, making it even better as an antibiotic and as a free-radical scavenger. It is very possible that water gives life to things because it resonates with the earth and this resonance makes it function as a catalyst for bioactive reactions. Water is water and should be taken straight.

Give yourself a section on silver amalgam fillings that are 50% mercury. If you believe amalgam fillings are safe in your mouth, find out why they must be disposed of as toxic waste after they are removed. Mercury is a deadly poison. Don't ruin your health by repairing your teeth with the wrong type of fillings. Don't believe that amalgam fillings are safe. There is far too much evidence to the contrary. How can mercury be a deadly poison everywhere except in your mouth?

Give yourself another section on margarine, and saturated fats if you still believe these chemicals and toxins are good for you. Give yourself a section on cholesterol if you believe it is a significant cause of hardening of the arteries. Remember that cholesterol is only made from carbohydrates by the liver. Eggs do not give you cholesterol, nor does meat or protein in reasonable amounts. Take time to read books that teach you how to balance your carbohydrates, fats and protein intake. All are essential to good health for most people.

Read the book by Barry Sears *Mastering the Zone* to learn how to balance meals for protein, fat, and carbohydrates. Don't rely on the Canadian or American food guides for proper balance. These guides have commercial influences. Millions of people live healthy lives without following these food guides.

Sears writes about the marketing of processed foods as a war between consumers and producers (Page 263):

It's a war out there. In fact, every time you enter the supermarket, consider it a war zone. It's you versus the food industry. And it's not fair. The food manufacturers have the high-tech weapons (e.g., marketing and packaging). You don't. They have the resources (e.g. advertising). You don't. The only thing you have in your favor is knowledge. Put that knowledge to work, and you can win the battle and the war.

The war-zone extends far beyond the grocery store. The whole health service industry is a war zone. There is so much conflicting information attached to health services, it is next to impossible to make rational decisions. Take one step at a time. Don't simply give up.

Researchers have found that cholesterol serves to protect our health by binding mycotoxins and microorganisms so they do less harm to the body. High levels of cholesterol may indicate a high level of mycotoxins in the body. Millions of people are taking cholesterol-lowering drugs with toxic side effects. Get the facts about this great American rip-off.

Give yourself a section on amino acids. Learn how to get them in food and supplements. Learn how vital they are for all life processes. Dr. Abram Hoffer's book, *Hoffer's Laws of Natural Nutrition*, provides an excellent source of nutritional data. When a food element is considered essential, doesn't it make sense to ensure you are getting an adequate amount in your diet? Doesn't it make sense that you know something about all of the essential nutrients? No one can do this for you.

Add other sections on vitamins and minerals. Many vitamin and mineral supplements are just toxins in our body. Our body digests food, or nutrients that have been taken up into plant membranes and given life or processed from bacteria or other life forms. Minerals such as ground-up calcium mined from the earth are not assimilated, and could be toxic to your health. Be careful with low-cost mineral supplements. All supplements with labels saying USP are manufactured chemicals. They may do more harm than good.

The Master Formula, my preferred supplement, is made from a combination of grains and all essential nutrients required by the body. Check it out on the Internet or see SOURCES for a booklet on this fabulous supplement. I am willing to endorse this product sold by multi-level networking, because I use it myself and it offers a convenient well-balanced nutritional package.

Remember your daily needs for supplements are always changing. Recommendations on bottles do not cover all situations. RDAs are recommended daily allowances to prevent death. What you need is the ODA, or optimal daily amount for you at this time in your life. Vitamin B6, for example, is an essential vitamin for production of energy. The harder you work, or exercise, the more you need. When taking supplements, review and record your body's response. The book *Young Again* by John Thomas gives you an outstanding self-test to score your biophysical age and observe your response to changes in nutritional supplements and lifestyle.

The Multi-Versa health strategy course

If all of the above research sounds like too much for you, most of it has all been done for you in one book by Penelope Coville and Kathleen Briglio. The material is presented in a 16-chapter self-instructional course that comes with a 45-minute video. The video focuses on specific exercises to cleanse the lymphatic system by exercising those muscles that pump lymph out of the intracellular spaces and lymph nodes to the colon for elimination of wastes. The video also teaches you how to maximize your time on a rebounder so that you exercise effectively. See Internet at www.trafford.com and go to the health section for details.

The course is based on the experience of a group of women in Victoria, B. C. who were successful in overcoming chronic fatigue. It is called The Multi-Versa Health Strategy. Multi-versa means *many ways*, and you can easily adapt the material to fit your needs.

Alternative health specialists can use the guide as a textbook for group discussions, along with a group exercise program similar to aerobic classes and weight-loss clinics. Alternately, individuals and families can use it for family activity and disease-prevention program. If you do not have Internet access, contact Feel Better Books for details. (See glossary.)

Before you can improve your health through lifestyle changes, you must identify where change is needed. Take all of your most cherished and fundamental *good-for-health* beliefs and question them. Ask yourself: "Why do I believe this? Look for answers. Make notes. If you do not enjoy good health, try something different, based on the data you have for your body.

Give heed to the statement that if something sounds to good to be true it probably is. In health care, if something sounds fishy (illogical), it probably is, such as oxygen is a dangerous free radical.

Be prepared to ask every caregiver these four important questions.

1. Why should I use your products or service at all?

2. What special features make your product or service better than that of your competition?

3. Why should I buy now?

4. Why should I believe you?

Of the four questions, the last one is the most important. Do not rely entirely on medical degrees or stature in medical circles. Do not be afraid to question health professionals who tell you oxygen therapies are dangerous, defective genes cause cancer, you need more toxins in your system, mercury fillings are safe, cholesterol causes heart attacks, or that you have an autoimmune disease. Remember that modern medicine is closer to applied mythology than to applied biology. There is a tremendous amount of misinformation indoctrinated into our health-care system. Look upon health-care services as a business. You are a customer. Successful businesses require repeat customers. The value of a health service business is based on the number of active patients, not the number of cured patients.

It wasn't that long ago that medical doctors were bloodletting to cure disease and using mercury to treat patients. The derogatory expression *Quack* was used originally by doctors against other doctors who continued to use *Quicksilver* (the first name for mercury) after the majority of doctors recognized the error and had changed their approach. It wasn't that long ago that ulcers were thought to be caused by stress, even though most doctors now recognize ulcers are caused by bacteria. Over 90 per cent of what modern medicine claims, as scientific medicine has never been scientifically proven. This text illustrates some of the more significant errors now accepted as dogma.

Embrace the metabolic theory

The metabolic theory states your body can heal itself providing it is given all the natural ingredients it needs, providing it can absorb, assimilate, and synthesize these ingredients, and providing metabolic wastes are removed in time.

Enzymes are the key to metabolic functions, and essential minerals and other nutrients are required to maintain your enzyme supply. Essential food nutrients include macro minerals and trace minerals, fatty acids, proteins, sugars, and vitamins. Exercise, water, sunlight, oxygen, rest, sleep, and lack of stress are all factors in metabolism and waste removal.

One might add Acidophilus and other friendly flora that must be replaced after taking chemotherapy and antibiotics. These bacteria are the first step in the digestive process that leads to complete assimilation of food nutrients to avoid trapped blood proteins. Plenty of pure water and fresh air are also vital. With good food, properly prepared, digested, and assimilated, you probably have all of the vitamins your body needs. However, most natural-health caregivers recommend mineral supplements and, in many cases, supplements are needed to rebuild and repair damaged cells.

Follow a lymphatic cleansing program

Dr. Samuel West, D.C. has established how to get the maximum use from time spent cleansing your lymphatic system. He recommends use of a rebounder in his book, *The Golden Seven Plus One*. On page 36, he writes:

> The importance of the function of the lymphatics cannot be stressed too strongly, for there is no other route besides the lymphatic system which excess (trapped) proteins can return to the circulatory system.

Dr. West establishes the chemistry of disease by showing how trapped blood proteins increase the sodium levels outside of cells so that transfer of electrons and oxidation cannot continue. In order for cells to function as electric generators, the cell wall must have sodium ions on the inside and phosphate ions on the outside. Cell walls must allow food nutrients in and waste particles out. During these processes, some of the cytoplasm or cell proteins seep out of the cell and into the cellular environment. He explains how these trapped blood proteins result in pain, loss of energy and disease.

The key to lymphatic exercises is to understand how the lymphatic system pumps lymph rapidly during an up-and-down motion of the body and breathing, which causes lymph to flow against gravity if necessary, from one valve to another. The lymph system does not have a heart or pump. It relies on gravity and muscle contractions to pump liquids through the system.

Bouncing on a rebounder, fast walking and jogging cause the body to move up and down, leading to increased lymph flow. Since lymphatic cleansing is so vital to health, it makes sense to follow professional advice rather than to rely on hit-and-miss exercises. Lying on a slant board with the feet and legs up is another way to increase flow of lymph from the legs.

Develop a health-oriented daily routine

If every day is a success, you cannot help but succeed. Every day will be a success, if every hour is a success. Every hour will be a success, if you make the right choices and do the right things during that hour.

Good health doesn't follow from making a few major changes in your life. It follows from making small but important choices all day long such as drinking enough water and avoiding contaminants. Right choices follow from knowing what to do, and doing it with enjoyment. Committing yourself to a daily routine makes it possible. Build your routine around suggestions made by numerous health advocates. Introduce one or two steps at a time until they become routine. Don't expect too much. It takes time to cleanse the body of toxins, excess weight, and habitual cravings.

Dr. Budwig and essential oils

Dr. Budwig's cancer therapy has a vital place in all cancer prevention and treatments. The only visual difference between normal cells and cancer cells is the lipid-layer in the cell and cell wall. The only difference needed to make a cancer cell is to modify the lipid layer so that it will not knit or bind to existing normal cells. To follow her main food supplement recommendation, put 2 to 3 tablespoons of fresh flaxseed oil in a bowl of cottage cheese. Mix, add a bit of honey if desired, and enjoy.

From a functional point of view for preventing and curing cancer, eliminating parasites, establishing a favorable mineral balance, and building effective cell-wall membranes are the three keys to success.

The body's main defense mechanism is production of interferon, which are proteins manufactured in cells when cells are under attack by fungi or virus. Interferon interferes with the ability of fungi to multiply in the body, possibly by destroying their growth hormones. Interferon and Interleuken-2 are two well-established interferon proteins, although there could be more.

Dr. Budwig's recipe of fresh flaxseed oil and cottage cheese provide the essential ingredients the body needs to make more interferon. Make one of her recipes twice a week and you will be amazed by your good health.

Supplementing with essential fatty acids and eliminating French fries and all deep fried food makes sense. Every cell has a membrane that gives the cell its form. This membrane allows nutrients to enter the cell and waste to leave the cell. If we do not provide cells with the proper fats and oils, we destroy the ability for cell walls to function properly. We create trapped blood proteins and pollutants that lead to fermentation. Several books on good and bad fats show a direct relationship between cancer and lack of unsaturated fatty acids. In addition, these essential fatty acids are significant to the cell for production of human energy.

Conclusion to developing a healthy lifestyle

There are many other products and systems that are effective for treating and preventing cancer. Cancer is a metabolic disease, dependent on toxins, enzymes, proteins, and lipids from microbes and parasites. We can eliminate these pollutants from our body to prevent and cure cancer, as well as most other diseases. Since we can be reinfected at any time, we must maintain a parasite cleanse and maintenance program to ensure against parasites. We must also strive to replace the nutrients the body uses as soon as required by the body.

In conclusion to the health-related theme, I hope this information will bring you some peace of mind over the fear of cancer and will also direct you towards preventing cancer for yourself and loved ones. The cure for cancer is to help the body grow healthy cells to repair a membrane injury or bone fracture. As soon as the injury is repaired, replication will stop.

In order to improve our personal life-style, we need the support of others and they need our support. We need to approach the problem in a new way. We have to reinvent our political-economic-medical system.

Now, lets look into the politics and economics of health care.

Section THREE:
Misinformation,
suppression, and cover-up

20. Historical documents on suppressed cancer cures

We are losing the war on cancer

because the *Cancer Establishment*

does not want to win.

In the following chapter we will deal with the problem of obtaining freedom of choice in health care so that effective cancer diagnoses and treatments will become available through mainstream medicine.

My personal experience with FDA and HPB suppression

I first realized in 1994 that Canada's Health Protection Branch of the federal government (HPB) suppresses alternative cancer cures. After researching the four-herb Canadian cancer remedy developed by Rene Caisse called *Essiac*, —*Caisse* spelled backwards, —I packaged these herbs in a low-cost, easy-to-use kit for home use. I called the herbal package *Caisse's Herbal Tea* and started selling kits and refills across Canada and into the USA to our customer base. Within a few months, the U.S. Food and Drug Administration (FDA) seized our shipment at U.S. customs. Shortly after that, our Health Protection Branch regulated me to stop using the name *Caisse's Herbal Tea*. The name was not permitted in Canada because it was *"an indirect reference to a non-approved treatment."* It was permissible to sell the product, due to previous court challenges in which HPB had lost its attempt to stop others from selling the herbs, but not permissible to use the name *Caisse's Herbal Tea.* The FDA gave the same ruling for the U.S. market.

It is important to realize that the HPB staff who enforced these regulations did so reluctantly. It appeared to me that they were just doing their job due to pressure from above. In fact, the Canadian Health Protection Branch did not restrict our business until they were notified by the American FDA about our exports. In my opinion, the whole problem was FDA-driven. I have always been treated reasonably by Canadian HPB staff and Canadian customs inspectors.

At the time when I was regulated, major Canadian and U.S. distributors of Essiac were permitted to continue selling the same herbs trademarked as *Essiac (a direct reference)* and advertise the product with Rene Caisse's picture. Direct references to Essiac™ from larger corporations were permitted seemingly without question on the basis that essiac was a common household word in Canada. HPB knew they could not win a court challenge to stop use of the word essiac. It seems strange that the Health Protection Branch would prevent me from marketing the product with reference to Rene Caisse while allowing others to do so simply because they could not face a court challenge to stop them.

In the U.S. market, the trade name Essiac™ was also permitted, and several smaller U.S.-based companies continued to market the herbs with indirect and direct references. One had preprinted bags marked Caisse's Herbal Tea and sold this product openly at health shows in USA. Another version combined with another herb called Cat's Claw, was being sold by a medical doctor at major U.S. health fairs, and is now available in Canada.

You can verify our close relationship with the FDA by looking up what we jokingly call the *Essiac Home Page* as maintained on the Internet by the FDA. (Search under FDA Essiac Import Alert 1A6664).

Why were we singled out for regulatory action? In addition to changing the product name, we also had to drop all references to these herbs being antifungal and antiparasitic. In addition, we had included a few photocopied pages in the kit. One was *The Prime Cause and Prevention of Cancer* contained in a speech given by Dr. Otto Warburg in which he established that cancer cells result from reduced respiration. I now suspect that we were singled out for regulatory action because we promoted the true cause of cancer.

At that time, I did not realize Dr. Warburg's research was being suppressed. In fact, I wasn't even sure he was right. My critical error was not really an indirect reference to an unapproved treatment. My error was a *direct reference to unapproved knowledge.*

After meeting with HPB officials in Toronto and Ottawa, I was allowed to continue marketing the herbs and tea-making kit under a different name, providing I did not have any written material other than minimum instructions on how to make the tea. Their real concern, which was never discussed, was to remove the suppressed information. I believe that is why no one else selling this product was stopped from doing so.

The historical facts that Nurse Rene Caisse healed thousands of people with this historical native Indian formula, that no one had experienced any bad side effects; and that it was very affordable, meant nothing. While personally researching essiac in Bracebridge, Ontario, I talked with people who say they watched forty years of Rene Caisse's records burned in barrels in her back yard. The medical establishment at that time did not want documentation of successful cancer cures by essiac to be known and published.

Since reading Dr. Hulda Clark's book, *The Cure for All Cancers,* I have added other well-known herbs to the product line which helps replace essential minerals, helps eliminate fungi and parasites from the body, and provides trace minerals for production of essential oxidative enzymes. Hardly a day goes by that we do not hear about amazing health benefits from this valuable self-health program. This protocol works because it provides essential trace minerals, helps eliminate fungi and parasites, and helps support the oxidative process. I know from first-hand experience that cancer and most other diseases are caused by conditions we create for cells in our body. Removing conditions that cause cancer can cure cancer. Without living proof from numerous cancer patients that cancer can be beaten, I could not write this report, nor would I be motivated to do so.

In my opinion, based on personal experience, the Canadian HPB and the U.S. FDA abuse their authority by creating regulations to suppress effective cancer cures and knowledge about them. As increasingly more people turn to natural products, the HPB increases suppression of them, especially if they can be used for alternative cancer treatments. Take dehydroepiandrosterone (DHEA), for example. The 1996 Regional Bulletin on DHEA stated: *"The unlawful distribution of DHEA or any product merely represented as containing DHEA can be viewed as trafficking".* Importing the harmless food enzyme that supports the immune system and capacity to produce vital oxidative enzymes results in imprisonment and fines based on severe narcotic penalties. Even importation of DHEA for personal use is not permitted. Can you name any other products that *"merely representing as containing"* constitutes trafficking? Banning distribution of other hormones, amino acids, and ozone therapy provides other examples of misuse and abuse of authority.

It is estimated that the proposed Dec. 18, 1996 Health Canada *Guidance Document on Establishment Licensing* for all alternative health product suppliers, importers, and retailers would have wiped out 75% of the Natural Health Products Industry in Canada. The regulators didn't back down until millions of Canadians signed petitions to stop implementation of the proposed regulations. In addition, the Minister of Health was presented with court order #499/97 to justify his department's proposed actions. The fact that government is now establishing a *Third Category* to regulate natural health products differently from foods, on one hand, and drugs on the other, attests to the misguided regulations being enacted by our infamous Health Protection Branch.

Licensed medical doctors are the only specialists permitted for testing and licensing a product or service for coverage by Health Canada and Medicare. This self-interest group is thus the only organization in Canada allowed to control its competition and regulate it out of business. This unconstitutional arrangement is the fundamental problem stopping advancement in medicine and health care in Canada. It is impossible to write about the cause and treatment of cancer without also discussing how existing cancer cures are being suppressed. Profit, power, propaganda, and politics go hand in hand.

Not all doctors are involved in suppression

I do not wish to blame all medical doctors for suppression. Far from it! My friends and providers who are medical doctors are dedicated, hard-working health-care specialists caught in a trap. Their medical association suppresses freedom of thought and choice. Individual doctors must either fit in or get pushed out. They are doing the best they can within regulations and available resources.

Historical data on essiac show that Rene Caisse worked with medical doctors and they supported her in her quest to have essiac brought into mainstream medicine. Those who supported her were forced by the association to stop supporting her. Medical doctors have technical knowledge that is not easily marketed outside of mainstream medicine. They are not free to practice medicine using the best methods available. Medicare pays only for prescription drugs and liability insurance protects them for only standard medical procedures. Medicine should be considered as applied biology and biochemistry, but modern medicine has become *Applied Pharmaceutical.* Doctors often prescribe drugs against their better judgement because the public demands treatment for their condition and they have nothing else to offer. A simple electronic device like a zapper to reduce infection could save millions of dollars in the cost of drugs and provide a far better answer for most microbial infections.

Many medical doctors are active community service members and many receive awards indicating their service-above-self attitude to the community. They have dedicated their lives to helping people through the field of medicine. They often struggle with teams of dedicated staff to save a child's life by replacement of a defective liver or kidney. What they do is so remarkable. It makes them fully deserving of our esteem. One cannot imagine the frustration they endure, knowing that chemotherapy is not effective for treating cancer and that they are not allowed to practice medicine as they wish. Most cancer clinics in Mexico or the Bahamas are operated by well-trained American and Canadian medical doctors. They have gone there for the freedom they need to practice medicine and to use methods not allowed in Canada or U.S.A. due to suppression.

If your opinion on Mexican cancer clinics is based on what you see on national TV, you have been falsely indoctrinated. Our news media does not report on any of the thousands of people who have recovered from cancer after mainstream medicine had given up. If Canada opened the doors to similar free choice in medicine, we could have a thriving industry treating cancer patients from foreign lands where regulations do not allow alternative therapies. Medical doctors would lead the way.

If viable options were permitted, most medical doctors would embrace an opportunity to practice medicine with less emphasis on drugs. The Province of Alberta recently passed legislation aimed at protecting doctors from their own medical association for using non-approved remedies. The act gave doctors the right to use any treatment that is known to be less toxic than the conventional drug therapy. The act protects doctors from things like loss of medical license for prescribing an alternative therapy

Think about this for a moment. Why don't people and politicians take court action against the medical associations for defrauding the public of their right to alternative health care?

Another reason why I believe that the majority of doctors are not involved in suppression of cancer cures is that doctors also die of cancer and the treatments. We have one customer of our natural health products who is now 75 years of age and doing well. He came to us in severe pain from bone cancer several years ago. When he was first diagnosed with cancer, his doctor at the time confided in him that he too had the same type of cancer. His doctor followed medical protocol and died three years after starting treatments. Obviously, this doctor was not aware of suppressed alternatives or did not have any confidence in them. Moreover, he did not have private access to effective alternative care. There is probably a large middle ground where the medical profession knows alternatives are suppressed but they would lose their license to practice medicine if they spoke up. Individual doctors are as powerless to stop it, as we are powerless to stop it. They just live with it and do the best they can.

Dr. Fibiger initiated cancer in the laboratory in 1913 using larvae

The most amazing evidence that cancer research is ignored and suppressed is that of Dr. Johannes Fibiger. The Nobel Prize in Medicine, was awarded to him in 1926 for initiating cancer in the laboratory with growth hormone from parasitic worms. Not one of my medical textbooks even mentions his name or discusses his research. I consider that as proof of indoctrination of medical students which has been ongoing since at least 1926. This information is only available on the Internet home page for Nobel Awards, webmaster@www.nobel.se. During the presentation speech the method for initiating cancer by using parasites was made public. The method was as follows:

> He achieved this feat although thousands had already failed to do so, by feeding *larvae of spiroptera*, (a parasitic worm in horses) to cockroaches from a sugar warehouse and then feeding the cockroaches to mice and other rodents. In 1913, Fibiger succeeded in producing cancerous growths in the stomachs of a large number of animals. This was the first time that cancer was provoked and controlled by a man-made stimulus.

Why do doctors say they do not know the cause of cancer, and deny the microbial cause of cancer, when Fibiger actually discovered the cause of cancer in 1913? Why is this information not common knowledge? Cancer was initiated by infecting the mice with parasites. The Nobel Prize was awarded based on significant contribution to the future study of cancer rather than the immediate significance.

Fibiger found mice with naturally occurring stomach cancer in a sugar warehouse. He realized immediately he had discovered something very special. Cockroaches were also abundant and he assumed the combination of sugar, mice, cockroaches, and parasitic worms from horse excreta could demonstrate the required conditions leading to cancer.

Here's how mice Fibiger's mice developed cancer. Horses infected with *Spiroptera* worms were used to deliver loads of sugar into the warehouse.

These worms lay eggs in the horse's colon and the eggs are expelled with excreta. Cockroaches eat the horse excreta with the eggs, enabling the eggs to hatch. Mice eat the cockroaches with *Spiroptera* in the larvae stage, The larvae damage mouse intestines, creating a current of injury, replication of cells, mutation, and cancer. We now know that stomach cancers arise from ulcers, and ulcers are caused by bacteria. It all fits.

Larvae contain high concentration of DNA polymerase enzymes and other growth factors. Fibiger realized that the parasitic worm *Spiroptera* required an intermediary host in order for eggs to hatch and larvae to develop. A study of parasite life cycles show that most parasites require an intermediary host, normally a plant used as food, to invade a new host. If parasitic eggs did not spread through the food chain, parasites could not survive.

Why is the sugar warehouse so significant?

Mice and cockroaches had unlimited access to sugar, and the mineral imbalance developed by excess sugar consumption turned their metabolism in favor of microbial enzymes and fermentation. The minerals needed to digest sugar include chromium, manganese, cobalt, copper, zinc, and magnesium. Sugar depletes the mineral balance and leaves the body with toxic levels of phosphorus.

Cancer occurred in the stomachs of mice and other rodents because the stomach became the first animal tissue to come into continuous contact with the larvae and the related growth factors. When we see people who are in excellent health suddenly develop stomach or colon cancer, it is probably through ingestion of parasitic larvae that causes the problem.

Dr. Fibiger's research and discovery have been totally ignored by mainstream cancer researchers. Why? I find it hard to believe Fibiger's peers would have selected him for this Nobel Award without first carefully investigating his research. Fibiger's research could have opened the door for effective cancer treatments and saved millions of lives.

There is significant historical proof that mainstream medicine in Europe, the USA, and Canada has also ignored all other research that indicates microbes cause cancer. There can be no doubt that mainstream medicine has been adequately informed about the nature of cancer microbes and growth hormones but has suppressed the information and discredited the researchers.

Cancer microbes observed in cancer cells by Russell, 1890

Alternative health care suppliers have many different books describing microbes observed in cancer cells and successful cancer cures based on cleansing cells of microbes. The following is a reference to medical observations of cancer microbes over 100 years ago.

In his book, *The Cancer Microbe*, Dr. Allan Cantwell, Jr. M.D. provides numerous references to cancer microbes such as that of Dr. William Russell in 1890 (Page 105):

> When bacteria were discovered in TB and other infectious diseases, it was thought that bacteria might also be involved in cancer. In 1890, William Russell (1852-1940) first reported "cancer parasites" in cancer tissue that was specially stained with carbol fushsin, a red dye. Russell, a distinguished pathologist and Professor of Clinical Medicine at Edinbourgh University in Scotland, identified microbes in almost every cancer tumor he examined. The "parasite" was present inside the cells (intracellular) and outside the cells (extracellular). The smallest parasites were barely visible microscopically, and the largest parasites were as large as red blood cells. Russell also found similar parasites in tuberculosis, syphilis, and skin ulcers.

Dr. Russel observed cancer parasites over 100 years ago, their various sizes were known, and Russel also found similar parasites in skin ulcers.

Coley's vaccine used successfully 100 years ago

According to Dr. Abram Hoffer, M.D., Ph.D. in an article published in *Journal of Orthomolecular Medicine,* Vol. 7, 1992, several vaccines have been produced to treat cancer. One of the most successful was that of Dr. Coley, which was used successfully more than 100 years ago.

Recovery rate of 51% exceeds modern drugs

> Dr. Coley prepared a vaccine from heat killed streptococci mixed with the toxin of bacterium *Serratia Marcescen*. This was the first use of a mixed vaccine in medicine.... Dr. Helen Coley Nauts assembled 896 cases treated by this mixed bacterial vaccine (MBV). She found that of 523 inoperable patients, 238 recovered (46%), while from 373 operable cases, 190 or 51% recovered.

> Considering how little was known about optimum use of the vaccine, the results obtained are remarkable and surpass the results obtained by any modern treatment using surgery, chemotherapy and radiation.

Scott's vaccine cured hopeless cancer patients in 1925

In 1925, Northwest Medicine published two papers by Dr. Michael Scott, a Montana surgeon who had learned about the cancer microbe. Scott's microbe was a parasite which had a life cycle composed of three stages: a *coccus*, a *rod*, and a *spore sac*. Cantwell's book, *The Cancer Microbe* (Page 108) gives us these details:

> Scott detected the cancer microbe in cancer tissue and insisted the parasite secreted a toxin that made the body's cells cancerous.

> Scott believed an effective vaccine against cancer could be developed. He devised a promising treatment that cured some hopeless cancer patients, **but his treatment methods were quickly suppressed by the medical establishment.**

Here we are 75 years later saying the same thing. History shows that Dr. Scott fought until he died to get his vaccine accepted by the medical establishment but failed. By 1925, mainstream medicine was already suppressing the microbial cause of cancer and suppressing all effective vaccines. The effectiveness of microbial vaccines proves that cancer is a fungal disease. Vaccines do not cure defective genes. Vaccines kill fungi and other bacteria. The suppression of this type of successful cancer cure for over 100 years is an historical fact. Vaccines are not suitable for use by the cancer industry because they cannot maintain the myth of defective genes and the excuse for lack of progress.

Royal Rife described cancer microbes in 1930s

The following information is taken from the book *The Cancer Cure that Worked, Fifty years of Suppression*, by Barry Lynes, first published in 1987.

In the 1920s, Royal Rife of San Diego, California, developed a high-powered microscope capable of enlarging images by 1,500 times, far more than any other known instrument. He was later successful in identifying cancer microbes, proving they are pleomorphic (capable of changing form) and that cancer could be cured by killing these microbes with a vibrational frequency in the range of ultraviolet light.

Since the principle used by Rife to destroy microorganisms is still being suppressed, and this is the same principle at work in a zapper and other electronic devices that could save medicine billions of tax revenue dollars, let's review the following brief description. (*The Cancer Cure that Worked*, Page 6):

Biophysicists have now shown that there exists a crucial natural interaction between living matter and photons. This process is measurable at the cellular (bacterium) level. Other research demonstrated that living systems are extraordinarily sensitive to extremely low-energy electromagnetic waves. This is to say, each kind of cell or microorganism has a specific frequency of interaction with the electromagnetic spectrum. By various means, Rife's system allowed adjusting the frequency of light impinging on the specimen. By some insight he learned that the light frequency could be 'tuned' into the natural frequency of the microorganism being examined to cause a resonance or feed-back loop. In effect, under this condition, it can be said the microorganism illuminated itself.

This equipment was developed long before we had the benefit of modern electronics, and Rife-like machines are now available for only a few thousand dollars. Once the frequency of resonance is known, the microorganism can be identified specifically by the resonance frequency, and destroyed by increasing the voltage. Microorganisms simply explode much like a strong voice can shatter a crystal glass.

The resonance concept is also capable of being modulated so that it can be heard by the human ear. This is the principle upon which Dr. Hulda Clark has built a diagnostic device capable of identifying the presence of parasites in human tissue. Her 'syncrometer' allows for identifying toxins, pollutants and microorganisms inside living tissue by producing a resonance which is amplified through a speaker system. This device will resonate only if the item on the test plate of the syncrometer is also inside the body of the person being tested. The speed and ease with which microorganisms can be identified has enabled her to develop a therapy against parasites, for example, and test its effectiveness quickly and easily. In order to prevent these inventions from being suppressed, she has described the printed circuits in her books.

History shows that Rife's equipment was destroyed and research suppressed by Morris Fishbein, Director of the American Medical Association at that time.

Rife demonstrated and recorded the appearance of cancer microbes observed in his microscope. The following quotation is taken from *The Cancer Cure that Worked* (Page 50) *(My emphasis on fungi added)*.

Rife's laboratory notes for November 20, 1929 contain the first written description of the cancer virus characteristics. The cancer virus was indeed small. The length was 1/15 of a micron. The breadth was 1/20 of a micron. No ordinary microscope, even in the 1980s, would be able to make the cancer virus visible. In time, Rife was able to prove that the cancer microorganism had four forms:

1) BX (carcinoma)

2) BY (sarcoma – larger than BX)

3) Monococcoid (a round single-celled organism) form in the monocytes of the blood in over 90% of cancer patients.

4) *Crytomyces pleomorphia* FUNGI —identical morphologically to that of the orchid and the mushroom.

Note that cancer did not develop until the microorganism reached the fungi stage in which it could invade human cells. In the round monococcoid form it parasitized the red blood cells. That is why cancer can be diagnosed accurately long before tumors form. This vital information has been ignored and suppressed for over three generations. Consider the financial and human consequences of these facts.

There can be no doubt that Rife's system worked both to diagnose cancer before tumors formed, and to cure cancer after tumors were evident. On pages 60-61 of *The Cancer Cure that Worked*, we read:

Rife cures 14 of 16 so-called hopeless cases in 1934

In 1934, sixteen hopeless cancer cases were treated using Royal Rife's frequency generator. After fourteen months, fourteen of these so-called hopeless cases were signed off as clinically cured by the staff of five medical doctors.

Pause and think for a minute about the futility of donating money to cancer research for a cancer cure. If they will not use the perfect cure, what are they looking for? Even if they could develop a drug, would they use it?

The text continues to describe how well the cancer treatment worked (Page 60).

The treatment consisted of three minutes duration at three-day intervals. With the frequency instrument treatment, no tissue is destroyed, no pain is felt, no noise is audible, and no sensation is noticed.

It was found that the three-day elapsed time between treatment attained better results than the cases treated daily. This gave the lymphatic system an opportunity to absorb and cast off the toxic condition that is produced by the devitalized dead particles of the 'BX' virus.

Similarly, people who are very ill, and are using any of the available cancer cures not yet suppressed by the authorities, consideration should be given to start cautiously in order to avoid a problem with devitalized dead particles from parasite cleansing.

Parasitic flukes cause liver and bladder cancer

During the 1950's, in a series of medical texts called *Animals Parasitic in Man*, Geoffrey Lepage describes cancer caused by flukes. This book describes hundreds of human parasites and establishes a direct relationship between some parasites and cancer.

Not many parasitic animals are able to cause them (tumors), but cancer of the liver has been attributed to the Oriental liver fluke, *Opisthorchis sinensis*, and to its relative, *O. felineus*, and cancer of the bladder of man to the urinary blood fluke, *schistosoma haematobium*; and there are instances among hosts other than man.

Here again we see the direct connection between cancer and parasites. There is substantial proof that hundreds of leading doctors were introduced to the truth. That is why it is so hard to determine where the line is drawn between the suppressor and the suppressed.

Dr. Beigelson is able to detect cancer long before tumors form

American born Dr. Harvey Beigelson operates a cancer clinic in Mexico where he has helped thousands of cancer victims by using alternative cancer therapies based on the cancer microbe concept, darkfield microscopes, and homeopathic remedies developed and used in Germany. He has written a book called *Your Cure For Cancer* in which he describes his methods. He writes:

The use of very high resolution darkfield microscopes today permits the detailed examination of a single drop of (fresh) blood in a manner that provides more information about the health of the patient and the condition of his or her cancer, or other disease, than has been available in the past by using any other of our Western technological tools.

Further, due to the dynamics of the pleomorphic cycle we can now detect the approach of a cancer two to ten years before any symptoms (tumor, or organ system dysfunction) are present... Cancer can now be stopped, long before it becomes visible.

Two essential points emerge from the above reference. Dr. Biegelson had to leave United States and set up his practice in Mexico, and he is using data supplied to and suppressed by the U.S. cancer industry. Cancer can be identified before tumors exist by reviewing the life stages and quantity of microbes in the body. There is no need to wait for cancer to develop tumors before one is diagnosed with cancer. Cancer can be diagnosed before it creates serious health problems, pain and suffering. It can also be treated before it costs Medicare many thousands of dollars.

Dr. Biegelsen's successful cancer diagnosis, prevention, and cures are based on information given to the American Cancer Society more than 30 years ago. Dr. Virginia Livingston-Wheeler and colleagues presented a paper to the New York Academy of Sciences in 1969 entitled *"Microorganisms Associated with Malignancy"* in which she demonstrated with slides. The following reference is taken from *Your Cure for Cancer* (Page 60)(Emphasis on fungi, added.)

Microorganisms of various sorts have been observed and isolated from animal and human tumors, including viruses, bacteria, and fungi. There is, however, one specific type of highly pleomorphic microorganism that has been observed and isolated consistently by us from human and animal malignancies of every obtainable variety for the past 20 years...**Its various phases may resemble viruses, micrococci, ditheroids, bacilli and FUNGI.**

It is interesting that fungi are the last stage of observed microorganisms in the research of both Royal Rife and Virginia Livingston Wheeler. Fungi are also the microorganisms isolated by Dr. Costantini in his research on the cause of cancer. If we accept the concept that bacteria and fungi are different life stages of the same organism, the observation of both bacteria and fungi in cancer cells is obligatory. Conversion of human cells to fermentation units is beneficial to the microorganisms that control metabolism and replication cycles.

The fact that fungi are seldom, if ever, mentioned in mainstream medicine as a possible cause of cancer is a breach of public trust.

Naessens demonstrates complete cancer microbe life cycles

The Canadian Medical Association has suppressed several cancer cures. One prime example is recorded in the book *The Persecution and Trial of Gaston Naessens: The True Story of the Efforts to Suppress Alternative Treatment for Cancer, AIDS and Other Immunologically Based Diseases,* written by Christopher Bird, in1991.

Gaston Naessens of Rock Forest, Quebec, used a high-power darkfield microscope to study cancer microbes and successfully cured thousands of cancer patients with a special formula he developed called 714-X. Naessens developed a microscope, independent of the Rife model, and far more powerful, magnifying objects to 4500 times their normal size. With this microscope, he observed a life-form which he called a somatid. These life-forms go through one of two cycles. If a cell is healthy, the life cycle takes 3 forms. In case of cancer, the life cycle takes 13 forms.

Simply by identifying stages of the 13 life-forms in the blood stream, one can identify whether or not cancer is imminent. That is why cancer can be detected long before cancer tumors form and costly life-saving procedures are necessary.

Starting in 1972, Gaston Naessens with his wife, lectured and demonstrated the pleomorphic nature of cancer microbes to Dr. Y. E. Perey, assistant professor of pathology and surgery, at the McMaster University Medical Center in Hamilton, Ontario. The microbial cause of cancer was demonstrated to them.

Canadian medical authorities have been informed about the fungal cause of cancer, but refuse to use this research for the prevention, diagnosis and treatment of cancer. In Bird's book, we find information of the report by Perey to the Canadian Medical Association (Page 87):

> The report contained many other details, one of the most important of which was Perey's having seen, "beyond the shadow of doubt," that whereas "normal bugs," the first three stages of the somatid cycle, had appeared in the blood of "normal" rats unaffected with cancer, "abnormal bugs," the successive thirteen stages in the cycle, had appeared in the blood of rats that had received transplantable cancer tumors.

> Part of the same amazement applied to *specific mycelial forms,* which, because they looked and behaved like common fungi, should in Percey's view, have been susceptible to, and therefore annihilatable by, fungicidal antibiotics. But, as he reported to Stewart: "In spite of the extremely high doses of such drugs applied to them, the 'bugs' grew happily. They must therefore be considered not only resistant to the killing drugs, but also be quite different from what appear to be their first cousins.

While each of the separate forms show some characteristics of organisms well known in standard micro-biology – bacteria, fungi, and viruses – the big difference was that, far from living

independently, one from another, they had all seemed to derive from one bug.

Several significant conclusions can be drawn from the full report. The most significant fact is that the fungal life-stage of the cancer microbe is indestructible by chemotherapy and antibiotics because they continue to form from life-stages that are not affected by these antibiotics. It is comparable to trying to stop a flooded basement from a broken water pipe by removing the water faster than it comes in. To prevent flooding, one must turn off the water. To prevent cancer, one must interrupt the life cycle of the cancer microbe. One must return the cellular conditions to that which will stop the cancer-cycle of microorganisms in the body. Chemotherapy will never achieve this goal permanently due to reinfection. Cancer is caused by the invasion of human cells by fungal mycelia, and cancer will be cured by eliminating the fungal mycelia from the body, through metabolism and cleansing.

The significance of a growth hormone to control replication cannot be overlooked. DNA cannot replicate without some form of DNA polymerase. In his research, Naessens found that cancer patients had an abundance of growth hormone in the body. He wanted researchers at McMaster University to identify the source of this growth hormone. This research was never performed for him.

In addition, The Naessens wanted the University to research the chemistry of the somatid. This life-form appears directly related to the DNA crystal. DNA crystals form due to electromagnetic forces in the atoms just as any other crystals, such as salt form. Research on the somatid could lead to greater understanding of life itself. It appears that the great medical universities of our time, such as McMaster in Hamilton, do not have the freedom to research the true cause of cancer.

Let's leave *The Persecution and Trial of Gaston Naessens* with a brief review of what might have been. On page 95-96, we read:

> The McMaster effort, which had so much promise when overseen by Daniel Perey, finally ended in complete failure. What the Naessens, as they told me, always hoped was that, with David Stewart's support, an official university team of scientists, capably instructed, and honestly motivated, would be able to replicate the easily performed isolation and culturing of somatids.

> Following that, what the Naessens wanted determined, with lab equipment and methods more sophisticated than those available to them in Rock Forest, was, first of all, the exact chemical composition of the somatids, to reveal the connection with DNA, a finding that, if confirmed, might be as important to

science as the discovery of the nature of DNA itself, reported many years ago in John Watson's scientific thriller *The Double Helix* (New York: Antheneum, 1968)

Here they were with an opportunity to possibly identify the secret of life, itself or perform research with potentially significant benefit for all mankind. Imagine the let-down the Naessens must have felt when they were persecuted by the medical establishment for their efforts.

The action taken by the Canadian Medical Association to destroy and persecute Dr. Naessens sends a powerful warning to Canadian doctors. Don't mess with an effective cancer cure!

It should be noted that the Quebec Superior Court threw out all of the trumped up medical charges against Dr. Naessens and he continues to operate his clinic. Latest estimates are that over 100,000 people have been successfully cured of cancer or other diseases, including AIDS, by this method, but mainstream medicine still refuses to use his research and methods.

Gaston Naessens and his wife should receive the highest award Canada has to offer, as well as be nominated for a Nobel prize in medicine. The selection of projects for cancer research using publicly donated funds and tax revenues should be taken from the cancer establishment to stop the fraudulent use and abuse of public funds. A means should be established that public funds are dispersed according to an unbiased public group without hidden objectives.

Dr. Costantini identifies fungi in cancer

The World Health Organization has access to an outstanding source of research information that proves microbes cause cancer. As head of the World Health Organization's Center for Mycotoxins in Food, Dr. A. V. Costantini is privy to worldwide reports implicating fungi in all major degenerative or autoimmune diseases.

Three books of a series of fourteen are now available and can be reviewed on the Internet by using the search word *Fungalbionics*. About eighty pages of information describe the close relationship between fungi and breast cancer as well as Atherosclerosis. Fungi produce mycotoxins, which are the cause of all human degenerative and autoimmune diseases. Books can be ordered on the Internet.

A third book called the *Garden of Eden Longevity Diet* provides information on how to avoid toxic fungal foods.

Let's focus on *Fungalbionics The Fungal/Mycotoxin Etiology of Human Disease, Volume II, CANCER* by A.V. Costantini M.D.; Heinrich Wieland,

M.D. and Lars I. Qvick, M.D. 1994 edition. For sake of brevity, a reference to Costantini will include reference to the other co-authors of these books.

Viruses do not cause cancer directly

Costantini destroys credibility in a direct viral cause of cancer. He writes (Page 31):

Michael J. Bishop (1985) stated it quite clearly, 'Viruses have not been causally tied to the origins of any human cancer, although several candidates are under active study. If viruses are oncogenic in humans, it seems likely that predisposing factors are operating." Obviously, the postulate that viruses alone cause cancer in humans remains an unproven postulate.

It should be noted that there is no evidence that any antiviral drug has ever been shown to cure or regress any cancer which is postulated to be due to a virus; a clinical reality which must be taken into consideration whenever viral researchers postulate a viral etiology of a cancer.

The viral connection to cancer has been established. You will recall that virus cause benign growths. The rupture of a benign growth turns on the current of injury and causes cells to multiply. Microbes resident in these cells also multiply and mutate the cell wall. Rejection of mutated cells leads to cancer and tumor growth.

Untreated tobacco does not cause cancer

Dr. Costantini also explains why smoking cigarettes causes cancer but smoking cigars does not. It's a result of the fermentation process used to cure tobacco for making cigarettes. He writes (Page 67):

Bock also found that *cured* tobacco leaf caused numerous cancers in animals. It was neither the heat factor, nor the tobacco paper, for unburned tobacco caused as many cancers as burnt tobacco.

In 1968, Van Duran found Mycotoxin producing fungi *Alternaria* and *Aspergillus Niger* in six brands of cigarettes but none in cigar tobacco. It is well known that cigarettes (cut tobacco to which is added yeast and sugar for flavor enhancement), cause cancer. Cigars made of rolled tobacco leaf do not cause cancers.

Smoking causes cancer indirectly because sugar curing of tobacco (a fungal process) for flavor enhancement laces tobacco with fungi and fungal produced toxins. Smoking reduces the capacity of lungs to remove carbon dioxide and supply oxygen to the cells. In addition, ammonia from ammonia treated tobacco and other toxins increases pollution, stops the citric acid cycle, and initiates replication in lung tissue through the current of injury. None of the carcinogens in tobacco or smoke can cause DNA to replicate, so smoking is still an indirect cause of cancer.

Fungi and mycotoxins cause virtually every type of cancer

Towards the end of his text, Costantini writes a brief conclusion that should be noted by anyone concerned about the cause of cancer.

Conclusion:

Data collected and presented here documents that fungi and their mycotoxins cause virtually every type of human cancer in either animals or humans or both.

Equally important, the series also documents that each and every dietary measure or drug found to be effective in treating diseases share nothing in common except that they are all antifungal and/or antimycotoxic.

The above statement has significant implications. Here is a highly qualified medical researcher saying that the only drugs or remedies that work to heal cancer are antifungal or destroy fungal enzymes. Herbs and natural health products are antifungal and can cure cancer. According to Dr. Costantini, drugs used in chemotherapy that are not antifungal cannot cure cancer.

Thousands of different drugs have been used on cancer patients, like human guinea pigs, without any real hope that they will address the true underlying cause of cancer. If drugs were first tested on fungi, rather than cancer cells, the value of the drug could be determined without animal and human testing. In simple terms, if the drug does not kill fungi, it will not work. In order for our NAP products to qualify for import into China, we increased the anti-fungal qualities based on this research. Unfortunately, fungi are ubiquitous in our bodies; we can never eliminate them entirely, and the fermentation of glucose feeds fungal growth. Treating cancer by treating fungi is not adequate. We must also eliminate parasites that are host to fungi, and eliminate conditions that lead to fermentation.

Dr. Clark identifies parasites in all cancers

The Cure For All Cancers by Dr. Hulda Regehr Clark Ph. D., N.D., was first published in 1993. Although the title suggests there is now a cure for all cancers, I believe that author means there is a cure for all types of cancers, because there is really only one type of cancer. If all cancers are caused by replication of infected cells, it follows that there is only one cure for all cancers. That cure is to remove all pollutants and parasites from the body and enable the cell to replicate normally.

Dr. Hulda Regehr Clark is the only cancer researcher I know of to recognize the significance of parasitic microorganism growth hormones in the cancer process. She should be awarded a Nobel Prize for her work in cancer research. Allow me to quote this momentous statement first published in 1993 that has already benefited many thousands of people.

> **In 1990 I discovered the true cause of cancer. The cause is a certain parasite, for which I have found evidence in every cancer case regardless of the type of cancer.**

In the revised 1998 edition, Dr. Clark also identifies excess DNA in tumors and cancer cells (Page 56):

> **But, in spite of all these tumor-promoting forces, a tumor could still not grow unless it had sufficient DNA to grow on.**

> **In tumors, the Syncrometer detects DNA all the time. Only in tumors and ovaries does it show up, leading me to believe that when I do detect it, it is out of place and out of control.**

> **How can DNA be continually supplied for cell multiplication? The answer is bacteria.**

The DNA of bacteria and fungi is not bound within a nucleus. Consequently, during the replication process, free microbial DNA could be found in the cells.

The Syncrometer is a measuring device that uses the capacity of electrical waves to resonate whenever two identical frequencies are imposed one over the other. By placing a test substance in circuit with the body, resonance occurs if something in the body matches the frequency of the substance on the test plate. This device has placed Dr. Clark far ahead of conventional researchers because she can treat patients, test, and verify her work quickly and accurately. With this device, she is able to identify the presence of DNA molecules not bound up into cells. For further information on the Syncrometer, please review information in her books.

Dr. Clark is also the only researcher I know of who has identified a method to inspect for growth factors and unbound DNA crystals. Close to one million copies of her books have been sold without the benefit of any major television talk show host or national advertising program. Word of mouth recommendations have been the major source of sales. That is why her program is gaining popularity worldwide, including China.

Dr. Clark writes (Page 8):

As if these parasites were not fiendish enough, as soon as there are adults in the liver something NEW happens. A growth factor, called ortho-phospho-tyrosine appears. A monster has been born! Growth factors make cells divide. Now YOUR cells begin to divide too! Now you have cancer.

...Other growth factors are produced, too. There are: epidermal growth factor (EGF), platelet derived growth factor (PDGF) insulin-like growth factor (IGF), fibroblast growth factor (FGF). These can also be made by bacteria. But only Fasciolopsis makes ortho-phospho-tyrosine.

Ortho-phospo-tyrosine is one of over two dozen "cancer markers" (indicators); it is present in cancerous tissues. The enzyme that makes it can be inhibited by genisteine. Genisteine can be isolated from red clover blossoms! Red clover blossoms are one of the best known traditional anti-cancer herbs!

I find that Dr. Clark's theory that all cancers are caused by the same fluke parasite difficult to accept, as any large parasite can damage cell-wall membranes and turn on the current of injury. I also disagree with the statement that microbial growth factors make cells divide. Microbial growth factors only mutate the cell wall. If she is right, my theory is wrong. This is definitely a good time to say: "Why should I believe you?"

The important thing to realize about what I consider to be an error in Dr. Clark's theory that microbial growth factors cause cells to replicate is that it doesn't really matter in regard to the cure for cancer. She claims microbial growth factors cause cells to replicate and mutate. I claim that the current of injury causes cells to replicate, and the growth factors only mutate the cell-wall membrane. Curing cancer by eliminating parasites is the same in either case.

What is so special about this one particular parasitic fluke called Fasciolopsis? Is this the only source of ortho-phospho-tyrosine in the body? Since, in my opinion, this is not the cause of DNA replication, it follows that this fluke need not be present in the body. Perhaps the body makes ortho-phospho-tyrosine due to microbial infection of the thymus.

To learn more about ortho-phospho-tyrosine I checked out the medical textbooks. According to Dr. Guyton, in the *Textbook of Medical Physiology* the major component of hormones produced by the thymus gland is made up of the amino acid tyrosine. Tyrosine is distributed throughout the body and an abundance of tyrosine is essential for control of body temperature through metabolism and production of ATP.

The presence of ortho-phospho-tyrosine in cell tissue is possible without the parasite *Fasciolopsis* being present. According to *Harper's Review of Biochemistry*, tyrosine is classed as a non-essential amino acid because it is easily produced from the essential amino acid phenylalanine. I am not convinced that any one parasite is responsible for all cancers, because all parasites can damage human tissue and create a current of injury. As mentioned earlier, bladder cancer has been attributed to the urinary blood fluke. Moreover, large parasites are not necessary for all cancers. If anything creates a current of injury, replication will take place. Cancer follows when replication of infected cells takes place. How the injury is created is more or less irrelevant.

If tyrosine is combined with phosphorus perhaps due to microbial enzymes, our body's control of metabolism would be reduced and fermentation increased. If molecules of phosphorus combine in a straight-line molecular structure to the amino acid tyrosine we get *Ortho-phospho-tyrosine*. It is recognized as a cancer 'primer' because the combination with phosphorus makes it a high-energy molecule, like pentose-phosphate, serving as an energy source for assembly of stable purine and pyrimidine molecules in DNA.

Dr. Bigelsen's book, *Your Cure For Cancer*, talks about the current of injury from medical treatment (Page 29). According to Bigelsen, a Canadian study of more than 50,000 women showed that women of ages 40 to 49 who were given annual mammograms showed a 36% increased breast cancer mortality compared to those given physical examinations only. A similar study from Sweden showed a 29% higher mortality rate. Due to the pressure put on the breast during the mammogram, and subsequent biopsy, the current of injury theory would account for the increased death rate for those who underwent regular mammograms. Parasites and microbial growth hormones alone do not account for this difference.

Dr. Clark has followed mainstream thinking that enzymes control all bodily functions, included DNA replication. This error does not significantly reduce all the other amazing benefits she has given mankind. Indeed, if she hadn't pointed out the connection between parasites and cancer, and if I hadn't seen the benefits of her program time and time again, I would never have started this research.

Ralph Moss has written a book called *Herbs Against Cancer* (1998). Moss is author of two other cancer-related books called *Cancer Therapy, The Independent Consumers Guide to Non-toxic Treatment and Prevention*, and *The Cancer Industry, The Classic Exposé of the Cancer Establishment*. Several references to his research, such as the importance of arginine are taken from his books. Moss was assistant director of public affairs at Memorial Sloan-

Kettering Cancer Center. In his book, *Herbs Against Cancer*, Chapter 16 is dedicated to a review of Dr. Clark's program.

Moss comes down very hard on Dr. Clark and destroys the safety of taking the recommended herbs, destroys the parasite theory of cancer and destroys the concept that ortho-phospho-tyrosine is a recognized cancer marker. He also destroys the credibility of five cases Dr. Clark uses as testimonial backup for her cures and completes his review without making any points which support Clark's program.

Although I tend to agree with his views against a single parasite causing cancer, I totally disagree with his view that parasites are not involved in the cancer process. He also claims that these herbs are too toxic to be taken safely and that Clark's program is not effective. It is obvious from his writing that Moss has never tried Clark's parasite cleanse program or else he is purposely trying to discredit the program. He claims that Dr. Clark recommends taking 80 capsules of wormwood to kill the parasites and another 80 capsules to kill the worms. The reader understands by the context that this is one dose equal to half a cup of fresh leaves. Such a large dose would, of course, be far too much.

The truth is that 80 capsules are taken over a three-week period, which amounts to about four per day. To ensure safety, Clark's program specifically instructs to start with one capsule on day one, go to two capsules on day two, and advance slowly. If any toxic effects are noted, return to the previous day level. Similarly, the additional 80 capsules are used as a maintenance program after the first bottle is used, and the second bottle of capsules is part of a three-month program. Since I have sold thousands of these kits, without hearing of any undesired side effects, and have sold more than 3 million capsules to a Chinese pharmaceutical distributor, I know this program is both effective and safe. It has been tested and proven by qualified medical cancer specialists in China.

Moss's chapter destroying credibility in Dr. Clark is a full 12 pages in length. Why would someone devote 12 pages of a book on herbs against cancer to destroying the credibility of another researcher who recommends using herbs to treat cancer?

In my estimation, Dr. Clark has given a great deal to the world. She has established the fact that parasites cause cancer, after mainstream medicine has rejected the idea. She introduced the concept that parasites have life cycles in our body, just as fleas and lice have life cycles outside of our body. To kill lice and fleas you should eliminate all life-stages simultaneously. You schedule treatment to kill the eggs and the adults, otherwise one or the other will maintain the infestation.

The same principle applies to parasites inside our body. To kill fungi and parasites with herbs, we treat them for a minimum three-week period to kill all life cycles. We need herbs or agents that kill eggs, larvae and adults simultaneously, and attack each stage for a three -week period. Even then, if we are living with a spouse or pets with the same infection, we can be easily reinfected. To be successful we have to improve the immune system and eliminate the possible sources of reinfection. We should also build up our mineral balance and ensure that all trace minerals are available for healthy cell-wall membranes.

Since fungi and bacteria can multiply in less than an hour, we must saturate our bodies 24 hors a day with these agents. We do not need a massive dose. We need continuous small and safe doses over a long period of time. In Clark's program herbs are taken four times a day for three weeks. As I said earlier, Dr. Moss did not appear to know that Dr. Clark's program was more than one big dose, which goes to show how little he knows about the program.

Dr. Clark has also given humanity the concept of using a simple low-voltage vibrational frequency to destroy microbes. We all know that we cannot have an electric current without a corresponding magnetic field. In physics, the study of electricity is called the electromagnetic spectrum. If you induce a small electric current into your body, you must also induce a small magnetic current through your body. If you cause the electric current to pulsate, the corresponding magnetic field will pulsate. If this magnetic field pulsates at a frequency that interferes with the natural bioradiation of microbes, they die. Enzymes have magnetic and paramagnetic properties, substrates have magnetic and paramagnetic properties. These magnetic properties can be increased by sleeping on magnetic pads, wearing magnetic devices, sunbathing, color therapy, sound therapy or zapping. It all makes perfectly good science.

Royal Rife established the concept in the 1930s and the theory is consistent with reality. Life is an electromagnetic phenomenon, and electricity is an electromagnetic phenomenon. It is inconceivable that one does not influence the other. Chemical bonds that require a sharing of electrons or an exchange of electrons at the molecular level, is an electromagnetic phenomenon. Free radicals are electrically charged particles making free-radical damage an electromagnetic problem. The use of an electrical device to measure pollutants in the body, or to check for the bioradiation of them, is a perfectly logical extension of the electromagnetic function in living things.

Life is considered by some researchers as an electromagnetic resonant frequency with the earth's electromagnetic field. If so, a fundamental understanding of living things can be known by the study of the unique resonant frequencies that distinguish one living thing from another. Rife proved that cancer microbes exist and that they can be destroyed by the proper resonant frequency that caused them to explode, much like a strong voice can shatter a crystal glass.

I have personally met with Dr. Clark on several occasions. What a fine, warm-hearted person! She is truly dedicated to helping cancer victims. In her books, she freely publishes information that now makes it possible for people with cancer and many other diseases to eliminate the cause of disease. Anyone who does not believe this statement should at least try her program. I am now a believer because I have witnessed the good results far too often to have any doubts.

Dr. Clark lectured in Toronto in 1995 to a group of about 450 ardent followers with several medical doctors in attendance. Following her speech, several people gave powerful testimonials about cancer cures using her methods and a lively question-and-answer period followed. A videotape of the event is available. See SOURCES for details.

Dr. Costantini presents overwhelming evidence that fungi and mycotoxins cause cancer, but he does not mention the DNA polymerase enzymes or flukes. He suspects that fungi cause genes to become defective, but cannot trace a pathway for that to happen. Comparison of DNA from normal tissue to tumor tissue shows cancer-cell DNA to be poisoned with aflatoxin but no other changes. Costantini cannot explain why the DNA would replicate out of control. He concludes that this research only "implicates" aflatoxin as a cause of breast cancer. Genes p53 and p16INK4 are implicated as mutated due to aflatoxin. However, the mechanism of mutation is still missing. Dr. Costantini assumes fungi cause genetic defects that lead to cancer. He does not look for other options such as the cell wall and its incapacity to knit with normal cells.

Our minds become a product of our education. It becomes difficult to question fundamental beliefs and look beyond them. The concept that genes control replication is so bound into medical education that the concept is not questioned. Research is being wasted to prove a false premise.

When we develop faith and confidence in people, we accept what they say without question. The position of authority in medicine carries a lot or respect. When authorities are wrong, who is there to question their error? The monopoly in medicine ensures that fundamental errors are not questioned.

21. Exposing indoctrination, deception and fraud

The purpose of this chapter is to illustrate how the cancer service industry maintains favorable public opinion even though, behind the scenes, they suppress effective cancer cures and thwart honest men who try to change the system. The simple truth is that perception is reality, and perceptions are controlled by dominating communication in the public media.

In 1998, Oncologist, Robert A. Weinberg, Director of Oncology Research at the Whitehead Institute in the U.S., published a summary of the gene theory of cancer in a book called *One Renegade Cell*. References to this book were used in Chapter 6. This easy-to-read narrative summarizes all the significant genetic research findings of the century and discusses numerous problems for research during the first decade of the next century. An endorsement on the back cover flap, by the director of the National Cancer Institute adds credibility to the book.

In this text, there is not one word about the possible fungal cause of cancer or the known characteristics about cancer cells having reduced respiration. The major conclusion is that genes cause cancer through interaction of genes for replication and lack of brakes called suppressor genes. Same old theory expressed as fact and dogma (Page 83):

> *Hence, the activation of oncogenes cooperates with the inactivation of the suppressor genes to create cancer.*

He also describes the close similarity between cancer cells and normal cells and the failure to discover any significant difference capable of causing cancer. As a result, early detection is not possible. He writes (Page 157):

> In spite of these failures, the most attractive approaches to tumor detection still derive from identifying genes and proteins that are unique to cancer cells. Mutant oncogenes, tumor suppressor genes, and their proteins come to mind.

Information such as this continues to convince the public that defective genes cause cancer, there is nothing one can do about it, early detection is not possible, and only a cancer specialist can help you.

There is significant evidence in alternative medicine that cancer can be detected before tumors form by studying life stages of fungi in the blood, or by measuring the electrical vibrations of the cancer cells. Why are early diagnoses by other methods ignored by the National Cancer Institute?

Billions of dollars have been wasted on gene study looking for genetic changes in normal cells that cause cancer. None have been found. Why don't they simply look for external causes in the cellular environment such as fungi and parasites, microbial growth hormones and lack of essential minerals required for maintaining the oxidative process? They know that cancer cells do not knit to human tissue. They know that bone growth is increased by an electro-magnetic stimulus. They know how to measure the damage of a heart attack by measuring the current of injury. They know that infectious agents may cause the current of injury. Through the research of Robert Becker and others, they know the current of injury causes replication of cells. The DNA polymerase chain reaction is cancer in a test tube. To claim they are looking for the genetic causes of cancer while millions are dying is incomprehensible.

At the present rate of increase in frequency of cancer, I wonder how many millions of men, women and children will die of cancer during the 21st century. More than one-half million Americans now die annually of cancer. That would be 5 million every ten years, or 50 million in the next century. What a frightening thought for the future of our children, grandchildren, and great grandchildren. Consideration must also be given to the fear of cancer during life, and the quality of life for those who survive treatment. In addition to death and suffering, consideration must be given to amputations and surgery that maim or disfigure cancer victims. In addition, the cost of treatment destroys the capacity of governments to maintain other essential services. The world-wide death rate from cancer is now 6 million annually and death rates are increasing.

Preventative mastectomies are a disgrace to medicine

The following report by Doug McConell on the Internet (*www.chroniclbooks.com*) describes the medical practice of removing healthy breasts in order to prevent future cancer due to defective genes. This "do no harm" form of treatment fits right in with mercury poisoning and blood letting as sheer ignorance.

Researchers at the Mayo Clinic in Rochester, Minn. studied the cases of 639 women who underwent the procedure (removal

of healthy breasts) at the clinic between 1960 and 1993. Doctors rely on genetic screening. Those who are carriers of BRCA1 or BRCA2 (genes that can lead to breast cancer) are of greater risk of developing the cancer.

The report goes on to illustrate how effective this treatment is as only two patients died of breast cancer after their healthy breasts were removed (due to missed tissue). Of course, these operations are relatively successful as no additional fermentation can occur. But what a price to pay.

Various publications now show that this practice continues to be used as a form of treatment to prevent breast cancer. What a horrible medical error! How could it happen? Why would medically trained cancer specialists have so much confidence in an unproven gene theory that they would operate and remove healthy tissue to prevent cancer that hasn't even appeared? Is indoctrination the whole story? What ever happened to the Hippocratic oath to "do no harm"?

Medical textbooks as a source of indoctrination

The *Textbook of Medical Physiology* by Dr. Arthur Guyton, used by the huge majority of medical students, is probably the primary reason for worldwide medical belief in the defective gene theory. This textbook is available in seven of the world's major languages, covering most of the world's population (China excepted). It has been used in medical universities since at least 1956. My copy is the 1981, 6th edition. Medically trained professionals believe in the defective gene theory because they have been taught to believe in it. This is what you would probably have been taught if you attended medical school.

Basically all of the misinformation that we have discussed in this text can be found in this one major textbook. The following quotations come from the section on cancer entitled *Genetic control of cell function, protein synthesis, and cell reproduction* (Pages 38-39):

Cancer is a disease that attacks the basic life process of the cell, in almost all instances altering the cell's genome (the total genetic complement of the cell) and leading to wild and spreading growth of the cancerous cells. **The cause of the altered genome is a mutation (alteration) of one or more genes; or mutation of a large segment of a DNA strand containing many genes; or, in some instances, addition or loss of large segments of chromosomes.**

Here is the cause of cancer, as taught to medical students, according to Professor Guyton:

Thus chance alone is all that is required for mutations to take place, so we may suppose that a very large number of cancers are merely the result of an unlucky occurrence.

Chance causes cancer because chance causes defective genes. The defective gene theory is just assumed correct. It has never been proven. Like the 'big bang' theory in creation, it serves a purpose. **The concept of 'chance' answers the need for a cause.** The outstanding value in promoting chance as the cause of cancer is that individuals have no control over cancer.

If we combine the above dogma with the dogma that genes control function of the cells by determining what substances will be produced, there is no reason to question the indoctrination. It all starts with the fatal flaw in the defective gene theory quoted earlier from Guyton's *Textbook of Medical Physiology*, Chapter 3.

The genes control function of the cell by determining what substances will be synthesized within the cell—what structures, what enzymes, what chemicals.

No other theory on the cause of cancer is taught or even discussed in this key medical text because 'chance' provides the only logical conclusion for a person trained to believe in the mechanistic concept of life. The only conclusion is defective genes cause cancer.

Medical students do not have an opportunity to evaluate alternative ideas. They are indoctrinated!

In all other fields of science, the development of a theory consists of evaluating a body of related observations and developing an explanation for the observations. Proof of the theory entails developing scientific, chemical or mathematical formulae that can be applied to all observations, without exception. If a series of formulas and equations can explain all observations, the theory is proven correct. If no such formula or equation exists, the theory has not been proven.

It is impossible to prove that chance causes cancer. More important, the frequency of cancer in the human population, as compared to animals in the wild, proves cancer is not due to errors in replication of DNA. DNA is a stable crystal formation of only four nucleotides, A to T and C to G.

If you read any educational publications and handouts provided by the American or Canadian Cancer Society or mainstream medicine for public education of cancer, you will not find any significant references to growth hormones, or fungi and parasitic infection as a possible cause of cancer. These references are conspicuous by their absence. Any honest and straightforward attempt to find a cure for cancer must consider other alternatives. One-sided, biased information is nothing more than deception and propaganda.

For example, the Canadian Medical Association's *Everyone's Guide to Cancer Therapy* (700 pages) does not have the word 'microbe' or 'parasite' in the 24-page index. A six-page section on genes and cancer does not mention the essential enzyme DNA polymerase required for replication of cells. The only reference to fungal infection is a brief reference to problems cancer patients may experience due to low resistance after chemotherapy. The only reference to growth hormones refers to diseases of the pituitary gland causing over production of growth hormones that lead to excessive growth or to cancer tumors that produce growth hormones.

Public perceptions are formed by publications such as these, and these perceptions are false. People who read this information and place their trust in the medical authorities are victims of fraud and injustice.

Deceptive claims abound in medical publicity

Take a moment to review any long quotation from the cancer establishment about the cause of cancer, oncogenes, carcinogenic bullets and multiple hits. Notice how deceptive they are. These cancer specialists do not commit themselves by making any positive statements.

From the following statement, for example, does the text say oncogenes (cancer-causing genes) exist or simply may exist? From *Everyone's Guide to Cancer Therapy* (Page 243):

> Some of the more *exciting discoveries in the past* is that *some of our normal genes may be activated* in various ways and transformed into genes capable of changing a normal cell into a cancer cell. These activated and cancer-causing genes are called oncogenes.

Statements such as "These activated and cancer-causing genes are called oncogenes" imply they exist. One is led to believe they were discovered "in the past." However, the whole paragraph is qualified by saying they "*may be activated*." The statement is deceptive and written with the intent to deceive because it only implies oncogenes exist.

Similarly in the section under what causes cancer (Page 5), we are told: "we *may soon be able* to test individuals, for example with a blood test, to discover whether a specific oncogene is present and if the suppressor gene is defective or absent."

And again: "The presence of certain oncogenes *may even give us* information about how likely it is that a cancer will spread."

The only reference to discovery of an oncogene that I can find relates to the 1976 discovery of the first 'cancer-inducing-gene' by Harold E. Varmus and J. Michael Bishop. There is no evidence that this discovery has been of any significant value, and I cannot find any details of the location of this gene in description of genes and their function. The current of injury that causes DNA crystals to separate is still the only known source of ionic energy required for stimulating repair to damaged tissue. There is so much misinformation printed in mainstream information, that it is difficult to take anything seriously.

If you look for it, almost every sentence on the causes of cancer is hedged with words like "may" and "it is thought" or similar disclaimers. I have yet to find any documented proof that an oncogene exists or that the Cancer Establishment has committed itself stating oncogenes have actually been proven to cause cancer. What exactly was the *"exciting discovery in the past"* that *"may be activated"*? Who discovered it? When? Did he or she receive a Nobel Prize for this significant discovery? Why not? Why should I believe you? Show me the proof.

In the modern (1997 edition) textbook *Human Genetics,* in the glossary oncogene is defined as a medical fact:

> **Oncogene** A dominant gene that promotes cell division. An oncogene normally controls the cell cycle but leads to cancer when overexpressed.

Where is the dominant gene that is overexpressed? Is it inside the cell with cancer or outside of the cell? Why hasn't the DNA polymerase chain reaction and DNA profile been used to identify it? Why has it never been tested and proven to cause cancer?

Cancer information is filled with references to oncogenes and proto-oncogenes. Here is another typical example:

> Oncogenes are also activated when a proto oncogene moves next to another gene, and the gene pair is transcribed and translated together, as if they form one gene. The double gene product, called a *fusion protein, somehow lifts control* of cell division.

The above section carries on like this for several paragraphs. It is hard to believe that there is not a shred of reality in the whole thing. It is all supposition expressed as fact to baffle and confuse the public. Try to explain how genes can fuse, and take control of cell division. Saying they do is not adequate. Genes are specific crystalloid structures. Genes don't fuse. Saying the gene pair is transcribed and translated must be a private joke. In medical jargon, DNA is *replicated*, RNA is *transcribed*, and proteins are *translated*. I wonder what he is talking about.

The concept that genes do not control replication of other genes has been adequately discussed in previous chapters With the knowledge about genes expressed in previous chapters, we can now recognize the lack of any value in genetic research into the causes of cancer.

Cancer is not caused directly by chemicals

In the public information booklet *Science and Cancer,* as published by the U.S. National Cancer Institute, we have reference to the first chemically induced cancer according to author M. Shimkin, M.D.:

> In 1915, however, two patient Japanese investigators, Katsusaburo Yamagiwa and Koichi Ichikawa, continued to paint the ears of rabbits with tar for many months, and were rewarded by the conclusive development of skin cancers at the site of the application of the tar. By 1933, British scientists under the leadership of Earnest Kennaway isolated a pure chemical benzopyrene from tar, and showed that it produced cancers at the site of application in mice.

Two facts should be pointed out about initiating cancer with chemical carcinogens: (1) An explanation as to how the carcinogen causes DNA to replicate is not available; (2) It takes a considerable length of time, as in months with repeated application, for cancer to be initiated. Why is so much time required?

The most logical explanation as to how many known carcinogens cause cancer can be found through the microbial process of fermentation. The carcinogenic substances become concentrated inside living tissue, where they stagnate and ferment or destroy cell-wall tissue. Heavy waxy products could also block the flow of ionic energy and imitate an injury to the cell wall. If the chemical damages cell-wall tissue, a current of injury will develop, initiate replication for repair, and allow parasitic life-forms to contaminate the repair process. Toxic chemicals are just another source of injury to cell walls leading to the natural process of repair.

I have not seen and reference to someone successfully initiating cancer in the laboratory from defective genes or by using known carcinogens. The concept that chemicals could cause replication of genes is akin to expecting life to rise from a batch of nucleotides. If chemicals could cause DNA to replicate, the DNA polymerase chain reaction would not need microbial DNA polymerase harvested from hot-spring bacteria.

Obvious indoctrination of medical students

Continuous indoctrination of medical students leads to continued belief in the defective gene theory as the cause of cancer. Let's review what is being taught in the 1997 textbook *Human Genetics,* Chapter 16. *Cancer is a Genetic Disorder:*

> Cancer is a consequence of disruption of the cell cycle. The timing, rate, and number of mitosis depend on protein growth factors from outside the cell and transcription factors within.
>
> Because these biochemicals are under genetic control, the cell cycle perturbation that is cancer is also.

Three points from the above quotation should be noted. Taken together, they show how easily it is to teach false doctrine. The first paragraph identifies two significant biochemicals or proteins: (1) protein growth factors from outside the cell, and (2) transcription factors from within.

The next statement says that since *these biochemicals are under genetic control,* cancer is also under genetic control.

The last statement is the critical error. The possibility that the biochemicals or external growth factor comes from a non-human gene source is not considered. Human genes do not control production of biochemicals by microbes and parasites living in the cell. The biochemicals that cause cancer are under genetic control, but microbes control these genes. The last important point is not part of the course.

The statement implies that all "biochemicals (growth factors) are under human genetic control." This implication is false. Only some biochemicals in the body are under human genetic control. The key to understanding cancer pivots on this vital issue. All possible sources of growth factor must be investigated and microbial growth factors eliminated before the statement can be considered true.

The previous reference illustrates how mainstream medicine continues to twist details to indoctrinate medical students with belief in the defective gene theory of cancer.

22. Ruthless ongoing suppression of effective cancer cures

In this chapter, let's review effective cancer therapies that are being suppressed by the cancer establishment. Some of these are suppressed in U.S.A. but that results, for some unknown reason, in suppression in Canada as well. The only possible reason is greed, wealth, and power. According to astronomers, no information comes out of a black hole, because all matter and energy is sucked in. Your taxes and mine are being sucked into this black hole of greed called the 'health care' industry. In addition, no information leaks out.

According to an article on cancer in The Toronto Star, April 1, 1999, entitled *No magic bullet yet* a record 62,700 Canadians died of cancer last year. The same article goes on to describe cancer as a genetic disease. Same old stuff expressed in different terms. Damaged cells receive *"phantom signals"* and *"hear voices that aren't there."* These cells *"keep the accelerator to the floor ignoring red lights and stop signs."* Dozens of companies are trying to design new drugs that affect signaling systems in tumor cells.

No one is trying to cure cancer. It is more profitable to design new drugs to be taken regularly in order to control the signaling system. At last report there were 129,000 new cancer cases in Canada last year. That's 350 per day, nearly 2,500 per week or 10,750 per month.

In the meantime all of the following valuable proven effective cancer cures are being ignored and suppressed. I referred to patent 5,139,684 in discussion of methods to cure cancer by vibrational frequencies. Let's take another look at this amazing patent in discussion of how the Health Protection Branch accepts electromedicine to enhance bone growth but denies electromedicine to enhance cell growth. The statement that electro- medicine has not been proven to be effective to reduce infection of human tissue and blood cannot be considered valid in view of the existing facts regarding blood electrification.

Suppression of 1990 U.S. patent #5,139 684

Blood electrification. Patent 5,139,684, granted Aug 18 1992 (filed Nov 16 1990)

Electrically conductive method and systems for treatment of blood and other body fluids and/or synthetic fluids with electric forces

Inventors: Dr. Steven Kaali and Peter Schwolsky

Abstract:

A new process and system for treatment of blood and/or other body fluids and/or synthetic fluids from a donor to a recipient or storage receptacle or in a recycling system using novel electrically conductive treatment vessels for treating blood and/or other body fluids and/or synthetic fluids with electric field forces of appropriate electric field strength to provide electric current flow through the blood or other body fluids at a magnitude that is biologically compatible but is sufficient to render the bacteria, virus, and/or fungus ineffective to infect normally healthy cells while maintaining the biological usefulness of the blood or other fluids. For this purpose the low voltage electric potentials applied to the treatment vessel should be of the order of from about 0.2 to 12 volts and should produce current flow densities in the blood or other fluids of from one microampere per square millimeter of electrode area exposed to the fluid being treated to about two milliamperes per square millimeter. Treatment time within this range of parameters may range for a period of time from about one minute to about 12 minutes.

Do you find this unbelievable? Treatment time is from about one minute to 12 minutes. Here is a simple cure, developed by mainstream medicine doctors, patented, and effective for treating diseases such as AIDS and cancer. Why isn't it being used in all mainstream health-care facilities?

I first heard about this patent at a health fair from a speaker named Bob Beck. This patent appears to be suppressed because electromedicine instead of pharmaceuticals drastically limits cartel profits and re-empowers patients' sovereignty over all diseases.

Who is Bob Beck? Beck is a retired physicist who is trying to make a difference in health care. He is a frequent speaker at health fairs where he talks about suppressed cancer cures and demonstrates electronic equipment that is being used successfully to cure cancer and other major diseases. Beck describes how you can build your own electrification devise and use it safely and effectively. For the complete microbial cleansing program four easy-to-follow steps are recommended:

1. *Blood electrification* based on suppressed patent 5,188,738 to kill off microbes and eliminate their toxins and enzymes. In the patented method, blood is removed from the body, electrocuted with a small voltage harmless to the blood cells, and the blood is returned to the body. Zapping flowing blood within your wrists results in the same effect without medical intervention.

2. *Pulsed Kilogauss Magnetic Fields* break up microbial microspheres, release trapped blood proteins from the lymphatic system and disrupt microbial enzymes. It also stops fermentation and revives the oxidative process. Requires a device called a pulse generator costing a few hundred dollars.

3. *Drink Silver Colloids* to cleanse the colon of anaerobic microbes and avoid reinfection of body tissues from the colon. Silver colloid kills over 600 known microbes by attacking their outer membrane layer. Silver colloid can be made at home with a low-cost colloidal silver generator.

4. *Drink ozonated water* to provide extra oxygen for cleansing the body of waste, revive the production of ATP and the citric acid cycle. Ozonated water is highly paramagnetic and delivers oxygen to the cells, destroys anaerobic bacteria, oxidizes toxins and helps build human based enzymes.

The U.S. medical patent 5,139,684 proves the effectiveness of destroying parasites with vibrational frequencies. By zapping the blood as it flows in the arteries, medical intervention is not required. The only cost is replacement of a nine-volt battery from time to time. The only thing difficult to comprehend is why the patented medical invention is not being used to save lives and reduce medical costs by mainstream medicine.

There is a cure for AIDS! It is just not being used.

There is a cure for Hepatitis! It is just not being used.

There would be no need to fear a viral pandemic, if we were free to use the non-drug therapies available to us. There is no need to crowd our hospitals with flue patients. Roughly 10% of flu patients die from opportunistic bacterial and fungal infection. There is no need for this to happen.

Victims of blood transfusion diseases do not need to die. Viruses can be killed in the body or in stored blood. Why not cure all Hepatitis C victims of the Red Cross-tainted blood supply and save medicare millions of dollars? One and one-half billion dollars are allocated as compensation for the victims who are in a position to win a court case. The others are left out. They could ALL be healed for a small fraction of that.

If Canadian doctors or alternative health professionals could freely operate alternative cancer clinics in Canada, millions of dollars could be saved from Medicare expenses. Low-cost cures for other diseases would follow. If freedom of health care were established in Canada, and supervised by a caring mainstream medicine, or at least paid for by medicare, millions of dollars could be saved from health care. In addition, millions of dollars could be earned by treating cancer patients from other countries where freedom of health care has not yet been established.

Due to an overload of the Canadian cancer hospital facilities, Canadians are waiting weeks for treatment or being sent to costly U.S. facilities. It doesn't have to be this way.

Vibrational and magnetic energy destroy enzymes

One day, and the sooner the better, vibrational medicine will take mainstream medicine out of the dark ages.

Costs of treating patients will be reduced to a small fraction of what is common now. All degenerative diseases will be treatable. Toxic drugs will be classed along with blood-letting and mercury poisoning as Stone Age Medicine. Metabolic therapies along with vibrational medicine will bring about a new age of health and productivity. If we consider how much productivity is lost due to illness and untimely death that could be avoided, we must realize that the cost of suppression has a bearing on our country's productivity and GNP.

The basis for vibrational medicine is well known in science. Every microbial life form has a specific vibrational frequency that can be easily measured with scientific equipment. By producing a suitable counter vibration, like jamming a radio station, the microbe can be destroyed without harming any other good microbes or destroying human cells. This equipment exists now in the form of Dr. Hulda Clark's frequency generator or zapper. (Instructions on how to build them are published in her books.) A list of vibrational frequencies for all common parasites is also given.

Magnetic therapy is also well proven as a benefit to health. Several companies market magnets to be placed on your body or beds for sleeping on. Magnetic fields disrupt microbes, and pulsating magnetic fields disrupt trapped blood proteins making them easier for the body to cleanse. Oxygen and water are paramagnetic. They can carry a magnetic field into a cell and increase the vital energy of the cell. Low-oxygen microspheres created by fungi can be disturbed by using magnetic fields produced by magnetic pads and magnetic pulse generators. Mainstream medical doctors claim there is no scientific validity in magnetic therapy, yet it works and there is a scientific reason why it works. The lack of medical validity doesn't mean it is not effective. It just hasn't been researched by those who are in control and who do not want it to reduce drug sales and profits.

Magnetic fields are the central foundation for energy medicine. A negative magnetic pole is used for relief of pain, production of sleep, reversal of edema, inhibition of microorganisms, reversal of cancer, production of anabolic hormones, and prevention of Alzheimer's. Because of the blood-brain barrier to drugs, magnetic therapy should be used to kill brain parasites to help cure Alzheimer's.

Cell-Specific Cancer Therapy uses magnetic pulses

Since cancer cells vibrate at a different frequency than normal human cells, cancer cells can be identified electronically anywhere in the body by using a machine similar to Magnetic Resonance Imaging. Cancer cells can be located in minutes by their vibrational frequency. After locating the cancer by its vibrational frequency, a magnetic pulse in this frequency can be aimed at the exact spot to destroy the cancer cells without any harm to nearby normal cells. The microbial enzymes are destroyed by the magnetic impulse and the microbe or cancer cells cannot function. The principle applies to all microbial diseases. What could be more logical, safe and simple? This equipment exists now and could save millions of lives and billions of healthcare dollars if it were allowed to be used in Canada and the United States. For more information, see SOURCES.

The Hepatitis C scandal in Canadian blood-supply products could be partially corrected by curing all patients of the disease. Imagine what could happen in the field of vibrational medicine in 10 – 20 years, if full-scale development were allowed by trained medical doctors using government funds. Suppression of alternative cancer therapies must first be eliminated.

The amazing thing about magnetic therapy is that it has already been proven safe and accepted by the FDA and HPB in the use of magnetic resonance imaging. The FDA has stated that the exposure to a magnetic field is not essentially harmful.

However, claims cannot be made for magnetic therapy because tests have not been conducted and mainstream medicine has not approved their use. Nor is there any intention to do so. Without medical approval, use of magnetic therapy devices is limited to research purposes, and sold without claims. They are legal to manufacture, distribute, and use only for research or personal use. No claims can be made for them. The medical dictatorship is at work to protect you from good health.

Finding a cure for cancer is not a problem. Using it is. There is no scientific reason why cancer cannot be diagnosed and prevented long before surgery is necessary.

Gaston Naessen's 714X terminated in USA

Since 714X was introduced more than 20 years ago, more than 100,000 cancer patients in numerous countries have enjoyed varying degrees of success, without one instance of any side effect. Furthermore, 714X can be used to prevent disease.

Charles Pixley of Rochester N. Y. introduced 714X into the U.S. market. The FDA stepped in, laid-trumped up charges, destroyed his business and sentenced him to 19 years in jail. A compassionate judge allowed him out in one year. By then Mr. Pixley had suffered total financial ruin from legal costs. Americans can no longer receive 714X. For complete details try sending Email to Pix108@frontiernet.net.

Gaeston Naessens and Dietmar Schildwaechter, MD, PH.D., have spent the last 25 years perfecting darkfield microscope blood tests. They claim to be able to diagnose any type of cancer and immune system disorders up to two years prior to their onset, with a 1% margin of error.

In contrast, women are given mammograms to detect breast cancer, knowing there are many false positives, and the process, with a biopsy, creates a current of injury that causes replication of cells to repair the injury, possibly causing cancer, or causing existing cancer to spread more rapidly.

In darkfield microscope videos by Gaston Naessens, you can see for yourself how cancer can be detected long before tumors develop and vital organs are damaged. There is no valid reason why millions of people must wait for tumors to develop and then undergo emergency cancer therapy costing thousands of tax dollars per person. When you study your personal, live-blood sample, and observe parasites in red blood cells and blood serum, you become more highly motivated to cleanse your body of pollutants, do a parasite and liver cleanse, as well as get serious about good nutrition. It is a lot easier to change your lifestyle when you are highly motivated by your personal observations, and providing you know what to do and why to do it.

CanCell: The magic cancer bullet is being suppressed

Author Louise B. Trull's book *The CanCell Controversy* recounts the unbelievable 70-year and still ongoing suppression of a non-toxic cancer cure that works on the vibrational level.

The formula started out as produced by a Jim Sheridan in the 1930s and was called ENTELEV. After outstanding success with cancer patients, and 40 years of failure to get medical approval, he passed the formula and job on to Ed Sopcak. In 1992 the FDA placed an injunction against Mr. Sopcak barring him from making and distributing the formula. By then, more than 10,000 cancer patients had received free bottles of the formula, many experienced complete cancer remission, and no one had toxic side effects.

In a nationally televised TV talk show in June of 1993, host Maury Povich featured Ed Sopcak with a number of people who pleaded with medical authorities for continued access to CanCell. Obviously the majority of U.S. government officials are aware of the product but authorities are doing nothing to make it available to the people.

The formula is made up of the following chemicals, according to FDA analysis and report: Inositol, nitric acid, sodium sulfite, potassium hydroxide, sulfuric acid, and catechol. These ingredients are heated for the better part of a day (four batches in an eight-hour cycle), resulting in batches of a dark brown liquid.

While looking for clues on the function of these chemicals in cancer cells, I ran across one interesting clue. Scientists who analyze cells to determine the contents of protoplasm use chemicals to precipitate proteins out of solution based on their individual ionic charges. In a text by D. A. Coult, *Molecules and Cells*, we read (Page 54):

> The protein chemist wishing to purify his product by precipitation at this stage adds solid ammonium sulfate. This bivalent sulfate ion is a good 'precipitating ion', but the solid salt itself also competes for water with hydrophilic protein. Removal of water brings the macromolecules closer together and allows the short range forces to operate, with the result that the molecules aggregate and precipitate.

CanCell is the only man made chemical or drug that I have found with a reputation of curing cancer. When we realize parasites in the body are producing enzymes that are unique to microbes, we could possibly produce a formula that would attack only these enzymes or proteins. For example, a mixture to precipitate chitin, thereby eliminating the contamination of cell-wall membranes, could be an effective cancer cure.

Allow me to digress for a moment. The author goes on to write: "The killing of protoplasm can be accomplished by allowing heavy-metal ions like chromium, mercury, or osmium *(an oxide of platinum found in light bulbs)* to enter the cell and to precipitate the proteins of the protoplasm. Eating with chromium utensils and cooking or storing food in stainless steel pots also adds to our toxic overload. Here's how heavy metal toxins from dental fillings or industrial contaminants destroy our cells. It may take years before we notice any health changes, but the pathway is obvious. Toxic chemicals can kill protoplasm and render it less productive, leading to chronic fatigue and immune system dysfunction.

Coming back to CanCell, according to Sopcak, the mixture works vibrationally, and can be applied internally as well as externally. The concept for this product starts with the work of Otto Warburg, who established the anaerobic characteristics of cancer cells. Instead of just two types of cells, aerobic and anaerobic, Sopcak establishes a third type, based on the electrical potential of the cells. Because of the chitin incorporated into the cell-wall membrane, cancer cells have a lower level of plasma membrane. Cancer cells have a lower redox potential than normal cells. *(Redox potential is explained below.)*

I suspect the reason for this redox potential difference follows from a reduced amount of phosphorus in the cell-wall membrane. That is why they are cancer cells. Cancer cells require some oxygen but not as much as normal cells. If we further reduce the ionic energy in the cell-wall membrane, metabolism stops and they cannot survive. Reducing the redox potential of the cell-wall membrane does this. It's really that simple.

Redox potential is perhaps best described as a representation of overall electron activity in a cell. In a broad sense, redox potential could be considered as a measure of the ease with which a substance either absorbs, conducts, or releases electrons. This donation or acceptance of electrons is correctly termed oxidation and reduction. Simply stated, oxidation is the gain of oxygen with the loss of electrons. Reduction is the gain of electrons with the loss of oxygen. Oxidation can also mean the gain of hydrogen, with the loss of electrons, and reduction can mean the gain of hydrogen and the loss of electrons. The transfer of electrons is the basis for all oxidation-reduction reactions. Oxygen does not have to be involved in the process. Redox potential is the ease with which electrons can be made to transfer, or chemical actions made to occur.

Cancer cells have a lower redox potential than normal cells because cancer cells have reduced respiration. Otto Warburg proved that embryonic mouse cells reverted to fermentation automatically when respiration was reduced by 35%. CanCell proves that cancer cells die when oxygen is reduced by about 50% while normal cells do not suffer any side effects. Embryonic cells are cells that are multiplying naturally and are used in laboratories where a current of injury is not available.

CanCell works by blocking respiration of cancer cells

Let's review the main concept of CanCell as written in the book *The Cancel Controversy* (Page 26):

If we continue to damage cells until they are in the electrical voltage established by Otto Warburg as being between a negative .17 and a negative .21 volts, there appears a very small bacterium that Sopcak believes the medical profession misreads as a virus. It is classified as Progenitor cryptocides, isolated by Dr. Livingston Wheeler several years ago. **That bacterium aids in the transfer of the cell from being oxygen-using, or aerobic, to anaerobic, or in a state of fermentation.**

I suspect that this is the most common bacterium or fungus that provides the microbial cell-wall membrane proteins that mutate the cell wall. Other parasites could also be involved.

In order for the microbes and cancer cells to survive, the electrical potential must be maintained at the values of a negative .17 to .21 volts. CanCell works electrically on the cell's redox potential by reducing it too low for respiration to occur at all.

CanCell works by reducing these electrical levels even lower, too low for the respiratory cycle of the microbe and the cancer cell, causing the microbe and cancer cell to suffocate and die, and the cells to lyes or self-digest.

Isn't this incredible?

Destroy cancer cells by suffocating them. Suffocate them by reducing the total energy level of all cells so that we selectively eliminate only those with reduced respiration.

Why not? That's how microbes take over human cells. For example, microbial enzymes and toxins eliminate the capacity of iron- based enzymes to use oxygen. Dr. Enderlein discovered that lactic acid binds with iron to produce *lactic acid ferric oxydul* that causes human cells to die from lack of oxygen.

A simple, non-toxic solution, taken for three weeks, causes cancer cells and microbes to suffocate and die because they cannot maintain respiration needed for life. They wilt like a plant without water.

No side effects. No hair loss! It is ideal for children with livers too small to process toxic drugs. Just perfect for the Last Wish Foundation to give to children dying from cancer. Perhaps a group of Canadians should start a "First Wish Foundation" with facilities in Mexico. This would be owned and operated by Canadians to treat Canadian children with affordable alternative therapies not allowed in Canada.

CanCell is the magic bullet to cure all cancers. However, it is being suppressed now and has been for over 60 years. Millions of people have died of cancer unnecessarily because of this inhumane act.

It takes about 20 to 22 days for most treatments with CanCell to have effect. I find this time frame conforms with the time required by Dr. Clark's parasite-cleanse program. It takes three weeks to eliminate the production of growth hormones by destroying all parasites and their life cycles whether you use herbs and/or vibrational frequencies. Dr. Philpott's negative-field magnets take two weeks of continuous application to kill microorganisms and 12 weeks of continuous exposure to treat cancer cells.

Canadians are waiting longer than three weeks to receive cancer treatments from the overloaded cancer facilities. Doesn't it make sense to provide them with these alternative cancer treatments while they wait for conventional therapy? Doing so before cancer treatments can be given will not keep them from receiving accepted methods or interfere with it. What other reason is there for not doing so?

U.S. Court order stops distribution of FREE cancer cure

The CanCell controversy describes a clear and outright suppression of an effective non-toxic treatment for cancer in the U.S. Ed Sopcak never sold any of his formula. He simply gave it away to people who requested it in order to support his claims that it worked. He never advertised the product. All requests were obtained by word of mouth following from recovery of cancer and other diseases. No one complained about the product, although the FDA sought complaints by illegally tracing UPS shipment records and interviewing people using the product.

In the final analysis, the U.S. court injunction was issued to stop Sopcak from giving CanCell away and curing people with cancer for FREE. No one had been injured, no one complained, and nothing was sold. The U.S. Court decisions against Sopcak for CanCell, and Charles Pixley for 714X cannot be explained within the concept of an honest judicial system. Frightening, isn't it.

The court order by the Province of Saskatchewan to force amputation of body parts on Tyrell Dueck is similarly an injustice. Authorities have established a precedent to force individuals to take medical treatment against their will and personal judgement. Can we trust the Canadian Judicial System to protect personal rights?

Isn't that frightening? Think of the possible ramifications if compulsory surgery and chemotherapy is made standard medical policy for all children 13 years and younger? Why stop at 13?

If you believe that fungi causes cancer and you have a child who is denied antifungal treatment as well as the right to go elsewhere for it, what would you do?

Children with HIV are being forced to take AZT for treatment. If you have a child who tests HIV positive, and you must submit that child to AZT treatment, or lose your child to the authorities, what would you do?

In the next chapter, we will read about a Dr. Philip Berger who has been quoted as saying: 'Doctors have to be the absolute custodians of children's care,' he says. 'Once the child is born,' he says, 'I think the state has a duty to protect the child from any disease for which a parent is refusing treatment where the benefits are clear.'

Clear to whom? Who decides? Why should any self interest group become "absolute custodians of children's care" Doesn't parenthood count for anything?

Let's take this to another level. What if veterinarians were to say: "Once a cat or dog is born, veterinarians have to be the absolute custodians of all household pets." It seems to me that animal owners and animal right activists wouldn't allow such intolerance for cats and dogs, if it were proposed.

Since effective cancer cures are being suppressed, why should doctors have the right to impose surgery, radiation, and chemotherapy? If drugs such as AZT are deadly to others, why should anyone have the right to enforce this drug as treatment for a simple HIV viral infection?

BioPulse uses insulin to starve cancer cells

A recent new cure for cancer reduces the sugar levels in cancer patients by injecting insulin into the blood stream. By carefully eliminating all glucose from the body, rendering it hypoglycemic, for an hour or so, cancer tumors and fungi starve to death without any toxic side effects to human cells. A large number of additional cleansing and nutritional steps enter into the program but the use of insulin is the main step. You will recall that fungi live on carbon, and carbon must be available continuously for their needs. This new treatment is limited to a clinic in Mexico but additional clinics could easily be established anywhere that mainstream medicine would allow. Call 888-523-0101 or check the Internet at www.Biopulse. com.

The concept of eliminating all glucose in the body to starve fungi and cancer cells brings up an important question. What is the result of giving bed ridden cancer patients a glucose drip?

As you see there are many cures for cancer based on finding a functional difference between normal cells and cancer cells as well as by eliminating fungi and bacteria. CanCell reduces respiration, Biopulse reduces metabolism. Oxygen destroys anaerobic microbes and cancer cells. Arginine reduces fermentation. Zappers destroy microbial enzymes and microbes. Magnetic pulses destroy cancer cells. 714X cleanses the lymphatic system. None of these rejected cures destroy all rapidly growing cells. To do so would render them ineffective because new cells are required to heal an injury and shut down the current of injury.

In contrast, many of the approved chemotherapy treatments eliminate all rapidly growing cells, cancerous or not. In addition, increasing glucose levels in the body with a glucose drip feeds fungi and cancer cells. On top of that, they tell us to be wary of unproven methods such as herbal remedies.

Eliminating microbes with herbs is possible

If we compare the way essiac is made to the method for making CanCell, we find a significant similarity. The four herbs in essiac are boiled and left to process for several hours, providing time for plant enzymes to form new compounds in the tea. People who just take the herbs, as in capsules, do not report the same significant benefits as those who make up their own fresh tea. Rene Caisse insisted on a fresh brew and made it almost every day.

Mainstream medicine refuses to prescribe herbal remedies such as essiac due to lack of standardization and consistency in herbal remedies. This problem does not exist with CanCell, and still they refuse to use it.

Metabolic therapy: The Ludde Protocol

Frank Ludde operates a small metabolic clinic in West Vancouver, Canada. With metabolic therapy, one does not treat symptoms; one removes the cause of diseases. Mr. Ludde believes all diseases can be cured by metabolic therapy. Since 1988, Mr. Ludde has sent the following appeal to the Minster of Health for each province as well as the Federal Minister of Health. No one shows any interest. Frank Ludde writes:

> I am now appealing to Canadians to form an impartial committee to scientifically examine metabolic therapy. The committee should be selected by an independent panel, in a manner similar to the jury-selection process. Its findings should then be reported to the Canadian public so that they may choose whether they wish to have the therapy made available to all, by process of referendum or whatever other means necessary.

No province has taken steps to scientifically investigate an effective cancer cure now available in Canada. Nor has the federal Minister of Health accepted the challenge.

I would like to see a similar jury-selection process set up to test and evaluate cancer therapies. To do so, I am suggesting we establish cancer clinics that function as detox centers. This idea will be developed in the next Chapter

An excellent video is available introducing the Ludde Protocol, complete with testimonials from people representing a variety of diseases. Many of these people were so called hopeless cases. All treatments are on an outpatient basis. The average length of treatment is 12 weeks. Patients come to see him four days per week. See SOURCES for details.

Ludde explains how toxins and parasites enter the lymphatic system and many are carried into the cytoplasm of the cell. Inside the cell, they disrupt further metabolism. In order to cleanse the cells of toxins and waste, we must first clean the lymphatic system and then allow several more weeks to detoxify the cells. It takes years of pollution to destroy cells and it will take months, rather than days or weeks, to cleanse the cells of their load of toxic waste and parasitic infection.

Fasting helps detoxify and cure cancer by forcing cells to make use of whatever they are storing for emergency and have an opportunity to dump toxic waste. Consuming only fresh and raw vegetables for a few days per month is a low-cost form of metabolic therapy anyone can use.

Amino acids banned for sale in Canada

Numerous books on amino acids describe how amino acids help cure cancer. Some cancer clinics in Mexico use amino acids as part of their metabolic therapy. In Canada, our Health Protection Branch has banned resale of individual bulk amino acids in health-food stores and drug-stores. Drug stores sell numerous products more dangerous to our health than amino acids. Why have amino acids been banned for sale even from drug stores?

Amino acids are derived from food. Arginine is a concentration of one amino acid found in food. There is a possibility of taking too much of one creating an imbalance, but that possibility applies to all supplements. The fact that we can purchase them in the United States and bring them back for personal use supports argument for their relative safety. There are no reasons to ban amino acids from public sale in Canada without first having a hidden agenda.

None of the regulations Health Canada enforces on the Canadian public to protect us from 'good health' is more effective than regulations against distribution of amino acids and bioactive mineral supplements in natural health products.

What will it take to stop suppression of cancer cures? If people from a foreign land invaded our country with mercenary soldiers, plundered our wealth, and killed thousands of people, would you stand by and wait for your turn to die? I don't think so.

What is the difference if multinational corporations with mercenary politicians and mercenary bureaucrats do the same thing?

We cannot stop the cancer industry unless we introduce competition into the health-services field and stop the suppression of cost-effective alternatives. Only by breaking the grip of the medical cartel on our health-care system can we hope to advance effective cancer cures and reduce costs. We can no longer be silent.

As I concluded my research on the cause of and cures for cancer, I realized this information would be of far more value if it ended with a call for political action. Knowing the cause of cancer and how to treat it gains value if this knowledge becomes available to the public and is accepted and recognized by government policy and costs are covered by health insurance plans.

It became obvious that there is a great need to encourage people to take political action and demand an end to suppression of effective cures for all diseases. But how can this be accomplished?

23. Developing cancer clinics as detoxification centers

Cancer clinics should be modeled on drug or alcohol detoxification centers. You commit yourself for a period of time to detoxify your body of parasites and pollutants, stop fermentation and rebuild your oxidative metabolism.

There is an easy way for Canadian federal or provincial governments to prove they are interested in and willing to allow immediate health care reform. Do a comparison study.

Give a group of alternative health-professionals and businessmen with a history of integrity and high moral standards, a chance to prove that cancer can be treated more effectively and at less cost than by conventional cancer treatments. These people must be protected from medical or economic reprisals for participating in this research. Allow these groups permission to set up alternative cancer clinics using equipment and methods not approved by mainstream medicine and the Health Protection Branch.

That's the key to success. These alternative cancer clinics must not be limited and made ineffective by regulations that restrict use of any cancer cure, herb, or product the cancer clinic operators wish to use.

As soon as cancer or abnormal growths are observed, put these people on a program of parasite, organ and tissue cleansing. Since most cancer patients must wait several weeks for cancer therapy, this will not keep them from receiving medically approved methods. What do they have to lose? They could benefit by immediate remission of their cancer or benign growths.

Let's build upon this concept. Parasite and tissue cleansing could save lives, save taxpayers millions of dollars, and help maintain our universal health care system.

Establish cancer detoxification centers

Just allow groups of responsible citizens and alternative-health caregivers to operate one or more of the recently closed hospitals or a vacant wing. Reopen the facility as a cancer detoxification center. Provide funding for a minimum ten-year research project so that definitive results can be obtained. In order to do this, four essential steps are required.

1. Declare these cancer facilities free from all Health Canada and the Health Protection Branch regulations that restrict use of any cancer treatment the patient may desire to use or the board may decide to employ. That's the key minimum requirement. Eliminate HPB regulations against using natural health products such as amino acids or any of the available cancer cures with a good track record in other countries.

2. After a medical diagnosis of cancer or of a benign growth, have cancer patients live in the detox center full time for three to four weeks to have the conditions that cause cancer removed from their body. Consider this as a pollutant and parasite detox program similar to a drug or alcohol detox program. Ensure that the patients receive sound nutrition. Have the patient return for medical reevaluation from time to time. Operate, radiate, or apply chemotherapy only if deemed necessary by the board or requested by the patient.

3. Upon observing reduced benign growth or tumor growth, release patients from the detox clinic. **Have patients report for parasite and blood tests to** ensure they have not been reinfected with parasites and have not returned to a life-style that leads to cancer conditions. After three months, return checkups could be extended to quarterly and semi-annual checkups.

4. Provide these institutions with an effective operating budget to include education of patients to follow a cancer-free lifestyle. Give caregivers an acceptable income and provide **liability insurance coverage** as provided to mainstream medicine. *(There is always a chance of meeting people who will want to shut the facility down through legal action or take advantage of caregivers through frivolous personal damage suits)*

Just as alcoholics and drug addicts check into a facility to detoxify and break their dependence on drugs or alcohol, cancer patients should check into a hospital to detoxify their body of parasites and pollutants. If Medicare pays for alcohol and drug detox centers, it should also pay for parasite detox centers. While in hospital, patients could nourish their body properly, cleanse the lymphatic system, eliminate parasites and disrupt the pattern of ingesting chemical pollutants and junk foods.

Hospitals could be equipped with magnetic wave devices, as used in the Dominican Republic, which destroy existing cancer cells and tumors quickly and safely with a magnetic frequency without damage to adjacent healthy cells. This one therapy alone, if made accessible by our medical services, would destroy the need for all conventional cancer treatments in vogue today.

Vitamins and minerals would be taken to strengthen and repair cell-wall integrity so that internal problems such as ulcers and cysts would heal, and the current of injury shut down. Without microbes polluting the cells as they multiply, new cells would knit to human tissue to eliminate tumor growth, or white blood cells would form properly to eliminate leukemia. Bone repair would also be enhanced with electromagnetic current as recognized now in mainstream medicine.

All health professionals could be invited to apply their skills where needed. Medical doctors would be included for their diagnostic expertise, but their authority to decide treatment would not exceed that of other health professionals or the board of advisors. Medical doctors would also be protected from retaliation by medical authorities.

Dr. Hulda Clark's 1999 book *The Cure for All Advanced Cancers* presents an ideal starting point. Her book outlines a 20-day program to reduce advanced tumors. Her book uses photos of x-rays taken before treatment and after treatment showing tumor regression. Her program consists of using parasite cleansing herbs, nutritional vitamin and mineral supplements, removal of dental amalgams, zapping, and cleansing of bowels, kidneys, liver and lymphatic fluids. If cancer clinics would start with this basic 20 day program and add to it the benefit of more expensive equipment such as live cell blood analysis, mineral analysis, and cell-specific therapies, I believe the cure rate would be extremely high.

The clinic could also serve as a facility for a cancer check-up. We could check for cancer-causing conditions based on live-blood cell analysis. Cancer could be prevented before a tumor or new growth forms. One of the major reasons people do not have regular cancer check-ups is that they don't want to know. All of the options are equally frightening. By removing fear of cancer treatments, people would be more willing to have regular check-ups.

Operating and managing a cancer clinic based on these suppositions could be achieved without control by mainstream medicine. Naturopathic doctors would be more suitable as directors, because their philosophy and education would not clash with these metabolic therapies.

If mainstream medicine really wanted a cure for cancer, this concept would already be in place. American and Canadian doctors would not have to set up cancer clinics in Mexico. The news media would report on the successful cases of alternative-care cancer clinics instead of just the unsuccessful ones. Public perceptions could be changed about the value of alternative cancer cures from that of something to fear to that of something to embrace.

Do you think it is possible that about 30 Mexican cancer clinics survive and prosper without any successful cancer treatments? Of course not. Their business success is based largely on word-of-mouth referrals from satisfied customers. I have met several people who have recovered from cancer by going to Mexican clinics. Have you ever seen one such cancer treatment success story broadcast on national television? I know I haven't.

If cancer detoxification centers were allowed, the patients would be fed a combination of fresh foods and juices along with food supplements known to stop cancer. Pollutants and toxins would be removed from their environment, along with toxic cosmetics and personal-care products. During the day, patients could attend lectures or watch videos instructing them on proper nutrition and methods of parasite cleansing, enemas, colonics, kidney cleansing and liver cleansing. During their stay, they would also be guided through these cleansing processes so that pollutants and parasites could be cleansed from the body. A series of lymphatic exercises, for example, would help cleanse the lymphatic system and lymph nodes. Oral chelation could help cleanse the arterial system.

Before entering the hospital the patients could have their hair and body fluids tested for mineral deficiencies, have blood tested with darkfield microscopes for parasitic infection, and have tests for levels of ammonia and mycotoxins. By the time they arrive for treatment, a suitable personalized cleansing and nutrition program would be in place for them to follow. For example, people with prostate cancer would receive flaxseed; people with bone cancer would receive boron supplements. People with liver cancer would receive silymarin, an extract that is derived from a herb called milk thistle. These supplements are known to be organ specific and help cancer patients with cancer in these organs.

In the event this natural program is not effective quickly enough for a late-stage critical patient, the patient can be transferred to a regular hospital. The time spent at the cancer rehabilitation center would prepare him or her to have far greater success with surgery, radiation, and chemotherapy if deemed necessary. Since patients often have to wait several weeks for conventional treatment, there is no reason for medical authorities to argue that alternative therapies would deter use of conventional therapies. Waiting time used in detoxification and supplementation would be far better in a supervised clinic than stress-filled hours spent at home waiting for surgery, radiation, and chemotherapy.

Upon leaving the hospital, patients would be supplied with natural herbal remedies called maintenance programs to avoid parasite reinfection and patients could be instructed on how to maintain a lifestyle that would keep them healthy. The cost of treating patients for additional cancer cases could be largely eliminated.

Herbs such as essiac, compounds such as the amino acids arginine and acetimide as well as personal electronic or magnetic devises could be purchased by the patient to take home. Cancer patients could complete and extend the treatment at home and avoid future cancer problems. Follow up visits and darkfield blood tests would help ensure that the patient has not allowed conditions for cancer to return to his body. Every clinic should be equipped with a darkfield microscope and with people trained how to use it.

Compare success of alternative therapy to conventional therapy

If one were to compare the costs to Medicare for all of the above supplies and use of equipment, it would only be a fraction of the cost of present mainstream radiation, surgery and chemotherapy. Cures would be faster, more cures would result and fewer repeat cases would be experienced. Millions of dollars could be saved from Medicare, and fewer people would die the painful deaths related to cancer and drug therapy. The success of this program would lead to discarding the other medical myths that are wasting millions of tax dollars.

For comparison, a second standard hospital could be selected to serve as a base. Have the same certified accountants keep track of expenditures at both locations and compare expenditures and effectiveness of the two options.

After five years, and again after 10 years, tabulate and publish the results. Acceptable evidence of success or failure would be based on the observed benefits to people and fiscal data.

If alternative health programs failed to prove their value, which I doubt, how much will we have lost? Who will have been injured? No one. If alternative health proves its value, we could save billions of dollars in future generations. The benefits of darkfield microscopes, ozone therapy, vibrational medicine, chelation therapy, amino acids, herbal cleansing of parasites, nutrition, and amalgam removal could become Medicare's approved treatments for fungal and microbial diseases.

Anyone opting for radiation or chemotherapy would have to pay for it out of his own pocket!

The government should support only the most cost-effective option. Government publications should change false perceptions about drugs and natural health products. They both have a place; neither should be excluded from medicare. When public perceptions change and cancer patients realize cancer is a microbial disease, easily treatable without toxic drugs and radiation, they will refuse standard allopathic cut, burn and poison treatments. Mainstream medicine will follow with anti-microbial treatments due to public demand.

Give the people a credible option. As long as the majority of people do not know about alternative cancer therapies, they cannot opt for alternative treatments. As long as medical insurance does not cover these costs, they cannot afford to select them. Our medicare system will continue to fail. All Canadians for generations to come will suffer because of our lack of action.

According to newspaper reports, cancer patients in the Hamilton region must wait up to three months before they can be scheduled for radiation therapy. Some are being sent to the U.S. for radiation treatment. Newspaper reports say it costs about $6,000 in Canada for a treatment and over $16,000 for the same treatment in the U.S. That's far more than the cost of living in a rehabilitation center for a month.

If people with cancer were put on metabolic therapy and detoxification while waiting, the cancer tumor, if present, would be far easier to destroy. Why allow cancer to progress for three months after diagnosis when alternative therapies are available to stop the growth? Eliminate DNA polymerase enzymes and heal the injury so that mutated replication stops. What can be more scientific? What can be simpler?

With one bold but simple directive from the Minister of Health to Health Canada officials, billions of dollars could be saved from current medical abuses by making use of proven effective low-cost alternatives.

If mainstream medicine believes conventional treatments are better, they should welcome this chance to prove it. A direct comparison of conventional treatment versus alternative treatment would establish the most efficient and cost effective way to treat cancer. Who would not want that to happen?

Chemotherapy reduces life expectancy for cancer patients

Correcting the cellular environment to stop mutated replication of cells is the cure for cancer. Toxic chemicals just add to the problem by suppressing the immune system, reducing capacity of the liver to eliminate ammonia, and increasing fungal mycotoxins. Is it any wonder that chemotherapy creates so much devastation? According to Barry Lynes in *The Healing of Cancer* (Page 9), Professor Hardin Jones, PH.D declared that according to his carefully researched statistics, the cancer patient who received no treatment had a greater life expectancy than the one who received treatment. He writes:

> For a particular type of cancer, people who refused treatment live an average of twelve and a half years. Those who accepted surgery and other kinds of treatment lived an average of only three years.

Everyone's Guide to Cancer Therapy lists over 40 toxic chemotherapy agents. None of them work as well as many alternative therapies that are suppressed. The very fact that hundreds of toxic drugs have been tried WITHOUT MEDICAL SUCCESS should tell you something. The fact that these treatments provide tremendous financial success to the cancer industry cannot be overlooked.

One has only to review the dismal failure of conventional cancer therapy to realize more could be done. Any cancer treatment that does not eliminate the cause of cancer is not going to cure the problem.

There is no hope in relying on mainstream medicine. Drug and genetic research is now focused on maintaining cancer victims on drug therapy, just as diabetics are dependent on insulin shots.

Gene therapy is not a cure, but a treatment that must be repeated at great expense. Herceptin blocks growth factor receptors in breast tissue, but does not cure. Costs for treating cancer will continue to rise until the people force government to stop the waste, or democracy fails and a benevolent dictator takes over. Political action is needed now before it is too late and our medical system fails. Benevolent dictators do not exist.

The tobacco industry is being sued for billions of dollars on the basis the cigarette companies "knowingly conspired to suppress health care risks associated with smoking."

Why can't the medical establishment be sued for billions of dollars because it knowingly suppressed effective cancer cures that have destroyed millions of lives as well as misused billions of tax-revenue dollars?

24. The greatest tax grab and cover-up in history

I believe the three major themes of this book have been completed.

1. We know the cause of cancer. We know that parasitic living things in our body cause human cells to mutate cell-wall membranes during replication; either during normal growth and cell replacement, or to repai an injury. Nutritional and mineral deficiencies and toxins reduce immune system function allowing for fungal and parasitic infection. Infection leads to the substitution of microbial enzymes and proteins for human enzymes and proteins. All degenerative diseases follow this path.

2. We know that the cure for cancer lies in removing the causes. Cancer is caused by microbial infections.

3. We know there is a serious cover-up in progress. We have also reviewed several remarkable cancer cures that are suppressed, and we know why they work, because we understand the true cause of cancer. We know that the cancer epidemic is a man-made phenomenon, and controlled by authorities who are defrauding the public on a massive scale. The same fraudulent activities apply to the heart and stroke industry, autoimmune diseases, diabetes, AIDS, Alzheimer's —all degenerative diseases caused by nutritional deficiencies, fungi, and parasites.

The rest of the book deals with what to do with this knowledge. Topics discussed will establish the need for political action and suggest some possible alternatives.

Take a moment and reflect upon the previous chapters.

How has false medical dogma affected your life?

How much needless pain and suffering have you experienced due to suppressed cancer cures and other false information?

How much of your hard-earned income goes to perpetuate a cancer service industry that wastes your donations and tax dollars?

How will continued suppression of cancer cures impact on your future and the future of the ones you love? Consider what life will be like for people 50 years from now if nothing is done to start changing the direction of health care now.

Is the quality of life in general getting better, or worse for you? Do you find yourself working harder for less? If the billions wasted in health care were made available for other government purposes, or reduced taxes, would the quality of life improve for you?

According to the *Vanier Institute of the Family*, the real average family incomes have fallen 5.6% between 1989 to 1997. At a time of significant national prosperity, the real average family income fell from $48,300 to $45,600. It is time to end monopolies, such as that in health care, that hold back creativity and destroy the quality of life for millions of people. The medical monopoly on health care, being the largest user of tax revenues, is the greatest single threat there is to society. The exploitation of tax revenue resulting in reduced wealth circulating in public hands is destroying the economy and social system. With each new business merger, hundreds of employees are let go and the tax base reduced. Society is moving rapidly in the wrong direction.

What are you going to do with this information?

What can you do about suppressed cancer cures?

If you are a reader who is dependent on the cancer industry for employment and income, consider the consequences of what will eventually happen to your quality of life and essential freedoms. By denying effective cancer cures for others, you also deny them for yourself.

Governments exist to govern the people and provide essential services. No government can survive without money to provide the services people require and demand. We have all witnessed the destruction of communism, due mainly to an entrenched bureaucracy that failed to provide for the needs of their people.

The United States is the only super-power left and it is deeply in debt —5.7 trillion—an increase of 148 billion in 1999 (based on Internet search "debt U.S. Government"). The U.S. dollar is the world's strongest currency. The demand for investment security leads investors to buy U.S. dollars, not because the U. S. economy is that safe, but because the U.S. has the largest and most powerful arsenal in the world.

Armed forces can protect a country from an invasion, but what can armed forces do to help a government that cannot provide essential services for its own people? Did the Communist army save Communism from political disaster? No. Consider what could happen to the U.S. economy, if a really major catastrophe occurred causing millions of foreign investors to lose confidence in the U.S. dollar as a safe haven

Numerous authors have written about an impending financial crisis. The American economy cannot possibly continue endlessly compiling government debt at such a staggering rate. Sooner or later a major economic correction will occur, as planned, and the investment wealth of the middle class will be lost. Those with great wealth will have sufficient funds left over to take advantage of opportunities, but the middle class will have lost most of their wealth. The government will no longer be able to provide for essential services due to reduced tax revenue. The quality of life we now enjoy will be lost. Possibly forever. Probably forever.

For more information look for books such as:

1. *The Great Reckoning, How the world will change in the depression of the 1990's.* This book was written in 1991 by James Davidson and Lord William Rees-Mogg, authors of *Blood in the Streets.* Although their prediction of a 1990s financial collapse has passed, the logic in their predictions remains strong. When the interest on public debt reaches a point that is too costly to bear, either inflation will obliterate much of the value (as was used in the 80s) or an economic deflation will cause the economic system to collapse.

2. *Agents of Influence,* (1990) by Pat Choate. The book exposes how lobbyists manipulate America's political and economic system. The same problem applies to all democracies. Major corporations control lobbyists, and lobbyists control government decisions. Government of the people, by big business, for big business is the reality of modern times.

3. *Global Tyranny...Step by Step* (1992) by William Jasper. Jasper describes how the United Nations will become the control center for a new world order, and how all countries will give up political freedom to the one world power in order to have social stability.

As we watch the United Nations take on the role of protector —supplying food and shelter to refugees of war, and as NATO (North Atlantic Treaty Organization) takes on the role of enforcer —such as the bombing of Yugoslavia to destroy its economy and capacity for war, we can see the emergence of a new world power.

However, I think William Jasper picked the wrong organization for control of a new world order. The United Nations is not organized effectively to take control of the world's economies.

The most likely source of global control comes from the World Trade Association. Giving a group of humans economic power over all countries of the world, with the right to sanction countries for stepping out of line, is worse than giving the medical cartel a monopoly on health care and a key to the public purse.

There is too much power in the hands of too few people, and they are all governed by self-interest and business wealth. Thousands of people boycott the World Trade Organization meetings because they fear the worst. Maybe they know what they are doing.

Dictatorial power comes from economic wealth. Wealth enables one to make decisions, influence people, and turn events in one's favor. The World Trade Organization already shows signs of repressing natural health products through the CODEX regulations.

One of the most sinister programs established to destroy alternatives in health care is called *Codex Alimentarius*. This international movement strives to limit all natural health products to a near dysfunctional level, and coordinate worldwide production regulations to facilitate international trade. The public interest is not being served by globalization of alternative health products. The public is not driving this action because of any perceived threat to health. Big businesses are doing so for their financial benefit. Eliminating competition and controlling natural health products is the primary goal. By limiting the functional value of alternative health products by international regulations, they destroy the market for these products. Financial gain follows for the pharmaceutical companies from increased sale of highly profitable drugs.

As you watch the multi-million dollar corporations merge into larger conglomerates, have you ever wondered why the owners do so? American Home Products Corp. and Warner-Lambert Co. are in talks to merge in what is expected to be a $65 billion U.S. deal that would create the world's largest prescription drug maker. Why do the directors do this? Financial gain or more power? They already have all the personal wealth they can possibly use. Could it be that individuals are jockeying for position in the starting gates of a New World order? How soon will the gates open?

Keep your eye on world economic events and watch them unfold. Freedom is at stake, not due to the obvious force of a political upheaval, but due to the sinister force of an economic upheaval. When democracies fail to provide for the needs of the people, what is left but some form of dictatorship?

25. Government health agencies abuse their authority

If we ever had an outbreak of *good health*, millions of people would lose their source of wealth and influence. Is it any wonder the medical establishment maintains the cover-up?

What would happen to the billion-dollar cancer research industry if someone with medical or political credibility announced the following information to the public?

It has just been discovered that cancer is a cell-wall membrane disease caused by fungal infection. The cause of cancer is the normal repair process of injured tissue. If infected cells are made to multiply, infectious agents within the cell mutate the cell-wall membrane causing new cells to be rejected by the body because of defects in the membrane. All known phenomenon about cancer can be answered by this normal autonomic process of tissue repair. Cancer is not a defective gene disease as we previously thought.

Cancer can be prevented and cured by eliminating infection, and by supporting the tissue repair process with metabolic therapies and cleansing of body organs and tissues. The cost of treating cancer with parasite cleansing and electromagnetic devices will be covered by medicare. You no longer need to wait in line for chemotherapy and radiation. Surgery will be limited to emergency life-saving operations.

Can you imagine the director of any medical association saying this to the public? How could they do such an about face even if they wanted to? You can be sure suppression of effective cancer cures will never be willingly initiated or promoted by mainstream medicine.

Can you imagine a high-ranking government official making the above statement and then announcing a new government policy such as follows:

The Government will no longer support research for the genetic cause of cancer. All funds donated for cancer research will be used to develop early cancer diagnostic methods, evaluate existing cancer cures, which have been suppressed, and focus on eliminating benign growths before they develop into cancer.

Just as the automobile industry was mandated to reduce auto emissions and improve gas mileage back in the seventies, the cancer industry is being mandated to reduce cost of cancer treatment by 50% and improve rate of cancer cures by 50% within the next ten years.

To prove that these goals are possible, we are establishing and funding a number of cancer clinics based on eliminating the infectious cause of cancer. These clinics will be allowed to operate outside of restrictions imposed by Health Canada and the Health Protection Branch. If mainstream medicine cancer clinics do not surpass the success rate of these new competitive treatment centers, all government health-care bureaucrats will be replaced and medical associations outlawed. Government will no longer allow abuse of tax revenue through cancer treatments limited to radiation, chemotherapy, and surgery.

Would the federal government or a provincial government do this on their own initiative? How would they handle the medical backlash? What would the government do if all doctors threaten to go on strike? How would the people respond? I remember the medical backlash when the Province of Saskatchewan introduced Medicare. The medical association opposed Medicare by threatening strike action and many doctors left the province.

What if cancer could be more or less eliminated like small-pox and polio in the third world countries. All three are microbial diseases. Why not?

Thousands of people would have their livelihood disrupted if cancer were to be eliminated. As the historic documents mentioned in the chapter on suppressed cancer cures shows, successful vaccines such as that of Dr. Coley and Dr. Scott, have been suppressed for over 70 years. I believe cancer could be largely eliminated if remedies were advanced to eliminate fungi and parasites from the body and if effective nutritional life-styles education programs were provided to the public. Cancer cannot occur without some form of parasitic infection, mineral or vitamin deficiency, or toxic overload. Because these conditions are measurable, preventable, and correctable, cancer can be prevented long before tumors form.

Separate Health Canada from Medicare

There are thousands of dedicated doctors in the health care system. Steps should be taken to free all medical doctors from suppression of alternative health services. Why are they suppressed? Who makes this decision? Why doesn't Health Canada fight for freedom of choice in health care to save costs and reduce suffering? That's their job. Why doesn't Health Canada support medical doctors such as the Toronto physician Joseph Krop, who is being persecuted by the Ontario Medical Association for using alternative therapies?

In my opinion, Health Canada has abused their position of trust and deprived Canadians of the very health care the organization was mandated to provide. Health Canada must give up the right to select and authorize health care products, services, and the like. Just as the Red Cross was removed from control of blood services, Health Canada must be removed from controlling health services.

Only two steps are required.

Set up a system whereby a panel of individuals without hidden agendas, evaluate medical products and equipment. Members of the panel would be selected in a process similar to selecting an independent jury and replaced equal groups every 2 or 4 years. Manufacturers would present their data and decisions would be based on the proven merits. The panel could demand information regarding health benefits, cost effectiveness and side effects for years after acceptance. Allow free-market forces and competition into the health-service supply marketplace and ensure freedom of choice in health care.

Provide an effective definition of the word drug to exclude Health Canada from regulating food supplement and minerals off the market.

If alternative cancer clinics were allowed to operate in Canada, and alternative health services accepted by Medicare we would soon need more medical specialists and hospital staff than we have now to treat patients from foreign lands who would be willing to pay for their cancer treatments in Canada. Instead of sending cancer patients to U.S. facilities, they would be sending them to Canada. Individuals would also be coming on their own for special treatments.

Canada, not Mexico, would become the alternate source for cancer cures by Americans and people from other countries. Costly closed up hospitals and vacant hospital wings could be saving lives and earning profits.

Where is the medical will to do so?

Where is the public demand to do so?

Where is the political will to do so?

If you would like to do something effective in your community, here is a good place to start. Start organizing information on effective alternative health specialists in your electoral district. Create public awareness, credibility, and availability in alternative health services in your area. Push for a private or public funded cancer detoxification and cure center in your area. Help destroy false perceptions created by the cancer service industry by creating public confidence in alternative treatments. Start with people you know and work within your electoral district.

Establishing availability, value, and credibility

There are many effective low-cost cancer treatments available. If alternative health specialists and we (the people) made a concerted effort on our own, to test, use, and verify these alternative programs, we could establish alternative cancer clinics.

Credibility and availability are the two major problems for alternative therapies. Where is it available? Who can you trust? How much does it cost? A group of public minded citizens, providing local health care services not available through mainstream medicine would establish credibility and availability in spite of medical propaganda and dictatorship.

If we had a network of privately operated alternative-health clinics owned and operated by responsible, public-minded citizens, nationwide credibility and availability could be established. Proof of effectiveness would be established at the local level. Public opinion could be organized to influence the politicians running for office in that riding. Politicians could be made to realize that only those with a platform of health reform have a chance of being elected.

If the majority of elected Members of Parliament wanted to bring about changes in health care, they could do so. The influence of lobbyists and misinformation about cancer allows for misguided policies. Now that the true cause of cancer has been exposed, the situation is different. We have a right to use this knowledge. It can be defended in a court of law. The state does not have a right to deny use of alternative therapies just because the authorities do not approve.

By breaking the political problem down to individual ridings, and having the people of that riding take an active part in politics for freedom of choice in health care, the problem becomes manageable. Each of us can make a big difference. Each individual can only make a ripple in the system, but ripples become waves. Its time to start making waves.

In the 1997 federal election, the Minister of Health, David Dingwall, was surprised when he lost his election and was forced to retire from active politics. The driving force behind his election defeat was a localized concerted effort by those fed up with the proposed regulations on natural health products and establishment licensing fees. After losing the election, he was reported as saying he underestimated the significance of public opinion against proposed natural health product regulations. Obviously that message was heard, as we are now well into the process of new regulations for natural health products. Whether the result will be any different or not remains to be seen.

An organized electorate is the most powerful lobbyist group possible. An organized electorate can control those they elect. Otherwise, the industrial lobbyists control them. It's time for people to start thinking and working at the community level. Electoral districts are broken down into convenient communities called polling divisions and boundaries are determined by federal politics. Organization is easy if we follow government guidelines.

Organization starts at the community level. Use of polling district maps is a simple and effective way to start organizing powerful community groups to lobby elected officials. These groups are not political party focused. Community groups will be issue focused. The person elected should be made to deal with issues relating to public interests and demands of the people who elected him or her.

In a democracy, we believe in government of the people, by the people, for the people. What we have is government of the people, by big business, for big business. Lobbyists make the difference. The effect on government policy by business lobbying for 4 years between elections is far greater than disorganized public appeals received from the public during one or two months of public campaigning. With the help of mass media and control of perceptions, politicians with deep pockets are most often elected by swaying the vote. Public interests are secondary.

Most individual elections in Canada are won or lost with just a few thousand votes. The time is right. The Internet is available to communicate and organize. Thousands of people know there is a problem with health care.

Should you become involved in politics? Just answer two questions:

What have you got to gain/lose by doing nothing?

What have you got to gain/lose by doing something?

Consider the effect of your decision on your children and grandchildren. Why not stop those that control Canadian health care policy from suppressing cancer cures that allow thousands of men women and children to suffer and die of disease? There are probably only a few individuals in the Canadian cancer establishment responsible for suppression of effective cancer cures. Why can't they be identified and weeded out? The Canadian court system is in place to protect all Canadians. Why not use it to prevent unnecessary pain, suffering, and death from cancer?

Can suppression of effective cancer cures be anything except a criminal offense against humanity? If tobacco companies can be sued for recovery of medical costs due to smoking, why can't the cancer industry be sued for the suppression of effective cancer cures?

What good is political freedom if we don't use it?

Increasingly, it becomes obvious. The people must organize and take up the challenge to fight for freedom of choice in health care. Our parents fought and died for political freedom. We still have it. Let's use it. It all starts with organizing people at the grass roots level.

It is time for people and elected government officials to demand change.

Health providers who withhold vital information about potential cancer cures from terminally ill patients should lose their medical license. Health providers who deliberately deceive the public with false written statements should face criminal charges.

Withholding non-toxic cancer treatments from young children with cancer is the most tragic. Nothing is more pitiful to read about in the papers than young boys and girls bravely going through chemotherapy and then dying a few months later. It's so inhumane to restrict cancer therapy to toxic drug chemotherapy for children with undeveloped livers incapable of processing the toxins. No wonder they die. From time to time I do hear about successful cancer remission in children, but these are far fewer than the failures.

Have you ever donated to the Last Wish Foundation so those children on chemotherapy with late-stage cancer could enjoy one last wish? What does this tell you about their chances for survival?

Why not spare their lives by using other methods that are non-toxic, available, and accepted by thousands of alternative health specialists?

The *Last Wish Foundation* is formal recognition of the most common result chemotherapy has on children. When a child with cancer is put on the last-wish program, isn't it time to stop chemotherapy and try something else? Why not send them to Mexico and test an alternative therapy? Better still, why not set up alternative cancer clinics in Canada?

First Wish Foundation needed to save children's lives

Children with late stage cancer should be provided them with a *First Wish Foundation*. Why not take these children off chemotherapy and send them to alternative cancer clinics and possibly save their lives? Given a choice, if one of your children or grandchildren could have only one more wish granted, don't you think he or she would want to try an alternative therapy? Not just a new and different drug. A whole new approach. What do you have to lose?

The heroic effort by 13 year old Tyrell Dueck to try a Mexican clinic in order to save his leg caught the public interest because that is what he wanted to do. It was his life at stake. He knew the consequences. His only chance for a normal life was to not have his leg amputated. He didn't want to live with that handicap. It took a court order to stop him from going for treatment in a timely manner. He was allowed to go, only after cancer had spread to his lungs.

The fact that Social Services for the Province of Saskatchewan would force 13-year-old Tyrell Dueck to undergo surgery and chemotherapy against his will, and that of his parents, is frightening. What is the difference between forcing a young child to take chemotherapy than forcing a young adult to take it? Why not force everyone to take it?

If loving parents cannot decide the cancer therapy for their 13-year-old child, at what age do we draw the line? This wasn't a misguided religious issue or an attempt to commit euthanasia. It was a conscious loving decision to save his life and his leg based on his perceptions and free choice.

What ever happened to freedom of choice in health care?

After Tyrell's cancer spread to his lungs, he was allowed to go to Mexico for the cancer treatments he wanted and needed earlier. Why did he have to wait until cancer had spread to his lungs before he was allowed to go elsewhere? Have we also lost our freedom to travel if we have cancer?

The derogatory term *Quackery* is routinely applied by licensed medical professionals to Mexican cancer clinics, and non-licensed health care professionals in competitive fields. This term has a powerful effect on credibility of competitive cancer treatments and public perceptions.

We need to extend and apply the term to government officials and medical professionals who continue to support the defective-gene theory as the cause of cancer. Removing healthy breasts because they contain defective genes is quackery. Using costly gene therapy to block growth hormone receptors is quackery. Treating the body for autoimmune diseases by lowering the immune system is quackery. Raising funds for continued research on the genetic cause of cancer is quackery. Most of all, refusing to use effective cancer cures is quackery.

26. A history of wrongdoing through control of the media

In this chapter, I would like to review how propaganda and control of TV news and talk shows control public opinion. Public opinion in health care is the result of massive amounts of publicity, advertising, and damage control. We (the people) believe what we are told to believe.

The power of medical propaganda comes from the fact that medical associations control the news media. One cannot advertise a health product without permission from medical authorities. While this is a good thing to keep people from being scammed, it also ensures that good products that compete with medical dogma will not be made available to the public. It also ensures that one cannot criticize what they do.

Public criticism of mainstream medicine on major TV channels is not permitted. I have never seen a documentary program describing how cancer patients have benefited from any of the suppressed cancer cures discussed in this text or similar cancer treatments. If I wanted to advertise this book on TV in Canada, for example, I doubt if I would ever get permission to do so.

Modern medicine promotes unproven theories as explanations for medical conditions not explainable by the Germ Theory or other accepted concepts. These explanations are now medical dogma woven into the fabric of public belief and accepted medical treatment. For sake of a better word, I will refer to these unproven theories as modern myths.

A myth is a fictitious traditional story or legend embodying ancient or primitive beliefs to explain observed phenomena that could not be explained by other means, such as the forces in nature. The horoscopes published daily in every newspaper in North America and read daily by millions of people are myths. Truth is not important.

Myth: Defective genes cause cancer

Obviously, they (those who supply news clips and press releases) support a defective gene theory that has no validity in science and should not be promoted more than any other theory. There is no proof that defective genes cause cancer but this fact does not stop cancer information from saying so. Numerous examples have already been discussed, such as oncogenes and suppressor genes. Millions of dollars have been spent researching genes without finding any proof. Taking public donations amounting to millions of dollars for further cancer research of genes is fraud because other possible causes of cancer are not researched.

Obviously, most physicians do not promote any alternative therapy or even suggest it to a cancer patient. Withholding information about effective cancer treatments results in needless suffering and painful death. Refusing to treat children with safe non-toxic remedies is beyond human understanding. Hospitals fight to save lives of children on one hand, and refuse them life saving alternative cancer therapy on the other.

Obviously, they say they do not know a great deal about what causes cancer but they are very effective in banning effective herbs, food supplements and alternative treatments such as ozone therapy and arginine. The resulting suffering and loss of life appears to be insignificant to them.

Myth: Excess growth hormone receptors cause breast cancer

Obviously, they avoid all direct references to microbial growth hormones and microbes as a possible cause of cancer. Instead, they make the cancer process sound very confusing. In the U.S. publication, *PEOPLE Weekly*, (October 26, 1998) there is a detailed report on Herceptin and how it works. Let me quote exactly what is written and then discuss the misinformation and other propaganda features (My emphasis added in italic type.):

> Combined with chemotherapy, Herceptin has been shown to shrink tumors in women with an aggressive type of breast cancer that accounts for 30 per cent of all cases and involves a gene called HER2. *The gene produces a protein that acts like an antenna on the membrane of a cancer cell, transmitting and receiving the signals that tell the cell to reproduce.* Herceptin arrests the cancer by bonding to the protein that prevents the tumor from growing.

If you want a good example of doublespeak, compare this description to that of the Hamilton Spectator article describing the same product and process (Chapter 4). In the previous description, we had growth factors of unknown source and excessive numbers of growth factor receptors in the cell walls. Here we have a metaphorical expression of a radio receiver. We now have cells with antenna, transmitting and receiving signals that will tell cells to reproduce.

Is there anything in the carefully worded description that would give you hope that a simple cancer cure could be found? Notice too, there is no mention of the genetic defect not being inherited but caused by an unknown environmental factor, as in the newspaper article. In addition, the genetic defect is promoted as a medical fact, but the truth is it has never been proven.

The *PEOPLE Weekly* article (Page 71), goes on to point out the great success of the drug with reference to a Virginia Empey, who "for more than three years received weekly Herceptin infusions… **although Virginia is not considered cured** her hope is restored."

The report illustrates the deceptive propaganda of news releases by the cancer industry to promote confidence in defective genes as the cause of cancer and drug therapy as the cure. It also shows that the primary goal for cancer research is to produce drugs to maintain the life of a cancer patient, for as long as possible to maximize drug sales. Weekly infusions to block the growth hormone receptors are far more lucrative than killing the microbes that produce the growth hormone.

Myth: We don't control the news

In the court case over freedom of speech in America, reporters Jane Akre and Steve Wilson are suing Fox TV for being fired over controlled reporting on Bovine Growth Hormone. This court case gives us a clear illustration of how pharmaceutical industries control the press and the news. The Internet article, as written by Ronnie Cummins, reads as follows:

As reported by Jeanette Batz in the St. Louis news weekly, Riverfront Times, David Boylan, WTVT station manager, was blunt in demanding that Akre and Wilson tell the story about rBGH the way Monsanto wanted it told. "We (the Fox TV network) paid $3 billion for these television stations. We will decide what the news is. The news is what we tell you it is." So much for freedom of the press in the era of Corporate Power. Full details of the lawsuit and the BGH story are available at: http://www.foxBGHsuit.com.

Consider for a moment the advertisements you watch on TV that are drug-related to treat headaches, heartburn and back pain. How many millions of dollars do these networks take in from these pharmaceutical advertisers? If you owned the network, would you be willing to lose all this revenue by promoting the true cause of cancer and all diseases? If your job and payroll for hundreds of employees rely on this income, what would you do? Leave it to the next guy! Send it to committee!

Myth: AIDS is a disease caused by a specific virus

In 1993 American Dr. Willner, M.D., Ph.D. publicly inoculated himself with the blood of Pedro Tocino, an HIV positive hemophiliac. This demonstration occurred in Spain and was reported in all the major papers and TV stations in Spain. Willner demonstrated that he could not be infected with the so-called AIDS virus, not even by inoculation with contaminated blood. Willner proved the AIDS theory is wrong. This historic event was never mentioned in the U.S. press.

All of the following references are supported by documentation in a book called *Deadly Deception, The Proof That Sex and HIV Absolutely Do Not Cause Aids.* This 1994 publication by Robert Willner exposes the *AIDS industry* as a medical fraud. This book contains the following statement that applies equally well to the cancer industry (Introduction page XX)

> Yet, today, lies potentially more dangerous then Hitler's are being disseminated by unsuspecting governments, the World Health Organization, and a media power that couldn't even be imagined in Hitler's time.

Since information on AIDS is not pertinent to the main theme of this text, for the sake of brevity, I would like to just summarize some of the main points. There is a close similarity to the cancer industry and the AIDS industry as both are profitable monopolies which needlessly convert tax revenue into drug profits.

People who have reviewed the AIDS disease claim the disease was created by publicity and illustrates the awesome power of the press. The virus-AIDS hypothesis was announced in the press before it was checked by the scientific community and published in scientific journals.

The so-called AIDS virus does not cause death or weaken the immune system to cause death. It is the other way around. The weakened immune system allows the so-called AIDS virus or viruses to thrive. You are deemed to have AIDS if your body has a specific antibody that is used to destroy the AIDS virus or any other virus. Researchers cannot specify that a specific antibody attacks only the AIDS virus. The antibodies indicate acquired immunity to a virus. The so-called AIDS virus doesn't need to be present, just the antibody. In any other disease, if you have antibodies for the disease, but not the disease, you are deemed to have an acquired immunity. In AIDS, you are deemed to have the disease.

The AIDS virus served the purpose of creating a business opportunity from the loss of immune system function due to recreational drugs or the result of medical drugs and antibiotics. AIDS started out as a collection of 25 conditions characterized by an immune system dysfunction; hence the name, Acquired Immune Dysfunction Syndrome. The syndrome became the disease.

People do not die from the syndrome; they die from opportunistic infection. If they die from other diseases, AIDS is nothing more than a dysfunctional immune system? The cure for AIDS is to repair the immune system with nutrition and cleansing and eliminate opportunistic infection.

In AIDS we are being told that HIV, a retrovirus, is an RNA rather than a DNA virus. It encodes its RNA into human-cell DNA and is then capable of duplicating itself through a process called reverse transcriptase. It then commences to multiply and destroy the immune system, allowing opportunistic infection to kill the person. The concept is a highly promoted myth for the same reasons that the defective gene is a highly promoted myth. It confuses the public. Both of these diseases rely on the public misunderstanding of genetics. They both rely on a defective gene concept that has never been proven.

You will recall that the retrovirus disease concept does not fit the facts regarding DNA replication as expressed by *Harper's Review of Biochemistry* (See chapter 6). The RNA virus infect DNA but can only replicate themselves, like a mirror image, and do not produce enzymes to destroy the immune system. The immune system is weak before any viruses can invade the cells. The so-called AIDS viruses cannot invade a healthy cell any more than any other virus can.

AIDS represents an example of the awesome power of the press, propaganda and indoctrination. We are constantly told about the AIDS epidemic. How many people do you know who have AIDS? Do they fit into the group that includes pharmaceutical-drug dependent people or illicit drug users? Do you know any healthy people who suddenly developed AIDS? The Hamilton district hospitals reported only 12 cases of HIV infection for a 12 month period in 1998. That's not an epidemic.

The HIV virus as a cause of the AIDS syndrome is medical misinformation created by control of the media.

The AIDS hypothesis has resulted in the sale of millions of dollars worth of a toxic drug called AZT. The test for AIDS is positive if your blood has antibodies for virus. Over 200,000 people are now being treated for a disease that does not exist with a drug that has not been proven effective as a treatment for a dysfunctional immune system. Since AZT is toxic, people taking it die of AIDS. The disease is claimed to be incurable. If they don't die, they claim AZT saved their life.

The awesome power of the press can also be used to deny the existence of a disease created by chemical food additives.

Myth: Food additives such as Aspartame are safe

Due to control of the press, we must go directly to the Internet to research information such as this that follows. The following article is one of over 400 home pages that you will find by doing an Internet search under the words 'Aspartame Disease'. The article requests that we copy this information, and distribute it as widely as possible. Please do likewise.

February 4, 1999

WORLD ENVIRONMENTAL CONFERENCE and the MULTIPLE SCLEROSIS FOUNDATION -- THE FDA IN COLLUSION WITH MONSANTO

Article circulated by Nancy Markle, but which in fact is a transcript of a conference originally given by Betty Martini on 11/20/1997.

"I have spent several days lecturing at the WORLD ENVIRONMENTAL CONFERENCE on "ASPARTAME marketed as 'NutraSweet', 'Equal', and 'Spoonful'. In the keynote address by the EPA, they announced that there was an epidemic of multiple sclerosis and systemic lupus, and they did not understand what toxin was causing this to be rampant across the United States. I explained that I was there to lecture on exactly that subject.'

When the temperature of Aspartame exceeds 86 degrees F, the wood alcohol in ASPARTAME coverts to formaldehyde and then to formic acid, which in turn causes metabolic acidosis. (Formic acid is the poison found in the sting of fire ants). The methanol toxicity mimics multiple sclerosis; thus people were being diagnosed with having multiple sclerosis in error. The multiple sclerosis is not a death sentence, where methanol toxicity is.

In the case of systemic lupus, we are finding it has become almost as rampant as multiple sclerosis, especially in Diet Coke and Diet Pepsi drinkers. Also, with methanol toxicity, the victims usually drink three to four 12 oz. cans of them per day, some even more. In the cases of systemic lupus, which is triggered by ASPARTAME, the victim usually does not know that the aspartame is the culprit. The victim continues its use aggravating the lupus to such a degree, that sometimes it becomes life threatening. When we get people off the aspartame, those with systemic lupus usually become asymptomatic. Unfortunately, we can not reverse this disease.

On the other hand, in the case of those diagnosed with Multiple Sclerosis, (when in reality, the disease is methanol toxicity), most of the symptoms disappear. We have seen cases where their vision has returned and even their hearing has returned. This also applies to cases of tinnitus.

During a lecture I said "If you are using ASPARTAME (NutraSweet, Equal, Spoonful, etc.) and you suffer from fibromyalgia symptoms, spasms, shooting pains, numbness in your legs, cramps, vertigo, dizziness, headaches, tinnitus, joint pain, depression, anxiety attacks, slurred speech, blurred vision, or memory loss -- you probably have ASPARTAME DISEASE!" People were jumping up during the lecture saying, "I've got this, is it reversible?" It is rampant. Some of the speakers at my lecture even were suffering from these symptoms. In one lecture attended by the Ambassador of Uganda, he told us that their sugar industry is adding aspartame! He continued by saying that one of the industry leader's son could no longer walk - due in part by product usage!

We have a very serious problem. Even a stranger came up to Dr. Espisto (one of my speakers) and myself and said, 'Could you tell me why so many people seem to be coming down with MS? During a visit to a hospice, a nurse said that six of her friends, who were heavy Diet Coke addicts, had all been diagnosed with MS. This is beyond coincidence. Here is the problem. There were Congressional Hearings when aspartame was included in 100 different products. Since this initial hearing, there have been two subsequent hearings, but to no avail. Nothing has been done. The drug and chemical lobbies have very deep pockets. Now there are over 5,000 products containing this chemical, and the PATENT HAS EXPIRED!!!!! At the time of this first hearing, people were going blind. The methanol in the aspartame converts to formaldehyde in the retina of the eye. Formaldehyde is grouped in the same class of dmgs as cyanide and arsenic-- DEADLY POISONS!!! Unfortunately, it just takes longer to quietly kill, but it is killing people and causing all kinds of neurological problems.

Aspartame changes the brain's chemistry. It is the reason for severe seizures. This drug changes the dopamine level in the brain. Imagine what this drug does to patients suffering from Parkinson's Disease. This drug also causes birth defects.

There is absolutely no reason to take this product. It is NOT A DIET PRODUCT!!! The Congressional record said, "It makes you crave carbohydrates and will make you FAT". Dr. Roberts stated that when he got patients off aspartame, their average weight loss was 19 pounds per person. The formaldehyde stores in the fat cells, particularly in the hips and thighs.

Aspartame is especially deadly for diabetics. All physicians know what wood alcohol will do to a diabetic. We find that physicians believe that they have patients with retinopathy, when in fact, it is caused by the aspartame. The aspartame keeps the blood sugar level out of control, causing many patients to go into a coma. Unfortunately, many have died. People were telling us at the Conference of the American College of Physicians, that they had relatives that switched from saccharin to an aspartame product and how that relative had eventually gone into a coma. Their physicians could not get the blood sugar levels under control. Thus, the patients suffered acute memory loss and eventually coma and death.

Memory loss is due to the fact that aspartic acid and phenylalanine are neurotoxic without the other amino acids found in protein. Thus it goes past the blood brain barrier and deteriorates the neurons of the brain. Dr. Russell Blaylock, neurosurgeon, said, "The ingredients stimulates the neurons of the brain to death, causing brain damage of varying degrees. Dr. Blaylock has written a book entitled "EXCITOTOXINS: THE TASTE THAT KILLS" (Health Press 1-800-643-2665). Dr. H.J. Roberts, diabetic specialist and world expert on aspartame poisoning, has also written a book entitled "DEFENSE AGAINST ALZHEIMER'S DISEASE" (1-800-814-9800). Dr. Roberts tells how aspartame poisoning is escalating Alzheimer's Disease, and indeed it is. As the hospice nurse told me, women are being admitted at 30 years of age with Alzheimer's Disease. Dr. Blaylock and Dr. Roberts will be writing a position paper with some case histories and will post it on the Internet. According to the Conference of the American College of Physicians, 'We are talking about a plague of neurological diseases caused by this deadly poison".

Dr. Roberts realized what was happening when aspartame was first marketed. He said "his diabetic patients presented memory loss, confusion, and severe vision loss". At the Conference of the American College of Physicians, doctors admitted that they did not know. They had wondered why seizures were rampant (the phenylalanine in aspartame breaks down the seizure threshold and depletes serotonin, which causes manic depression, panic attacks, rage and violence).

Just before the Conference, I received a FAX from Norway, asking for a possible antidote for this poison because they are experiencing so many problems in their country. This "poison" is now available in 90 PLUS countries worldwide. Fortunately, we had speakers and ambassadors at the Conference from different nations who have pledged their help. We ask that you help too.

Print this article out and warn everyone you know. Take anything that contains aspartame back to the store. Take the "NO ASPARTAME TEST" and send us your case history.

I assure you that MONSANTO, the creator of aspartame, knows how deadly it is. They fund the American Diabetes Association, American Dietetic Association, Congress, and the Conference of the American College of Physicians. The New York Times, on November 15, 1996, ran an article on how the American Dietetic Association takes money from the food industry to endorse their products. Therefore, they can not criticize any additives or tell about their link to MONSANTO. How bad is this? We told a mother who had a child on NutraSweet to get off the product. The child was having grand mal seizures every day. The mother called her physician, who called the ADA, who told the doctor not to take the child off the NutraSweet. We are still trying to convince the mother that the aspartame is causing the seizures. Every time we get someone off aspartame, the seizures stop. If the baby dies, you know whose fault it is, and what we are up against. There are 92 documented symptoms of aspartame, from coma to death. The majority of them are all neurological, because the aspartame destroys the nervous system.

Aspartame Disease is partially the cause to what is behind some of the mystery of the Desert Storm health problems. The burning tongue and other problems discussed in over 60 cases can be directly related to the consumption of an aspartame product. Several thousand pallets of diet drinks were shipped to the Dessert Storm troops. (Remember heat can liberate the methanol from the aspartame at 86 degrees F). Diet drinks sat in the 120 degree F. Arabian sun for weeks at a time on pallets. The service men and women drank them all day long. All of their symptoms are identical to aspartame poisoning. Dr. Roberts says "consuming aspartame at the time of conception can cause birth defects". The phenylalanine concentrates in the placenta, causing mental retardation, according to Dr. Louis Elsas, Pediatrician Professor - Genetics, at Emory University in his testimony before Congress.

In the original lab tests, animals developed brain tumors (phenylalanine breaks down into DXP, a brain tumor agent). When Dr. Espisto was lecturing on aspartame, one physician in the audience, a neurosurgeon, said, "When they remove brain tumors, they have found high levels of aspartame in them".

Stevia, a sweet food, NOT AN ADDITIVE, which helps in the metabolism of sugar, which would be ideal for diabetics, has now been approved as a dietary supplement by the FDA For years, the FDA has outlawed this sweet food because of their loyalty to MONSANTO. [You can obtain Stevia now in natural foods stores in either cut sifted dried leaves or in powder form. I use it and it's great.

If it says "SUGAR FREE" on the label-- DO NOT EVEN THINK ABOUT IT!!!!!! Senator Howard Hetzenbaum wrote a bill that would have warned all infants, pregnant mothers and children of the dangers of aspartame. The bill would have also instituted independent studies on the problems existing in the population (seizures, changes in brain chemistry, changes in neurological and behavioral symptoms). It was killed by the powerful drug and chemical lobbies, letting loose the hounds of disease and death on an unsuspecting public. Since the Conference of the American College of Physicians, we hope to have the help of some world leaders. Again, please help us too. There are a lot of people out there who must be warned, *please* let them know this information.

The Sheep Station Dunsford, Ontario.

End of file.

e-mail fincham@peterboro.net."

Amazingly, we do not hear about this disease in any of the major information networks or TV newscasts. I only learned about it through membership in a U.S. organization called the National Health Federation. Another way to verify this information and enlarge upon it is to go to the Internet and type in "nutrapoison" for a list of 68 web pages. The Internet is not controlled (yet) so you will find hundreds of chilling case histories and warnings including increased cancer incidence.

In *Everyone's Guide to Cancer Therapy*, 'Adapted by the Canadian Medical Association' under Bladder Cancer we read conflicting evidence to any danger from artificial sweeteners. (Page 278):

The relationship of tumors to the use of artificial sweeteners such as cyclamates and coffee drinking is questionable. Recent studies have completely failed to find any risk above that of the general population.

One report on the Internet states that in the U.S. 85% of complaints to the FDA involve aspartame. Canada is probably about the same. In my opinion, public awareness of this obvious and serious health problem is being suppressed and government authorities are not taking these chemicals off the acceptable food additive list.

Why are valuable and safe food supplements such as arginine removed from the public without just cause while toxic chemicals such as aspartame are allowed to be sold as food additives?

How many other dangerous food additives pollute our daily food intake causing enzyme damage or other neurological diseases? Ammonia is toxic to living things, yet used in household cleansers, hair conditioners and shampoos. How can we possibly know what is safe and what is dangerous? We believe what we are told in the press, and we are told what not to believe.

Myth: Unproven cancer therapies are dangerous

In *Everyone's Guide to Cancer Therapy, Adapted by the Canadian Medical Association'* we have the primary source of medical information available for Canadians who have been diagnosed with cancer and want to inform themselves about the treatment process. After describing in detail all of the accepted methods of treating cancer, we find Chapter 13,

Questionable and Unproven Cancer Therapies.

Obviously, the Canadian Medical Association should warn Canadians to avoid unproven cancer therapies. That's why they enjoy a monopoly in health care. What if they abuse this monopoly to warn people with cancer to avoid competitive treatments that are very successful? Would that be a breach of public trust? If not, what is?

Metabolic therapy, for example, is based on the principle that the body can repair itself, provided it is given all the natural ingredients it needs, and provided it is enabled to absorb, assimilate and synthesize these ingredients. You cannot harm yourself with metabolic therapy. Nevertheless, here's why metabolic therapy is dangerous according to the Canadian Medical Association. (From Everyone's Guide to Cancer, Page 98)

Metabolic Treatments: these are offered by practitioners and clinics in the United States and in Tijuana, Mexico. Metabolic procedures vary according to the practitioner, but they generally include:

♦ "Detoxification," typically cleansing of the colon

♦ Special diets

◆ Vitamins

◆ Minerals

◆ Enzymes

Metabolic treatments sound appealing. They emphasize "natural" therapy with treatment directed at "cellular detoxification and restoration." *But these treatments are neither natural nor safe. Many people have been harmed by them.* Like most unproven treatments, metabolic therapy is based on an *invented principle: that toxins and waste material interfere with metabolism and healing.* Cancer and other diseases are seen as a result of degeneration of the liver and pancreas or of degeneration of the immune or "oxygenation" systems.

The educated consumer will know that there is no such thing as an oxygenation system. Nor is there any such thing as cellular detoxification and restoration.

Isn't this unbelievable? They claim there is no such thing as 'cellular detoxification'. In my opinion, the action of medical advisors publishing false information warning desperate cancer victims to avoid the one therapy that will help them the most is a breach of public trust. What does that tell you about who is behind the misinformation regarding cancer? It's not a simple mistake, as if they don't know the truth. "*Questionable and Unproven Cancer Therapies,*" demonstrates a direct and conscious effort to keep desperate people with cancer from trying any effective cancer treatment.

How can any medically trained person argue against metabolic therapy? Dr. Guyton teaches medical students about the dangers from buildup of blood proteins in the intracellular spaces. He explains how blood proteins are continually fed from arteries into spaces between the cells to nourish human cells. Any unused material must be returned to the circulatory system within hours via the lymphatic system, or it will stagnate and ferment as well as block off oxygen from the cells. Dr. Guyton writes:

> If it were not for continual removal of proteins, (by the lymphatic system) the dynamics of fluid exchange at the blood capillaries would become so abnormal within only a few hours that life could no longer continue.

It's hard to believe that a qualified medical doctor would write: "There is no such thing as an oxygenation system. Nor is there any such thing as cellular detoxification and restoration." How the body utilizes oxygen is a significant portion of a course in medicine. In Guyton's Textbook of Medical

Physiology, we learn all about it in Chapter 8. entitled *Respiration* Pages 476 to 558.

Don't doctors have a moral obligation to tell the truth? If he or she presents himself as a trained person with specialized skill and knowledge, such as a cancer specialist writing a book for people lacking this specialized knowledge, shouldn't this be considered a criminal act? Does it not harm innocent victims who have placed their trust in recognized and approved authorities? Take for example the case of the Montreal mother fighting to save her children from being forced to take AZT.

HIV-positive mom refuses AZT for kids.

A Quebec court will decide whether a Montreal mother must give her children a potentially risky drug cocktail—or lose them to a foster home.

The Hamilton Spectator (Thursday Dec. 9, 1999) published a full page article written by Alyson Mead, on the right of a 37 year old mother to refuse giving her children, who are HIV positive, AZT which is a highly controversial drug with horrendous side effects. The decision will decide whether the government has the right to mandate medical care.

A Dr. Philip Berger is quoted as saying:

'Doctors have to be the absolute custodians of children's care,' he says. 'Once the child is born,' he says, 'I think the state has a duty to protect the child from any disease for which a parent is refusing treatment where the benefits are clear.'

AZT is a very toxic drug. Thousands of people with AIDS and HIV infection refuse to take it because their experience show it has killed their friends who have taken it. There is no way that an objective person can claim AZT benefits everyone who takes it. Does it actually benefits anyone? I have not read of any good effects from taking AZT.

What is the medical pathway that makes AZT a functional product? My understanding is that the HIV virus is considered to be a retrovirus that attaches itself to strands of DNA. AZT functions to terminate expressed genes so that the virus cannot do so. You will recall that the Universal Genetic Code has 64 possible combinations. Three of these codes (ATT, ATC, and ACT) are used to identify termination points in genes. If we take the ACT terminator, and substitute Z for C, we end up with AZT. We end up with a toxic drug that destroys DNA.

AZT was first developed by the pharmaceutical giant Burroughs-Welcome to treat cancer but it was far too deadly for continued use. Why is it suddenly safer to use for HIV patients? Why is it recommended for children when there is a group leading a Class Action Suit in the United States to have it stopped as a drug for AIDS victims?

The Dec. 9th newspaper article goes on to say:

.... Dr. Mark Weinberg, is president of the International AIDS society in Canada and the inventor of an antiviral drug 3TC. He maintains that she (the mother) and other "AIDS dissidents" are comparable to Holocaust deniers. They are, he says, 'ill-informed, confused individuals who either do not or cannot understand the issues involved."

What issues are involved? It will be a sad day for all Canadians and the health care system, if the medical profession, representing the government, has the right to mandate toxic drug therapy on all children. Such a law would essentially mean that when a child is born, mainstream medicine has the sole right to treat that child for illness, based on the good of the state.

The fact that doctors, or someone in the group, own patent rights to drugs that are being mandated into use, such as antiviral drug 3TC, should be considered as grounds to destroy such proposed laws. The fact that the whole medical system is drug orientated, to the exclusion of more modern and efficient methods cannot be overlooked. The fact that mainstream medicine cannot be trusted, based on suppressed cancer cures alone, is obvious.

Let's consider the probability of a drug such as AZT being mandated for treating all HIV infections. The reason for discussing this here is that it represents the future possibility for cancer. If toxic drugs are mandated for HIV, the regulation will soon extend to other diseases.

The description of a virus in medical text books identify viruses to be free RNA and DNA nucleotides that cause disease by mutating or otherwise disturbing the DNA of the cell. In contrast, the scientific textbooks, describe viruses as mainly protein shells, with a tiny portion of DNA or RNA inside. The shells exist only in rod or ball shaped forms. The two descriptions, one medical, the other from science, are not compatible. One or the other is false information. Why would scientists describe viruses as rods and spheres if they were not rods and spheres?

The DNA structure is limited to combinations of precise nucleotides limited to only two combinations. These are adenine to thymine, (A to T) and cytosine to guanine (C to G). Viruses don't fit the DNA structure.

RNA of any type, if attached to DNA, can only reproduce itself, which is nothing more serious than viruses that reproduce in the cytoplasm of the cell. The theory that AIDS is caused by a virus is false. AIDS is Acquired Immune Deficiency Syndrome. A syndrome is a collection of conditions following immune deficiency. The HIV virus is secondary. HIV is an opportunistic infection that does not kill. The cure for HIV infection is to enhance the immune system. Toxic drugs like AZT destroy the immune system.

Viruses can be killed with electronic frequencies, or by enhancing the immune system with metabolic therapy. Making drug therapy for HIV infection mandatory serves only the drug industry.

It follows that giving mainstream medicine the power to enforce drug therapy on HIV positive children is not in the public interest, and therefore cannot be allowed to happen. Mainstream medicine should lose the right to treat HIV infected children with AZT until it has been proven effective, with proof established through a judge and jury system similar to that used in a court of law. In addition, the more effective suppressed systems should have to be proven less effective and more dangerous than the toxic drugs being forced onto an unwilling public.

There is some reason to agree with Dr. Berger who says: *I think the state has a duty to protect the child from any disease for which a parent is refusing treatment where the benefits are clear.*

It follows that the state has a duty to protect the child from unproven toxic drugs and demand that the latest scientifically proven cures for disease be used immediately, such as the suppressed U.S. medical patent 5,139,684, or any of the other methods described in this book or in public knowledge. Drugs are not the only cure for disease.

The state has the obligation to stop suppression of more effective treatments suppressed by mainstream medicine. There is no truth in the statement that: *'Doctors have to be the absolute custodians of children's care.'* Doctor's have misused and abused the trust and authority placed in them through the monopoly in medicine, and they should forfeit the right to be the *absolute custodians of children's care.* The elected government should take immediate action, to save lives, the economy, and the Canadian medical system. To do anything less is to be derelict in their duty as elected officials with obligations to protect the public.

Viral flu pandemics in the past such as the Spanish, Hong Kong or Asian flu, have killed up to 50 million people world wide and these pandemics repeat roughly every 25 years. As I write this text, Canadian hospitals are overflowing with patients from a relatively minor flue outbreak, but there is no movement toward using electromedicine to treat it. If a pandemic broke out today, threatening the lives of millions, would the medical authorities use electromedicine? I doubt it. It takes time to develop the equipment and expertise to use it.

Does the state have an obligation to mandate use of electromedicine now in order to be ready for an emergency? I believe it does. Anything less is criminal.

Myth: We need a double blind study

Some doctors I have met want to see a double blind study proving that cancer can be cured by alternative methods. Three major problems make this virtually impossible. First, no one will pay for a costly study using low-cost natural remedies that cannot be patented or otherwise controlled. Secondly, people who believe in natural health products do not want to deprive half the test population of health benefits in order to prove what they see as obvious. Thirdly, blind tests are not possible. With drugs, you swallow a pill and blind crossover studies are possible. With foods, you see, taste, and smell the product. It is impossible to create a realistic double blind crossover study based on a combination of whole natural foods versus drugs or other foods. The person who is eating good food will know. You cannot fool him with drugs. That's why it is so illogical to demand natural health products meet drug regulations and comparative studies before making claims. That is why the drug directorate must be removed from regulating natural health products.

If they want a truly valuable test, open doors to a cancer detoxification clinic and allow free use of all the suppressed cancer cures. Test these against your conventional treatments. Have an open study, one on one. Do not make it a blind study. Give people a choice to use one or the other.

Myth: Mainstream medicine is scientific

What is scientific about claiming the cause of cancer is chance and unlucky circumstance? The cause of cancer, according to Dr. Guyton, as taught to medical students is as follows (Page 39): "*Thus chance alone is all that is required for mutations to take place, so we may suppose that a very large number of cancers are merely the result of unlucky occurrence*"

How can chance and unlucky occurrence be the cause of cancer? These universal concepts exist only in the mind. What is scientific about the defective gene theory when it can be disproved by the atomic theory? What is scientific about suppressing all alternative theories? What is scientific about exclusive use of toxic drugs radiation and surgery for therapy? What is scientific in having spent 100 years and millions of dollars in cancer research and saying we still do not know the cause of cancer?

If you find yourself hanging on to medical dogma, ask yourself why you should believe the dogma. Modern medicine is becoming "applied mythology."

Health care should be a science based on biology. Health care is not a religion. Why is change so difficult? The same hypocrisy can be found in most, if not all, diseases treated by toxic drugs. One of the most devious lies has to do with the elimination of low-cost hydrogen peroxide and ozone therapy for cancer.

Myth: 'Ozone unsafe at any level'

The head of Health Canada's Air and Waste Section recently released a report on Ozone entitled *'Unsafe at any Level'* (Hamilton Spectator, June 24, 1999).

The report tells us that *"ozone is the largest component of smog, and it is the leading culprit for air quality advisories.*

That statement cannot be true. Ozone levels are measured in parts per billion. Ozone is not the largest component of smog. Smog in cities is low in ozone. The same report says so.

The report goes on to say: *"At 15 parts per billion science can detect health effects such as premature deaths, hospitalizations, and emergency room visits."*

That statement cannot be true. Ozone is seldom if ever *less* than 15 parts per billion in the air. How could they possibly detect health effects from ozone in smog? It's ridiculous to claim: *"At 15 parts per billion ozone leads to premature deaths."*

The next statement is similarly false:

Ozone is a pollutant for which it is now understood there is no safe level.

Ozone is part of the environment, is a relatively stable molecule keeping the sky blue, among other things, and protecting the earth from ultraviolet rays from the sun. There is a safe level.

The author explains that ozone is a secondary pollutant:

It is not emitted but is formed in the atmosphere from industry and the burning of fossil fuels in cars.

According to press reports, the chemical reactions that lead to formation of ozone are spurred by heat and sunlight. That is why ozone is a hot summer day phenomenon. It is also why ozone levels typically build through the day, reaching a peak in the afternoon, and decreasing through the evening.

The report goes on to say that ozone is a deceptive pollutant that defies some basic assumptions about air pollution. For example, it can be higher in rural areas and some of the lowest levels are recorded in the centers of big cities. Even Alert, in the high Arctic, recorded an average of 28 parts per billion over a three-year period. That's nearly twice the rate that: *"At 15 parts per billion science can detect health effects such as premature deaths, hospitalizations, and emergency room visits."*

I think it's time to pause and ask the authorities: "Why should I believe you?" What you say does not make any sense.

Ozone is mainly a byproduct of photosynthesis in plants

Ozone is a bluish gas and gives the sky its blue color. Smog creates a yellow haze across the horizon because we can see light reflecting from the billions of particles of noxious nitrogen oxides, suspended dust particles, and emissions from coal furnaces and fossil fuel motors. We do not see the ozone layer as a yellow cloud in the sky. Ozone measured at 60 parts per billion does not give smog its yellow color. Ozone has been around for millions of years, and did not destroy life on this planet. I wonder if the author of this report has ever thought that the health problems related to smog could come from the pollutants and hydrocarbons that darken the sky.

As for seeing higher levels of ozone in rural areas on hot summer days, has he ever stopped to think that plants produce oxygen through photosynthesis? During periods of rapid photosynthesis on hot sunny afternoons, ozone levels ebb and flow with the rate of photosynthesis. Rapid photosynthesis results in increased ozone. That is why there is more ozone in rural areas on hot summer days.

Industrial smog has very little to do with rural ozone or ozone levels would be more constant throughout the year. Ozone occurs with periods of high photosynthesis in areas of rapidly growing plants. Ozone levels increase during and after a rain because rainwater contains ozone as hydrogen peroxide, and plants grow faster and produce more oxygen. Oxygen is a light gas that rises up into the atmosphere where the ultraviolet rays of the sun split diatomic oxygen molecules allowing oxygen atoms to combine with oxygen molecules to form ozone. Ozone, is a heavier molecule than oxygen and drifts downward through the atmosphere, making the sky blue. Ozone is a natural component of our atmosphere, always has been, and always will be.

Due to traffic and volume of vehicles, inner cities have the highest amount of auto emissions. Oddly, inner cities have the lowest readings of ozone. Perhaps his theory is wrong. Has he considered the inability of concrete streets, sidewalks and buildings to produce oxygen through photosynthesis? Perhaps there is less ozone in urban centers because there are fewer plants and less oxygen being produced.

Ozone and other photo-chemicals are produced wherever plants produce oxygen through photosynthesis. Take a trip through the American Smoky Mountains and view the blue haze produced by photosynthesis.

Ozone in the high Arctic is made by bright sunshine splitting diatomic oxygen (O_2) into singlet oxygen, which then combines with two molecules of oxygen to form two molecules of ozone. It is generally accepted that the earth's ozone layer in the upper atmosphere is produced this way. Ozone is universal in the atmosphere and is not dangerous at any natural level. Lightning produces ozone during thunderstorms, leaving the air smelling fresh and clean.

Newspaper reports on smog continue to identify ozone as the major health problem in smog. For example, in the July 16 edition of the Hamilton Spectator we read:

> The Ministry *measures six pollutants* to determine air quality, although much of Southern Ontario's *bad air can be blamed on the ozone.* It is formed from industrial gases and the burning of fossil fuels in cars.
>
> Ozone produces inflammation in the airway, Pengelly said. "It makes it difficult for air to get in and out. The inflammation makes it harder for blood to flow through the lungs putting extra effort on the heart."

(Note: Pengelly is the specialist credited with making this report.)

What's wrong with this picture? Burning of fossil fuels in cars does not produce ozone. How does ozone at sixty parts per billion inflame airways so badly that it becomes difficult for air to get into our lungs?

If you check *Harper's Review of Biochemistry*, which details how oxygen functions in the body, ozone is not even mentioned in the index. Since when does an inflammation reduce blood flow? According to the medical dictionary under *inflammation*, we read that histamine increases blood flow:

> When a body tissue is damaged, specialized mast cells release a chemical called histamine. Histamine *increases blood flow to the damaged tissue,* which causes redness and heat.

I cannot find any biology or biochemistry text references that ozone produces inflammation. The claims are false.

There are six pollutants measured in smog, five of them noxious chemicals derived directly from fossil fuels. It is nitrogen dioxide that provides the smelly yellow and brown colour that is consistent with smog levels. It is the sulfur oxides that burn lung tissue (recall that mustard gas, used in W.W.I, was sulfur based). The dictionary describes mustard gas as 'a heavy, sluggish, blistering, irritant chemical gas. The word smog originated to mean a combination of smoke and fog. On a hot summer day we do not have any fog in the air. We have a heavy, sluggish, blistering, irritant gas closely resembling mustard gas. Why not blame the other five components of smog for the health problems? Why single out ozone at a mere fifteen to sixty parts per billion as the cause of health problems? I wonder why these articles never list the parts per billion of the other gases.

The connection between toxic gases such as mustard gas and cancer can be explained by the current of injury theory. Certain gases, such as mustard gas are referred to as being a vesicant, or capable of causing blisters in lung tissue. The U.S. Department of Veterans Affairs have a compensation program in which they are paying victims of a group of 4000 servicemen who participated in mustard gas experiments. The majority of servicemen have some type of cancer. See http://www.va.gov /pressrel/99mustd.htm.) Toxic gases cause blisters of lung tissue, blisters damage skin tissue and turn on the repair mechanism with replication of proteins or cells. Contamination of these repair proteins with microbial growth factors causes mutation, rejection, and blockage of the repair process. Continuous replication results in cancer.

What is the hidden agenda in blaming ozone for health damage of smog? Is the high incidence of lung cancer due to sulfur related toxins from petroleum products? Are they trying to protect the petrochemical industry from public outcry or just scare people away from ozone therapy?

How can we improve our environment by fixing the wrong problem? If burning fossil fuels creates ozone, why do we have a hole in the ozone layer? As pollution increases, there should be a corresponding increase in ozone. Obviously, that is not the case.

About 70% of the earth's oxygen is produced in the ocean, and about 30% by plants on land. Recall the public outcry against destruction of the rain forests because it led to the destruction of the ozone layer. Doesn't that tell you that ozone is produced by rapid photosynthesis? Everyone knows photosynthesis produces oxygen. Is it not likely that rapid photosynthesis produces ozone? Ozone is a natural product, without serious toxicity at normal levels.

Perhaps governments should build giant outdoor ozonators to replace the loss of rainforest ozone? An increase in atmospheric ozone will help reduce pollution and rebuild the ozone layer to protect our planet from the dangers of excessive radiation, heat and storm-related damage. While we are at it, why don't we use ozone therapy to cure cancer?

Over the years we have been told that the hole in the ozone layer is caused by the propellant and refrigerant gas, Freon, sprayed into the air from aerosol containers and leaking from refrigeration units and air conditioners. The theory is that Freon, a very light gas, rises into the atmosphere and ozone layer. Here it serves as a catalyst to destroy ozone and causes a hole in the ozone layer. To protect our environment, aerosol containers containing Freon have been banned, and all new refrigeration equipment uses something other than Freon. Billions of dollars have been appropriately invested to protect the earth's ecosystem.

It seems to me that the figures just don't add up. The earth's upper atmosphere is such a vast area that the amount of Freon available is insufficient to destroy the amount of ozone being produced by plants through photosynthesis. It would take a massive amount of Freon to accomplish this task. There must be something we are doing on a far more massive scale that is causing the problem. Internal combustion motors produce reactive carbon monoxide. Carbon monoxide converts to carbon dioxide with the bonding of an atom of oxygen. Millions of cars and trucks producing carbon monoxide account for the loss of oxygen in the atmosphere and the corresponding hole in the ozone layer?

Perhaps ammonia from liquid fertilizer in fields converts to nitrous oxide, and creates the smog we experience only on hot summer days. Could nitrous-oxide be a major contributor to the hole in the ozone layer allowing excess ultraviolet energy to reach the surface of the planet, increase heating, and cause the climactic shifts that are disrupting life on earth?

If you had to bet your life, or the life of your grandchildren, on the right answer, and in a way you may have to do so, would you accept statements claiming Freon, as the major cause for the destruction of our ecosystem?

Aerosols have been banned for years now, but the climatic conditions around the globe are getting progressively worse. Freon cannot be the only problem.

What are people doing on a massive scale that wasn't being done before the hole in the ozone layer first appeared? The answer is in the use of ammonia to fertilize plants and increase crop yield. They now estimate that 80% of the worlds crops are now fertilized with ammonia based products. Ammonia could be the answer. Ammonia accounts for increased plant growth and photosynthesis, which would help explain the increase in ozone during the peak growing season. But what happens to ammonia for the rest of the year? Nitrogen in ammonia combines with oxygen to form nitrous oxide. Nitrous oxide is a major contaminant in smog.

If we study how refrigeration units work, we learn that gases with a low boiling point, such as Freon can be cycled, under different pressures to evaporate, take on heat, and then be compressed into a liquid to give off heat. That's how refrigerants work.

In the book, *The Way Things Work*, by Simon and Schuster Publishers, under the topic 'refrigerators' we have reference to ammonia used as a refrigerant.

> ...so called refrigerants are employed. (these are liquids with low boiling points or liquefied gases, e.g. ammonia, ethyl chloride or Freon).

Millions of tons of ammonia are being placed in the soils around the globe as a source of nitrogen for plants, and massive amounts of ammonia are being introduced into the atmosphere. Perhaps ammonia is the problem that is disrupting the earth's ecosystem? The daily heating and nightly cooling of the atmosphere, with refrigerant-type gases somehow functions to break down ozone. Ammonia, being the reactive substance it is, may react with oxygen and ozone to destroy the ozone layer even without the daily-heating and night-cooling cycle.

Perhaps, too, this is why smog levels increase in summer. On a hot summer day, more ammonia is leached into the atmosphere from the fields. Modern smog could be largely the result of modern farming practices using ammonia fertilizer to increase crop yields. In that case, the destruction of the ozone layer and climactic changes could be the result of modern chemical farming.

This section on a relationship between ammonia and destruction of the environment is only speculation on my part because I cannot find any collaborating evidence. I introduce it here to suggest there must be a reason to mould public opinion and create false perceptions about the dangers of ozone. It seems that ozone is being wrongfully fingered as a health and environmental culprit to protect something else. Hopefully, someone will come up with the truth about what is causing the cancer epidemic and climactic changes on the planet before it is too late for normal life. The loss of oxygen seems to be the one common denominator.

The unregulated use of ammonia could well be a major factor in the worldwide cancer epidemic in industrialized countries. The incidence of cancer is low in Africa and Mexico, and the use of ammonia for chemical farming in these countries is limited by poverty and traditional farming methods.

Ozonators provide low-cost health care

There are several companies manufacturing and marketing room ozonators such as the Living Air Corp. of Blaine, Minn. These are sold as 'Electronic air purification systems' and generate ozone which is distributed by a fan into the room. In our home and office, we run room ozonators 24 hours per day. We believe low-levels of ozone purify the air of airborne microorganisms, reduces mildew, and slows the aging process. There are no signs of ill health due to ozone, because there are no signs of ill health. There is certainly no sign of inflammation of airways.

If ozone were unsafe at any level, why would thousands of people use room ozonators regularly and believe in them as a health benefit? The ozone in our home does not come with all of the hydrocarbons that make up modern smog. It is the chemical pollutants, not ozone that creates the health problems.

Bob Beck's cancer treatment features ozonated water to increase the supply of oxygen in the blood. Dr. Hulda Clark's recommendation includes ozonated olive oil to destroy virus, fungi and yeast. We can buy ozonators to put in fish tanks and aquariums to purify the water. We can also buy ozonators for hot tubs and spas. However, we cannot promote ozonators for better health and treatment of disease.

Ozone provides a low-cost do-it-yourself method you can use every day to clear your body of toxins and oxygenate the cells. Ozone generators, called PortaZone, costing around $300 in Canada are available from various sources.

As you can see, Health Canada and the medical advisors who inform the public about health issues, are either *lacking in scientific knowledge* and common sense or they publish *misinformation* for a hidden agenda. In either case, the popular media publish whatever they say and no one questions the content. Misinformation about the danger of ozone and hydrogen peroxide as well as oxygen free radicals is surpassed only by the misinformation about cholesterol.

Myth: Cholesterol causes heart disease

What is the true source of excess cholesterol in the body? Would you believe it is not from eating fats? Cholesterol is caused by excess processed starches and hydrogenated oils. Let's take a look.

In *Harper's Review of Biochemistry* (Page 240), we are told:

The greater part of the cholesterol of the body arises by synthesis (about 1g/d), whereas only about 0.3 g/d is provided by the average diet.

In other words, 3 times as much cholesterol is made or synthesized in the body than is ingested. The text goes on to say:

Cholesterol is typically a product of animal metabolism and occurs therefore in foods of animal origin such as meat, liver, and egg yolk.

The fact that cholesterol *occurs in animal products* does not equate with high cholesterol from eating animal products. Cholesterol is not absorbed as cholesterol through the colon wall nor is reformed from the breakdown of cholesterol. On page 243 we read: "Dietary cholesterol takes several days to equilibrate with cholesterol in the plasma and several weeks to equilibrate with cholesterol of the tissues." Animal products are mainly proteins and animal fats can be easily digested. Cholesterol is composed mainly of carbon from processed hydrogenated oils and carbohydrates that cannot be digested because these molecules are not natural. The genes lack the capacity to produce enzymes to process chemicals and processed food that does not spoil. Breakfast cereals, for example, have a shelf life of several years. White flour, hydrogenated oils and sugar do not require refrigeration because they do not spoil. Food that does not spoil is not easy to digest.

In *Harper's Review of Biochemistry* (Page 24), we read:

Virtually all tissues containing nucleated cells are capable of synthesizing cholesterol, particularly the liver, adrenal cortex, skin, intestines, testis and aorta...*Acetyl-COA is the source of all the carbon atoms in cholesterol*...Synthesis takes place in several stages. The first is the synthesis of mevalonate, a 6-carbon compound from acetyl-COA.

So where does acetyl-COA come from? Is it animal products or carbohydrates? On page 234, we learn that carbohydrates are the chief source of acetyl-COA and therefore the chief source of cholesterol in the body. In Chapter 18, *Metabolism of Lipids*, we read:

1. The liver has active enzyme systems for synthesizing triacylglycerols, phospholipids, cholesterol, and plasma lipoproteins...

2. The fatty acids used in the synthesis of hepatic (meaning liver) triacylglycerols are derived from two possible sources: (1) synthesis within the liver from acetyl-CoA derived in the main from carbohydrates and (2) uptake of free fatty acids

from circulation. The first source would appear to be predominate...

Biochemists discovered that excess cholesterol is produced in the liver from excess carbohydrates in the 1940s. Excess acetic acid, a byproduct from incomplete digestion of sugar and grains leads to acetic acid overload. The problem results from the lack of certain enzymes. The liver converts toxic acetic acid into non-toxic cholesterol.

In the Nov. 1966 issue of the alternative health magazine EXPLORE For the Professional, there is a relevant article by Dr. Amar S. Kapoor, M.D. FACD, President of the Heart Mind Body Institute. He writes (Page 32):

. . . Total cholesterol elevations are in epidemic proportions in the general population. It is estimated that 80 million Americans have hyperlipidemia. Should these people be treated? Before you treat them, it is prudent to know the side effects and toxicity of the two most prescribed groups of cholesterol lowering drugs, the fibric acid derivatives and the HMG-CoA reductase inhibitors or the "statin" drugs. . . Side effects include abdominal pain, vomiting, gallstones, insomnia, and increase violent behavior to name but a few.

Note that the health benefit of taking the 'statin' drugs is stated to inhibit the function of acetyl-CoA reductase, the enzyme essential for digestion of carbohydrates. Why reduce the function of this enzyme? What does it have to do with fats that cause cholesterol problems? Note also that you are advised to eat more carbohydrates to reduce cholesterol. Do you see any common sense in this procedure if the drugs destroy the enzymes needed to digest carbohydrates?

Dr. Costantini informs us in the book *Fungalbionics, Atherosclerosis* (Page 13) that the "statins" were "initially developed as an antifungal agents which just happened to have an effect on lowing blood levels of low density lipoproteins (commonly referred to as bad cholesterol)." According to Costantini, the statins are mycotoxins derived from fungi. They help destroy other fungi in the body, reduce granuloma, and thereby reduce the demand for more cholesterol to coat the arteries. This is also proof that Atherosclerosis is a fungal disease.

Preventative information from the heart and stroke industry appears to be designed to create business. Look at any cholesterol information pamphlet and it says to eat less meat and protein and more carbohydrates, such as processed grains. This information is wrong.

The fact that meats contain cholesterol does not cause cholesterol in the body. Cholesterol is broken down and used by the body. The fact that meats contain limited amounts of saturated fats, does not account for cholesterol in the body. Most of the fats in natural food consist of unsaturated fats that can be readily digested and used by the body. Hard to digest saturated fats found in the starchy foods recommended to reduce cholesterol cause cholesterol. Cholesterol is made from consuming processed sugars and hydrogenated oils.

Numerous books have been written by highly qualified medical doctors to inform the public about the truth of cholesterol, but their message is lost in the sea of medical propaganda. Dr. Richard Murray's *Basic Guide to Understanding Clinical Laboratory Tests* has the following summary (Page 52):

The book *Cholesterol Conspiracy* (Smith & Pinkney) attempts to establish that the American public is a victim of a fraud unparalleled in medical history. According to Dr. George V. Mann, "Saturated fat and cholesterol in the diet are not the cause of coronary heart disease. The myth is the greatest scientific deception of this century, perhaps of any century."

Advising people with heart problems to eat more grain products and pasta is either sheer medical ignorance or pure deception.

In the book *Fats and Oils* by Udo Erasmus (Page 62):

The body makes cholesterol. The cells of the body can make all the cholesterol they need for their membrane requirements. Cells manufacture cholesterol in response to demand. For instance, when someone drinks alcohol, the alcohol dissolves in the membranes, making them more fluid. In response, the cells will manufacture cholesterol, build it into the membrane, and thereby bring the membrane back to its proper (less fluid) state.

Udo Erasmus explains that cholesterol is vital for health. He then explains that cholesterol is a 27-carbon chain molecule and is derived mainly from food with a high content of carbon such as sugar and starches. He explains that metabolism of unsaturated fatty acids result in only a limited amount of carbon for cholesterol. Most cholesterol comes from foods that combine saturated fats (hydrogenated oils) with processed grains and sugars. All baked goods, cookies, muffins, and pastry provide acetate fragments the body converts to cholesterol. Then he states:

A diet high in non-essential fatty acids (hydrogenated oils) and refined carbohydrates produces an excess of acetate fragments in the body, and thus 'pressures' the body into increased cholesterol production. And there you have the reason for the high

cholesterol levels of most of the people in the 'processed foods' nations.

The Canadian heart and stroke industry is now costing about 19 billion dollars annually according to recent newspaper articles. In our market area, cardiovascular disease is the leading cause of death, at 36 per cent of all deaths. Drugs for cholesterol reduction and costly surgery and medical intervention are a tremendous drain of taxpayer dollars and a needless burden to medicare. The toxic effects of cholesterol lowering drugs just add to the Medicare burden.

The Minister of Public Works and Government Services produces a flyer called *Canada's Food Guide to Healthy Eating*. The flyer says to choose whole grain and enriched products more often. It then pictures, as wholesome foods to chose from, whole-wheat and white bread, muffins, hamburger buns, hot-dog buns, processed grains in cereals, pasta, white rice, crackers, pancakes and macaroni. The flyer also recommends 5 to 12 servings per day. Except for whole wheat bread and some bagels, all of the other products are cholesterol forming because they contain large amounts of processed fats, processed grains, and sugars.

The flyer also recommends 5 to10 servings per day of fresh or canned fruit and vegetables and 2 o 3 servings of meat or alternatives such as fish, beans, and tofu. There's no problem with that. However, the emphasis of the flyer—and the message one remembers —is to eat more cholesterol forming processed flour, sugar and hydrogenated fats.

Myth: Autoimmune diseases exist

The same hypocrisy pervades the autoimmune disease industry. The myth that the body's defense mechanism attacks human cells or that one defensive mechanism attacks another has never been proven. The recommended cure for autoimmune diseases is to provide toxic drugs to weaken the immune system so that the attacks will stop. Can you think of anything relating to better health that is more lacking in common sense?

Mistakes in the Germ theory, as discussed earlier, grouped a large number of human diseases as not being microbial. There was no other good explanation for them. Medical doctors are expected to have answers for the cause of disease. Consequently theories were suggested and the most plausible promoted as fact although there was no proof. These theories are now medical dogma or myths that have been woven into the fabric of medical opinion and treatment. Just like stress was once considered the cause of ulcers, it is now proven that the bacteria *Helicobacter pylori* causes ulcers. However, many people still believe that stress causes ulcers as well.

A brief search on the Internet under "autoimmune diseases" brings up the home page for the "American Autoimmune Related Disease Association, Inc." Over 80 diseases are now classified as autoimmune disease, including Addison's Disease, Diabetes, Chronic Fatigue Syndrome, Fibromyalgia, Multiple Sclerosis, Vasculitis, and Lupus. The common thread in these diseases is believed to be that the immune system misidentifies the body's own proteins as invaders and mounts an immunological attack against them.

The concept also assumes that as soon as invaders are defeated, the army of defenders may attack human cells. There is no evidence in biology that proves this happens or explains the pathway of chemical or enzymatic reactions in which human defensive cells or enzymes attack human cells.

In reality, each of these diseases can be traced back to a nutrient deficiency, or attack by toxins such as ammonia, fungal mycotoxins and microbial enzymes. Degenerative diseases suggest defects are worked into cell-wall membranes a bit at a time, in much the same way that microbial enzymes cause cancer. Our body is host to vast numbers of conflicting microbes that compete one against the other for space. Our foods contain fungi, yeast or mycotoxins as well as chemical sprays and food coloring. Aspartame and other chemical food additives break down into toxic chemicals.

Large parasites produce defensive cells and enzymes to destroy smaller microbes, just as human cells do. That's where vaccines come from. These defensive mechanisms and enzymes cause our so-called autoimmune diseases. Consider for a moment how many foods we eat that have been fermented or have been stored and fungal-processed before using. Mushrooms, for example, are the fruit of a fungal organism and contains spores for reproduction. Dr. Costantini advises strongly against consuming 'fungal foods'.

Well-aged beef, for example, is tender because the tissue has been softened by a fungal process while aging. Many people believe that gout is caused by eating meat. Dr. Costantini has observed that gout comes only from eating well-aged beef. Many farmers and ranchers eat excessive amounts of fresh meat without experiencing gout. It is the mycotoxins in meat that cause gout. This fact was discovered accidentally when chickens fed well-aged meat scraps suffered gout. When the meat scraps were removed, gout disappeared. Gout is a fungal disease.

A person who takes care of racehorses came to visit. While we were talking, he mentioned that his most successful and promising racehorse stopped winning even though he was feeding the horse properly and doing everything he could. It looked like a case of chronic fatigue.

I suggested we should check out his feed for toxins. We drove back to his stables with a bottle of hydrogen peroxide in hand. We took a sample of the grains and placed a couple of ounces in a container of hydrogen peroxide (35% diluted to about 6%). Within minutes, the container overflowed as the reaction of hydrogen peroxide on the fungi and yeast in the grains caused a tremendous release of oxygen. The feed was obviously contaminated with mycotoxins, fungi and yeast even though it looked and smelled normal.

Following that experience, he changed the feed and the horse won another race about two weeks later. The cost of checking the grain for fungal mycotoxins was less than two cents worth of hydrogen peroxide. He continues to use this simple, fool-proof method to check grains for mycotoxins, fungi and yeast. We use peroxide regularly in our home and keep a small spray bottle handy to sterilize counters, dishcloths, cutting boards and kitchen work areas. It is ideal for spraying on a sore throat at the first sign of a cold. Every home should be using peroxide to wipe out microbes and soak imported fruits that may contain dangerous bacteria.

Some mornings when you wake up with aching muscles, look back at your diet. Have you been eating fungal food? Fungi produce mycotoxins that cause many mysterious aches and pains. Ammonia is one of the most deadly toxins in the body and is produced by fungi and bacteria in the body.

Please note the difference between *autoimmunity* and *autoimmune diseases*. If the body develops defense mechanisms, such as resistance to measles, the body has *autoimmunity to measles*. However, if the body attacks normal healthy tissue or proteins, the body has an *autoimmune disease*. The autoimmune disease theory has never been proven, but it serves a purpose. It creates tremendous profits for the drug industry. If you suffer from an autoimmune disease, continue to take drugs for it without relief, and continue to lack good health, take time to investigate alternatives.

Medical students take courses in immunology from a text called *Basic and Clinical Immunology* by Dr. D.P. Stites and some 56 others. The 700 page textbook printed in small type looks like it could take five years to read —once. Obviously, immunology is a major course in medicine.

The concept of autoimmunity is treated rather lightly with only some 30 pages. In the introduction of this chapter, Stites describes the theoretical and possible microbial nature of the apparent autoimmune problem (Page 156):

In many instances, it is not clear whether autoimmune responses are directed against unmodified self antigens or self antigens that have been modified by any of numerous agents

such as viruses and haptenic groups (*substances that can react with antigens*).

There is as yet no established unifying concept to explain the origin and pathogenesis of the various autoimmune disorders.

The autoimmune disease concept has never been proven.

The text goes on to suggest that autoimmune diseases may be caused by viruses, bacteria, hormones, or abnormal genes. *The important point to realize is that the whole concept of autoimmune diseases has never been proven and that microbial toxins are highly suspected as the cause by the authors of clinical immunology texts.*

If you want to learn more about the autoimmune disease concept, a good place to start is with the book by James Carter, *Racketeering in Medicine, the Suppression of Alternatives.* You will find this book delightful, if you enjoy horror stories. Pages 175 to 180 describe how a woman doctor with mixed connective tissue disease took toxic drugs for a five-year period in order to lower her immune system. She believed her disease was caused by her immune system attacking her body. According to the autoimmune disease theory, her treatment was to attack her immune system with drugs to weaken it. She experienced tremendous pain and suffering to no avail. Her health just kept getting worse.

Finally she gave up on drugs and tried Chinese herbs. Chinese herbalists and alternative therapists attack so-called autoimmune diseases by strengthening the immune system, and do so with great success. They believe toxins and microbial enzymes attack human tissue and nerves. They cure autoimmune diseases by removing the causes, which are microbial mycotoxins and ammonia. To her great surprise, her autoimmune disease disappeared.

Dr. Costantini informs us in the text *Fungalbionics, Atherosclerosis* (Page 12):

> The mycotoxin cylosporin used for transplantation causes cancer and Atherosclerosis, complete with hyperlipidemia in ALL humans who have used it. Many others develop gout and other diseases.

Hyperlipidemia means high cholesterol levels. Cylosporin is used to reduce the immune system reaction in transplant operations to stop the rejection process. According to Costantini, impairing the immune system with cylosporin has resulted in cancer for all humans who have used it. I wonder how many other autoimmune drugs cause cancer? If you allow your immune system to be destroyed to benefit a 'so-called' autoimmune disease, and allow opportunistic infection to take over, you could cause cancer to occur.

The concept of autoimmune diseases has never been proven. There are no references in biology texts that outline the pathway that would explain how and why the body's defense mechanism would attack itself. Without competition to prove the concept is without merit, and with control of the press, mainstream medicine is raking in huge drug profits for treating the wrong cause of more than 80 diseases that plague mankind.

Alzheimer's now affects 5 per cent of the population over 65 years of age, and 25 per cent of those over 85 (based on 1997 figures). According to mainstream medicine, Alzheimer's is both a defective gene disease and an autoimmune disease. As with cancer, no research is being done to discover how microbes cause Alzheimer's.

The Hamilton Spectator Jan. 27, 2000 edition on Health and Science describes a $7.9 million dollar grant by the Federal Government to help fund research on drugs to cure Alzheimer's. The money will help Montreal based Neurochem Inc. to speed its drug Alzemed through pre-clinical and clinical development phases to licensing and the commercial market in about five years. There are 4.5 million North Americans with this disease, and the number is increasing by 10 percent annually.

The report adds that the government will be reimbursed by royalties on the drug's sale. This puts the government into business with the drug companies and ensures that methods of curing Alzheimer's by eliminating the cause will not likely occur.

In the same issue of this paper, there is an article entitled "The Vanishing Breakthroughs." This is a list of the many broken promises the Canadian taxpayer has financed through government funding. Numerous reasons are given for the lack of success for these new drugs. None of these reasons given suggest that diseases caused by toxins cannot be cured by adding more toxins. Millions and millions of dollars have been wasted!

Myth: Alzheimer's is an autoimmune or defective gene disease

Why is there an epidemic of mental disorders, hostility problems, and nerve diseases? Why are school kids attacking school children and teachers for the first time in history? Is this just the beginning of a new trend?

We have reviewed the damages to the nervous system from aspartame, but brain parasites are also involved. Fungi and bacteria have been found in brain cells. Fungal and bacterial waste produce ammonia. Shampoo and hair rinses contain toxic ammonia. Smoking loads the body with ammonia. Ammonia attacks nerve cells and causes various nerve-related diseases.

Microbes produce growth hormones in humans. What happens with microbial nerve growth factors produced by parasites resident in brain tissue?

Parasitic nerve growth factors would cause human brain cells to differentiate into a form not suitable for human use. The loss of a capacity to hold recent memory, but retain distant or early memory, can be explained by the concept that new experiences are recorded in new tissue growth or changes to existing growth. Microbial nerve growth factors, from parasites in the brain, would scramble new brain tissue growth and render it useless for recording new experiences. Ammonia in the blood from smoking, personal-care products, household cleansers, and fermentation of excessive amounts of processed foods will support microbial growth in the brain. The dreaded disease of Alzheimer's is a microbial disease and should be treated as such. Toxic drugs will not do the job.

One of the most important traits concerning DNA polymerase enzyme for cancer and nerve growth factor for Alzheimer's is how little is needed to have a profound effect.

Dr. Rita Levi-Montalcine, who was introduced in Chapter 5 on growth hormones discovered that a small amount of growth hormone produced dramatic effects. Her research applies to Alzheimer's as well as to other diseases. The information about her research says:

> In Rio she put mice tumor cells near a single nerve ganglion in a culture dish full of solution. Within ten hours the nerve ganglion gave rise, she said, to 'a dense halo of nerve fibers, radiating out like rays from the sun' **So powerful was the substance that one billionth of a gram in a milliliter of culture solution produced the effect.**

The significance of her research is that parasites and fungi may be the cause of far more diseases than we think. If microbial nerve growth factors mutate nerve growth, most, if not all of the nerve related diseases may be parasite related. We have seen dramatic improvement in people with mental fatigue and depression from zapping and parasite cleansing. The zapper crosses the blood-brain barrier with ease, whereas drugs and herbs do not do so as easily.

Cancer cells and brain nerve tissue must have a growth hormone from somewhere in order to grow and differentiate. The fact that human cancer cells do not develop human traits indicates that the enzymes and coenzymes are not of human origin. The fact that memory of Alzheimer's disease victims ceases to function first for recent memory indicates nerve growth is non-existent or non-functional. What possible source could there be other than parasites and microbes?

Dr. W. Philpott M.D. has connected ammonia toxicity directly to Alzheimer's, diabetes, amyotrophy (wasting away of muscle tissue) and amyotrophic lateral sclerosis (degeneration of the nerves, also called ALS or Lou Gehrig's disease). The relationship could be direct, as ammonia is highly toxic to neurons, or it could be indirect, as ammonia produces more mycotoxins through increased fermentation. Here's what Dr. Philpott has to say (Page 10):

> Ammonia is highly toxic to the neurons. When the spinal cord neurons are most affected, the disease is called amyotrophic lateral sclerosis. When the brain is the target organ, Alzheimer's disease develops.
>
> An institution specializing in Alzheimer's and senility case care asked for my ideas on Alzheimer's. I told them to feed an 80% protein meal and two hours after the meal, test for venous and arterial blood for ammonia. Twenty senile cases and twenty Alzheimer cases were tested by the process. All were diagnosed by neurologists. All twenty of the Alzheimer cases had hyperammonia and none of the senile cases had hyperammonia. My monitoring of ALS indicates the existence of hyperammoniemia. Amyotrophy, which has the same symptoms as amyotrophic lateral sclerosis is one of the complications of diabetes mellitus type II. The mental deterioration in a diabetic is attributed to different target organs. ALS and Alzheimer's is the same illness with different target organs.

The concept that Alzheimer's disease will become another profit center of drugs is really frightful.

In the 1997 textbook, *Human Genetics* (Page 63) we read: "Several genes have been identified as causing Alzheimer's disease".

Later, on page 182 we read: "The search for a genetic explanation for a severe form of Alzheimer's disease illustrates how discovering mutations can solve biological mysteries."

After listing all the defective genes already discovered we learn: "Normally the protein *probably somehow monitors* the cell's storage ...."

The defective gene theory of cancer and the defective gene theory of Alzheimer's have one significant feature in common. They are both false.

There is no reason why genes would become defective to cause Alzheimer's. Genes are stable molecular crystals with a history going back billions of years. Why would they suddenly become defective now?

In summary, ammonia is highly toxic to the human body and neurons and is directly related to cancer. You will recall that the four vestigal ionic hydrogen bonds include three with oxygen, found in the DNA molecules. The fourth type containing nitrogen, expressed as N—H...N is not found in DNA but is found in the body.

Ammonia is NH_3 and ammonia can form the vestigial ionic bond that disrupts the vestigial ionic energy that in turn makes up the autonomic nervous system controlling life functions. Alzheimer's, diabetes, and diseases related to malfunction of nerves and muscles are probably all ammonia toxicity diseases. We have seen people cured or improved of nerve related diseases by eliminating parasites from their body. By eliminating parasites, they also eliminate the major source of ammonia toxicity and fungal mycotoxins.

The enormous cost of medicare can only be reduced when millions of Canadians demand freedom of choice in health care, and support government action to end the medical monopoly of selecting and authorizing treatments for disease. Without competition, there is no control mechanism in place. The medical monopoly does not protect the consumer. It protects only those who take advantage of the monopoly to profit from human pain and suffering.

Myth: Diabetes is an autoimmune or defective gene disease

As already discussed, diabetes is a microbial disease which destroys the function of insulin and the pancreas. The autoimmune disease concept has never been proven. There are no explanations describing the metabolic process that would account for diabetes as an autoimmune disease. The medical knowledge that insulin is a transport mechanism for lipids, proteins and sugars is not common knowledge. Diabetes can be a result of protein or lipid deficiency due to microbial mutation of insulin.

The concept that microbial enzymes disturb pancreatic function makes sense. In her book *The Cure for All Diseases* (Page 173), Dr. Hulda Clark identifies the specific parasite found in all diabetics and describes how to eliminate them. She writes:

> By killing this parasite and removing wood alcohol from the diet, the need for insulin can be cut in half in three weeks (or sooner).

The autoimmune myth and treatment for 80 autoimmune diseases cost health insurance and medicare billions of dollars. Diabetes is becoming another man-made epidemic. The cost of insulin is a tremendous burden on medicare. Misinformation is a good part of the problem. The medical monopoly in health care is the other.

There are four major industries in Canada that are destroying the health care system. These are the tobacco industry, the cancer industry, the heart and stroke industry and the autoimmune-disease industry. They should all be sued by the government under the "Racketeer Influenced and Corrupt Organization Act", in order to recover millions of dollars wasted on controlled research and unnecessary medical expenses to the taxpayers. Reports show that the Ontario government is now suing the U. S. tobacco industry to recovery medical costs of smoke related diseases. That's a good start.

Rejecting dogma, myths and propaganda.

The significance of knowing the true cause of cancer enables you to reject the defective-gene myth and have real hope in beating the cancer problem. Women who are being advised to have their healthy breasts removed because they have defective genes can more seriously consider other options. In addition, people can have confidence in suggested remedies that eliminate parasites or destroy microbial enzymes.

The Germ Theory Part II makes more sense than any of the medical myths that are now costing human lives and overburdening our universal medicare system. It is time for people and governments to lead the way to a corresponding new health care system. We need Medicare Part II based on the microbial cause of disease without the domination by pharmaceutical interests.

Whenever you read medical propaganda about drugs and costly therapies, remember the truth about disease. All chemical reactions inside living beings are controlled by bioactive molecules we call enzymes or catalysts. Enzymes are either produced by the human body, resulting in better health, or produced by microbial parasites, resulting in disease. Our current health-care crisis is man made and dependent on propaganda for its continued economic success and exploitation of health-care funding. Defective genes do not account for the majority of human diseases as we area told. The success of propaganda is dependent upon maintaining the dictatorship of medical practice, exclusion of competition and control of the media.

Medical monopoly ensures public will be exploited.

Human nature is far from perfect. History has shown that dictatorships and business monopolies tend to corrupt people who attain too much power. The Canadian government is concerned about having one airline with a monopoly on air travel. Why not show the same concern about one medical association having a monopoly on health care? Health care is essentially a dictatorship because doctors can only prescribe products or services approved and dictated by authorities. Most doctors are even fearful to tell their patients about any alternative therapies, due to possible reprisals from medical authorities.

The late English Lord Acton was quoted as saying "Power corrupts. Absolute power corrupts—Absolutely." He was talking of political power and his statement applies to all monopolies.

Giving any group of human beings a monopoly on health care, with customers motivated by pain and fear of death, as well as giving this group a monopoly to exploit tax revenue and public funds for health care, is asking to be exploited. The monopoly provides far too much power in the hands of too few people, with no recourse by the public to address fraud and waste.

If Lord Acton were alive today, he would probably add: **Monopolies exploit. Absolute monopolies exploit—Absolutely.**

We cannot allow healthcare to be protected by a monopoly and run as a business to maximize profits. To do so is to have regulations that guarantee failure of our political, economic, and medical systems.

27. The helpless poor and homeless are the first to suffer

Medicare is a system whereby all Canadians have equal access to health care through public health insurance. Human nature being what it is, there is a tremendous amount of waste by some individuals.

The waste attributable to individuals can be minimized by photo I.D. cards and user fees. However, the waste from corrupt medical policy and suppression of alternative health care cannot be controlled. There is no mechanism in place to control the controller. Suppression of alternative cancer treatments indicates abuse of the health care system by those in charge of it. If we do not stop suppression, we will all have equal access to long waiting lines and insufficient service. The trend is just beginning. The safety net to protect the poor is coming unwound. When governments are forced into budget restraints, the people the people who rely on government services are the first to feel the pinch.

The ongoing movement to eliminate cost effective natural health products through establishment licensing and further import restrictions will just make matters worse.

Evidence of cancer cure suppression is worldwide

In 1989, Barry Lynes wrote in *The Healing of Cancer* (Page 87):

> The evidence that a vast conspiracy exists to prevent the use of new discoveries and known alternative therapies in treatment of cancer is overwhelming. The cancer industry has created a time bomb...

The time bomb is still ticking. The sooner it goes off the better. It's time for change.

Dr. James P. Carter has authored a large text entitled *Racketeering in Medicine, —The Suppression of Alternatives.* Dr. Carter doesn't only speak in terms of generalities. He presents names, events and facts, which prove that government agencies and 'kangaroo courts' suppress alternative therapies and destroy honorable men and women.

If anyone reading this book does not believe the cancer industry exists, please read a copy of Barry Lynes' book: *The Healing of Cancer —The Cures, the Cover-ups and the Solution NOW!* Peer reviews on the back cover of his book tell us:

He reveals how the American Cancer Society misleads the public in order to collect over three hundred and fifty million dollars a year in contributions, and how part of the money is used against innovative cancer researchers. Lynes also tells how the National Cancer Institute (NCI) and the Food and Drug Administration (FDA) conspire to stop promising cancer treatments.

The Healing of Cancer is a challenge to the doctors, bureaucrats and businessmen who are letting thousands die each week while a cure exists.

It is also a challenge to the average citizen to stop being silent while so many innocent victims undergo torture because of medical profiteering, outmoded thinking and a good deal of corrupt politics.

Lynes is making true statements that can easily be defended in court, if need be. That's why he was able to make them. The challenge to the average citizen to stop being silent wasn't heard. We are still letting thousands die each week while cures exist. Medical profiteering and corrupt politics are still driving the course of health care.

It seems to me that we are at a point in health care where the Negroes of America were when Martin Luther King rallied public support for a peaceful revolt against white supremacy. We are also at a point where the impoverished communist nations revolted against communism by the proven method of peaceful revolt. Millions of peaceful men and women standing for days and nights in front of government buildings presents a formidable foe. They cannot be ignored and they cannot be destroyed.

The AIDS victims marched on Washington with outstanding success. Victims of cancer, heart disease, and autoimmune diseases far outnumber the victims of AIDS. Perhaps it is time for the people of free democracies to block the streets of their government cities and health-edifices such as HPB and FDA, demanding an end to this evil in society.

Chemotherapy not effective against cancer microbes

Why does anyone maintain that chemotherapy and radiation are the most effective form of cancer treatment? Where is the proof?

The following quotation is from a medical doctor criticizing the value of chemotherapy, based on his study of corpses. Excerpted from a book by Dr. Allan Cantwell Jr., *The Cancer Microbe* (Page 115):

> When patients died from cancer, their tissues were overrun with cancer microbes. I studied autopsies of cancer patients who had been treated with massive doses of radiation therapy. I saw the microbe thriving in cancerous tissue that had been blitzed with chemotherapy; the cancer cells were destroyed, but the cancer microbe remained! Nothing fazed the cancer microbe; not surgery, not radiation, antibiotics, or chemotherapy. The cancer microbe was indestructible!

Autopsies do not support the value of chemotherapy to destroy microbes. Chemotherapy is not designed to eliminate parasites or microbial enzymes. Radiation leaves cells with damage that must result in a current of injury and repair of damaged cells surrounding the burn area. Radiation is too destructive to help heal membranes. Why should we be forced to take radiation and toxic drugs to treat cancer when more effective methods are available?

Barry Lynes, in *The Cancer Cure That Worked,* concludes his book with a personal note that expresses why mainstream medicine continues to suppress effective cancer cures. This note is a very meaningful statement and bears repeating (Page 126):

> A personal note: It took me years to realize that the people in control of the cancer treatment world today did not want a simple, quick cure for cancer. It was not in their economic or career interest. They wanted complicated disease syndromes and all the paraphernalia of techniques, expert analysis, peer group conferences, papers, discussions, research grants and clinical trials for years before a new cancer therapy might be allowed. It is a horrendous crime which serves only those "inside" who are playing the great, lucrative "expert" game.

Do you believe what you see or see what you believe? If you do not see suppression of cancer cures, you must only see what you believe and want to see. Saying, "I don't want to believe it", doesn't count. You cannot deny the holocaust and you cannot deny suppression of electromedicine.

The cancer service industry thrives on wasted tax dollars

The *cancer service industry* refers to all those who are in the noble business of treating cancer patients. The *cancer industry*, on the other hand, refers to all those who are in the horrific business of profiteering from within the cancer service industry by suppressing cancer cures.

Industry is defined as human exertion devoted to creation of wealth or capital (*Universal dictionary of the English Language*). In my opinion, the treatment of cancer has become the most lucrative industry ever developed by those who profiteer from human pain and suffering. The cancer industry is man-made and controlled at a highly profitable level, without regard for pain and suffering or death. The suppression of low-cost cancer cures proves the point. There is nothing wrong with businesses making a reasonable profit for the service of cancer care. There is everything wrong with businesses profiteering from cancer treatments at the exclusion of better methods. When these excessive profits are exported out of the country, all taxpayers suffer.

I believe the preceding material proves there is a cancer industry whose primary goal is the accumulation of capital and profit. Customer satisfaction is not a vital issue. Customers are just 'dying' for treatment. Fear, pain and suffering serve as powerful buying motives. Death and cures are to be avoided because income is lost when a patient dies or is cured. That is why use of low-cost effective cures cannot be permitted in conjunction with approved therapy.

In Canada, the monopoly is serviced by the Canadian Medical Association, enforced by the federal government's Health Protection Branch and controlled by the worldwide pharmaceutical industry. Through propaganda and control of the press, they maintain favorable public opinion.

According to the 1997 edition of **Human Genetics, Concepts and Applications**, "one in three people will develop cancer sometime in their lifetime. A million new cases of cancer will be diagnosed in the United States this year, and 10 million people are being treated for some form of the illness right now." According to *PEOPLE Weekly Magazine* over 178,000 American women will be diagnosed with breast cancer (in 1998) and more than 40,000 women will die from the disease. Breast cancer is now the most frequent type of cancer in women.

Canadian statistics say cancer is the leading cause of premature death, with 63,000 deaths, and 129,000 new cases. These are only statistics. Each one carries a sad and painful story.

The world's top-selling cancer drugs now generate more than $3-billion dollars in sales per year or more than $8-million dollars per day.

Customer satisfaction is not an issue. Competition is not allowed. Cancer patients have nowhere else to turn for help. Millions of health-care specialists rely solely on cancer treatment and research for their substantial incomes. Millions more work for pharmaceutical companies or have their personal wealth invested in pharmaceutical businesses. Millions more provide the cancer industry with facilities, equipment, education and training, publicity, insurance, publishing, legal and accounting services.

Millions of people with wealth, political power and medical authority do not want to see a low-cost cure for cancer.

The cancer industry continues to take in millions of dollars from private and public donations through various fund-raising cancer societies. They maintain public confidence by feeding the public with misinformation, regularly promising new cures that never develop and suppressing information about their failures. If any other organization did the same, it would be considered as fraud and stopped.

Propaganda is the only word to describe most of the one-sided educational information distributed by mainstream medicine regarding cancer. Every medical textbook on cancer that does not discuss the research of Nobel Prize winners Fibiger and Warburg are tools for indoctrination. Indoctrination and propaganda cannot be trusted, nor can the people who use it to sway public opinion be trusted.

The Canadian cancer service industry is looking for more money from the government. Press releases detail the urgent need for more funds. To support their argument for more funds, they released these statistics in the Hamilton Spectator, April 9, 1999. I have worked out the cure rate percentages and added them in italics.

On average, about 48 Canadians will die every day from lung cancer in Canada. This year, about 12,000 men will be diagnosed with lung cancer and about 10,600 will die. *That's 88% who die and only 12% survive.* For women with lung cancer, 8,500 will be diagnosed and about 6800 will die. *Another 80% will die!*

Out of 20,500 men and women diagnosed with lung cancer, 17,400 will die. *That's about 85% who do not survive.* After fifty years of fruitless research, why should medical researchers expect more donations or tax revenue for more research?

Success rates with prostrate cancer are not much better. In the 70 years-and-older group, expect 58,800 new cases with 36,600 deaths. That's a death rate of 62%. Cancer spreads most often to the bones, and they die very painful deaths.

The cancer industry is not an overnight commercial success. In this report we have seen references to effective cancer cures being suppressed dating back to 1913 and 1925, as well as more recent breakthroughs that are being suppressed and ignored at this time. There have been no significant changes in how cancer is treated in the last 50 years because all potentially better and less costly new treatments are ignored or suppressed. These costs are now destroying the Canadian Medicare system.

The cancer service industry affects all of society, whether we have cancer or not. The cost of cancer treatments and health insurance greatly increases the cost of personal taxes and the cost of everything we buy or sell. Small businesses cannot maintain employees due to the high cost of government taxes related to health care, health-care insurance, and the like.

Cannot save medicare by raising taxes

The Canadian Medicare system with universal coverage served the Canadian public well, but is now heavily overburdened with costs. We cannot expect it to survive the waste of people demanding excessive health care, as well as the waste of suppressed cancer treatments and other health care problems. An aging society in a polluted environment will greatly increase the incidence of disease. The bulk of the waste comes from suppressed cures and treatments. The true problem is with upper management.

Emergency health care in Canada is now in critical condition with long waiting lines for operations. Emergency vehicles are routinely shuttled to adjacent hospitals because the rooms and hallways are full. We fear the advent of a two-tier health system allowing the rich faster access to health service than provided to those limited to the public system. The Canadian Medical Association is pushing for billions of more dollars for health care. Billions more dollars for health care can only come from billions more tax dollars. Raising taxes reduces public incentive and reduces the economy, resulting in reduced tax revenues. Raising taxes is not the answer.

Health care expenses destroying government services

Health care is now costing Canadians more than 80 billion dollars per year and over 100 trillion in America. Every year, billions of Canadian tax dollars are paid to foreign based pharmaceutical businesses which supply the drugs for cancer treatment. Payments of tax dollars to the cancer service industry results in exporting tax revenues for health services. Exporting tax revenues creates a void in future tax revenues from local businesses. The true costs of health care goes far beyond the direct costs. The true cost of health care must include loss of tax revenues and employment by local businesses to fund other social programs. There is a limit to how much money a country can afford to export for health care.

The same financial problems apply to all countries where Western medicine is mandatory. That is why more than two-thirds of the world's democracies can no longer provide the level of service they did just a few years ago. Each time a cancer victim is treated at public expense, thousands of tax dollars are exported to tax-haven countries and future tax revenues are lost. The middle class is being bankrupted and destroyed through taxation that pays for the export of tax revenue.

One must realize that democracies are a middle-class institution designed to take power and abuse away from the elite minorities. Democracies are a fragile form of government and none have lasted for more than 500 years. As soon as the middle class is destroyed, democracies fail. Most democracies in the world are now failing due to elimination of the middle class. Taxation of the middle class with export of tax dollars for health services is the primary waste of tax revenue. Suppression of effective low-cost health care results in destruction of our democratic societies.

Billions of dollars are being wasted by our health-care system while more cost-effective ways to treat cancer and other degenerative diseases are being suppressed. The way for Canadians to save Medicare is to demand medical reform and break up the medical cartel that is suppressing competition.

Choices are based on perceptions; perceptions are molded by communication. In the final analysis, saving Medicare will only come about when millions of Canadians realize the Canadian Medical Association and the Health Protection Branch are destroying medicare by their suppression of alternatives. Public perceptions must change. Public opinion and outcry must cause government to introduce legislation that allows competition into the health care system.

At this time, just the opposite is occurring. The pharmaceutical industry is destroying the alternative health industry by instigating the Health Protection Branch to regulate competitive natural-health products and suppliers out of business. Public opinion is being led to believe that we must protect the public from alternative health products that are not adequately regulated and packaged, although there has never been one death reported due to use of natural health products in Canada. Even U.S. suppliers with high quality standards meeting FDA requirements must be inspected by Canadian inspectors at the importer's expense in order to 'protect' the Canadian public.

People often die from food related poisoning but nor from alternative health products. Why not improve regulations on foods first? Safety is not the issue. Competition for health care is the true issue.

Must eliminate suppression to have a cancer cure

Without first eliminating the suppression of effective cures, we will never have a cost-effective cancer cure within medicare. Public donations for cancer research are counter productive. Donations maintain false hope that a cure will soon be found. If you want a cancer cure in your lifetime, switch your donations to those organizations that are fighting to stop suppression of the effective low-cost cancer cures we already have.

The medical monopoly on human pain and suffering as a source of wealth must be broken. If unrestricted competition were allowed, no one would subject his or her body to chemotherapy and radiation knowing safer and better treatments are available. All that is needed is to eliminate parasites and microbes, and heal the injury to stop multiplication of cells. We don't need cannons to kill fungi. If competition were allowed, the economics of a competitive health-care system would reform the industry. If competition were allowed, propaganda would fail. Free competition is the key. Truth would have a chance. The medical dictatorship would be destroyed.

People must realize that a cancer victim is a victim of the medical establishment, as well as the disease. Cancer can be easily diagnosed at an early stage before a tumor forms; cancer can be prevented and cured in a number of cost-effective ways. The problem rests solely on the fact that one organization has a monopoly. There is no competition. There are no incentives to improve. Customer satisfaction is not an issue.

Why does government allow the Canadian Medical Association a monopoly in health care?

Reasons given for the monopoly are based on the need for highly trained medical professionals to prevent "snake oil salesmen" from "exploiting the public." The medical association also requires a monopoly to protect the public from would be product hucksters. But who is there to protect the public from the medical association? What if they are taken over by the pharmaceutical industry? That's the problem.

The pharmaceutical industry has captured the 'snake-oil market' and have become the most successful 'snake-oil salesmen' of all times. By 'funding' universities and hospitals they control education and indoctrinate medical students. The medical mind-set on drugs is controlled by education.

When life-saving treatments for cancer are neglected and suppressed, the fundamental reason for a medical monopoly has been destroyed. There is no longer any significant reason to maintain the monopoly in health care because the monopoly does not protect the public. Effective cures are suppressed in all disease specialties—including cancer, heart and stroke, AIDS, auto-immune, and diabetes. Indeed, the monopoly must be eliminated in order to *protect* the public.

Monopolies do not protect the public. Monopolies exploit the public, especially a monopoly with payments drawn from public tax revenue and public donations.

The existing medical monopoly on health care ensures the public will be exploited because there is no competition. Medical abuses cannot be recognized by comparison to alternatives or condemned in the media.

Aging baby boomers will pay the price

Recent statistics show that one in four people are now over the age of fifty. Ten years from now, if you deduct the unemployed and children, the capacity of the employed to support the youth, retired, and unemployed will not be sufficient to provide essential services. The Hamilton Spectator (April 9, 1999) gives us fair warning:

> **Aging baby boomers can expect cancer to extract a terrible toll on their lives as they head into their senior years. Dr. Barbara Whylie, the Canadian Cancer Society's director of medical affairs, says Health Canada's Cancer Bureau estimates that if current trends continue the number of new cancer cases will increase by 70% by the year 2010.**

The only real choice available to the public is to fight for freedom of choice in health care now! Reducing the cost of health care is the only variable that can be changed to save the baby boomers.

28. Summary and conclusion

The cause of cancer is not a mystery. Human cells have the capacity to function with or without oxygen, so they can switch from oxidative metabolism to fermentation. The life-force that created the body from a single fertilized egg has the capacity to cause DNA to replicate. During normal growth or normal repair of damaged tissue, the life-force causes cells to multiply by producing an ionic field known as the current of injury. This is not really a current but a stationery ionic field over the injury, or growth area. The current of injury initiates replication and stops as soon as a repair is made. Out-of-control growth occurs when the repair is not made because the cell walls are mutated by fungal proteins.

During the process in which new cells are assembled, microbial enzymes mutate the cell-wall membrane with primitive life form cell-wall tissue made of proteins such as chitin. These new cells do not knit to existing normal cells to repair the injury. As a result, the current of injury stays on and replication of cells producing more mutated cell-wall membranes continues out of control. These mutated cells form a cancer tumor if epithelial tissue is involved, or leukemia if leukocytes are involved.

Cancer is cured by proper nutrition, cellular oxidation, elimination of parasites, and cleansing of toxins and pollutants. Cancer cells cannot develop without DNA polymerase enzymes and proteins from microbes. That is why alternative cancer therapies such as vaccines and electromedicine work better than conventional profit-driven drug therapies.

Infectious growths are the chief cause of cancer. The medical establishment is wasting billions of dollars and destroying millions of lives by researching defective genes as the cause of cancer. There are many indications that the cancer establishment knows infections causes cancer.

We (the people) must eliminate the medical monopoly and the capacity to exploit the health care system by suppressing effective cancer cures while deceiving the public into donating millions for research on the defective gene cause of cancer. Political action is needed to make changes.

29. Fight for freedom of choice in health care

THE FOLLOWING EXCERPT WAS WRITTEN IN 1993.

The Need of our Time

As the mass media never lets us forget, the modern health care system has slipped into a deepening crisis. As this book goes to press, Americans are spending more than $800 billion a year on health care, nearly three times what they spend on national defense, more than 14% of the nation's gross national product. Management experts predict that within a decade, health care costs will cancel all corporate profits and bring the capitalist economy to a halt. (*Freedom From Disease* by Dr. Hari Sharma, M.D., Page 17).

Sharma doesn't give his sources for this statement, but it repeats predictions made in books such as *The Great Reckoning* by Davidson and Rees-Moog. What do you think will happen if the capitalist economy fails as predicted by these management experts?

This 1993 reference states medical costs of 800 billion. Recent estimates are now over one trillion dollars in the U.S. alone. That's a 200 billion dollar increase in less than 8 years.

Will there be a middle class to maintain a democracy, or will the elite take over and create some form of world economy totally dominated by those with the most wealth and power? Can we afford to take the chance? Can we stop the abuse of health care services before this happens?

The suppression of cancer cures and effective health care demands political action in order to stop the waste of tax dollars. ALL future generations will pay the price if we do nothing. The aging baby-boomer generation will pay a horrible price if we/they do not act immediately. It is in our hands. What can we do?

There are two main issues at hand.

1. To fight for freedom of choice to incorporate all effective cancer/health treatments, devices and services.

2. To destroy credibility in medical propaganda that distorts the truth and sustains favorable public opinion in the existing medical monopoly.

The goals are complementary. If government allows some effective cancer cures to be recognized and permitted within Medicare, success of these programs would destroy credibility in medical propaganda and conventional treatments.

Even if we opened only one government-sponsored cancer detoxification center in Canada, treated cancer patients for removal of the cause of cancer, and provided for early recognition and prevention, we could publicly challenge conventional therapy. After one successful center is established, more could be started. Millions of dollars could be saved and the economy stimulated by tax reduction to the public.

The issue revolves around motivating Canadian government officials to act and make this happen. Low-cost, effective cancer cures are available now. Public knowledge of them and availability to the public is the problem. The government must demand access to the media and force health-care bureaucrats to act in the public interest.

The same situation exists worldwide. What is said here about the need for public action in Canada can be applied equally to all countries even though specific issues may be different. The plan that I am proposing can also be implemented worldwide.

In 1995, Ross Perot, an American politician with concern for public needs, wrote a book entitled *Intensive Care —We Must Save Medicare and Medicaid Now* In this book he details the skyrocketing costs of American health care and the immense drain on tax revenues. Perot writes (Page 74):

> The Hospital Insurance Trust Fund, Medicare Part A, will be bankrupt within the next ten years. Under current conditions the fund will technically run out of money by the year 2002 or sooner.

In his book, he outlines several reforms to control spending, and reduce waste. Then he writes (Page 178):

> Local assemblies of citizens constitute the strength of nations.
> A nation may establish a system of free government, but without

the spirit of municipal institutions, it cannot have the spirit of liberty.

If people want a true spirit of liberty, they must have freedom of choice in health care. People will have to do so by taking action at the community level. Curing cancer has become primarily a political issue. Form and organization and keep the organization active year round as a business to generate profits and provide important services. Use some of the profits to lobby elected officials and to prevent business lobbyists from excessive control and influence. Fund the organization through business activities and reward those who make it profitable. Retired business executives and directors can come together to form a management team. In Spain, groups of people have formed such publicly owned and operated businesses with great success. Employees are paid. Management is largely volunteer. The big difference is that a public group is the owner and profits are used for public purposes. People with business skills and experience supervise the business; employees run it.

Organizing people on a national scale to write petitions and defend an issue has considerable merit, but the organization does not have any capacity to maintain an ongoing political presence. Organizing people to march on government offices is a quick fix. It is an effective way to polarize public opinion and start reforms.

Quick fixes have their place. The Federal Government of Canada is introducing a new category to take natural health products out of the control of the Drug Directorate. This step is due to recent public outcry, petitions, and legal action against proposed establishment licensing regulations that would have eliminated the natural health products industry in Canada. That's a good first step and we must wait to see how the process unfolds. We cannot let down our guard. As I see the new regulations taking shape, the capacity of the pharmaceutical industry to introduce drugs, containing molecules based on nature, will allow them to bypass the former drug inspection process.

A series of new regulations have been proposed that are closely similar to the ones that were rejected earlier. It seems to me that imposing the same regulations under a different authority will produce the same results. The majority of small natural health product suppliers will be out of business and the cost of natural health products will skyrocket. Health care costs will increase in all areas as alternative health care products become less available or more costly.

The new category does nothing to stop suppression of numerous cancer treatments now available. Nor does it do anything to suppress waste of tax revenues through mismanagement of tax revenues. Here is where the best solution to health care lies and where public action must be taken to force change. The failure of Health Canada to do its job is the main problem. The legal and justice departments provide means to stop the obvious abuse of tax revenue. We have to use other government departments to correct the failure of Health Canada and the Health Protection Branch.

Introduce laws to stop suppression of alternative health care

We need laws to reduce Medicare costs and improve health care. We should hold a health-care provider/healer just as legally responsible for failing to disclose and offer to use alternative treatment methods to a patient as we would if that health-care provider failed to mention the use of perceived worthwhile conventional treatment.

No profit-orientated business should have a business monopoly with customers driven by pain and fear of death from disease. No profit-orientated business should be financed by tax revenue and have a monopoly at the same time. Government should not be in charge of a business monopoly in health care.

People are dying needlessly because information is withheld and available cures are suppressed. Doctors who warn cancer victims to avoid safe alternative therapies, such as oxidative and metabolic therapy, should have their medical licenses removed for breach of public trust. Medical associations that persecute doctors because they use or recommend alternative devices should face court action for defrauding the public of taxes and healthcare. Organizations of professionals who collectively exploit tax revenue should be treated as criminal organizations. The tobacco industry is now considered a criminal organization with a history of harming the public and suppressing knowledge about the dangers of smoking. Smoking is not as harmful to the public as suppressing cancer cures.

Provincial Medical Associations as well as federal government agencies such as the Canadian Cancer Society should be held accountable for fraudulently seeking donations for cancer research and other diseases while suppressing effective treatments and valuable knowledge.

The Canadian Medical Association must stop demanding billions more dollars for health-care services while ignoring billions of savings available by alternative treatments the public would prefer to use if the public new they existed.

Class-action suits for access to cancer cures

Both the U.S. and Canadian governments have fined Swiss drug Giant Hoffmann-LaRoche for their part in an international price-fixing conspiracy of vitamins and food supplements. According to the Hamilton

Spectator, Oct. 26, 1999, Canada's competition commissioner Konrad von Finckenstein is reported as saying: "This conviction sends a clear message that foreign nationals, non-resident in Canada, who engage in illegal activity that affects Canadian consumers, will be held liable for anticompetitive offences." Bravo!

Now let's go after the suppressors of effective cancer cures and effective treatments of other diseases.

In my opinion, more freedom of choice can easily be won by class-action suits based on Canadian Anti-Trust Regulations through the Supreme Court of Canada. We must take the suppressors of alternative health care to court and stop them from illegal activities that affect Canadian consumers in health care. Since suppression of alternative therapies is worldwide in scope, those responsible are probably both Canadian and non-Canadian. If the Federal Government has convicted foreign nationals for price-fixing of food supplements, why not convict them of suppressing cancer cures?

Just as the Red Cross was dumped from distribution of blood products, we must dump Health Canada from suppression of health products and services. The Red Cross destroyed the lives of thousands of Canadians through distribution of tainted blood. Health Canada has destroyed the lives of millions through suppression of cancer cures.

The Province of Ontario is suing the tobacco giants for $40 billion U.S. to pay for smoking-related health care. Several American states have already done so and won. Ontario has obtained legal counsel in the U.S. as part of its plan to be the first Canadian jurisdiction to sue the industry for damages under the American Racketeer Influenced and Corrupt Organization Act. So many other countries sued the tobacco industries before Ontario completed its legal work, we must wait for the outcome of other decisions.

A claim under the Act is based on the law's distinct definition of a criminal conspiracy, defined by the act as *a pattern of wrongdoing which results in injury.*

Could the same American law be used to sue those who are responsible for suppressing ozone therapy in the U.S., as this is a pattern of wrongdoing that results in injury to Canadians? The U.S. government will not likely sue another branch of the U.S. government, but foreign governments could do so. Perhaps concerned Americans could help fund such an action from within Canada. Directors of Health Canada and the pharmaceutical giants should be sued for damages. Their actions demonstrate a pattern of wrongdoing which results in injury.

Class-action suits are actually the most effective and least costly way to influence government decisions in the profit-driven field of health services. Court action has an immediate effect. The individuals who create the problem are publicly identified and they must defend their actions in a public court. They cannot escape into 'the nebulous government'. In the final analysis, decisions are made by individuals and these individuals must be held accountable for their decisions.

Public information about class-action suits makes bad publicity and destroys political careers. Class action suits against individuals in charge of government policy initiates a response. Consider for a moment the Federal Government's decision to compensate Hepatitis C victims due to tainted blood. Only those who were infected between 1986 and 1990 will be compensated.

Why only these victims and not others? Because individuals in the government are vulnerable to a class-action suit from this group. The government is not responsible. Someone is responsible. Perhaps a group of people are responsible. A class-action suit would make them accountable for their actions. By paying out billions of dollars to the victims who could win a class-action suit against those who are responsible, the government protects those who are responsible for wrong-doing. The tax payers compensate those who were injured. The system survives and the wrongdoers continue to function.

Compassion or compensation for damage has nothing to do with political wrongdoing causing death. The compensation package *(payoff)*, protects those who are liable to court action. Not only is it totally unfair to those before and after these dates, the payoff costs Canadian taxpayers millions of tax dollars without correcting the problem.

Without a class-action suit, the 'nebulous government' is responsible, not the individuals who make the final decisions. With a class-action suit, the people who make the final decision for that department become responsible and their careers are placed in jeopardy.

A threatened class-action suit costs taxpayers millions of dollars, if those who have been injured are bought off with tax revenues through a settlement. We, the taxpayers, are the only losers. Class-action suits must be started by taxpayers for waste of tax revenue so that the injured cannot be bought off by additional tax revenue.

Court orders and class-action suits can save taxpayers billions of dollars by reducing waste and government inaction. Ultimately, the Minister of Health is responsible for continued suppressed cancer cures. Politicians must rely on the bureaucrats who run the departments for advice, but in the final analysis, the Minister of Health is responsible for decisions in his or her department to limit access to alternative cancer treatments.

Elected officials tend to react more strongly if court action threatens their political career, People working as a community can become a more powerful force than the most powerful lobbyists, if we organize by political districts and vote strategically. If we form publicly managed businesses to fund the organization, and the organization functions as a lobby group made up of the voting public, we could gain back the concept of democracy. Instead of government of the people, by big business for big business, we could have government of the people, by the people, for the people. Court action for a class-action suit sponsored by public organization from within an electoral district would be meaningful to elected officials in that riding. It would threaten his career, if his actions in government were not consistent with public needs.

Class-action suit to reorganize medicare

A class-action suit should be filed to determine the constitutionality of the system in place for approval and payment of health care products and equipment under Medicare.

If taken to court, the present system would not meet Canadian Anti-Combine Regulations. It should not be legal for a self-interest group such as mainstream medicine to disapprove competitive products simply because they are competitive. Increased use of electromedicine could be saving taxpayers millions of dollars.

A class-action suit should remove the medical profession from the Approved-for-Medicare process regarding what qualifies for Medicare payment. An independent body should approve all health care products. Anyone wishing to have a product approved would present the research data and facts, leaving it up to the independent panel to approve or refuse approval. Many people cannot afford alternative health products because they are not covered under Medicare. If a person chooses to treat a disease with herbs, magnets, or electromagnetic devices, why should he or she be penalized? They have paid their taxes into the system and warrant equal coverage.

When people send in their income tax returns, and can prove that they invested money for health care not approved by Medicare, they should be able to deduct money spent for all alternative health care products and services as a taxable expense.

Immediate action should be taken to establish cancer detoxification clinics and allow people with cancer to treat their cancer with natural therapies, within Medicare. Medicare can save millions of tax dollars, and reduce unnecessary pain, suffering, death and loss of family members. Why not do so?

Cancer cells requires microbial enzymes and proteins to cause cell-wall mutations that fail to knit with existing membranes. Elimination of microbes will stop the cancer process. Why not adopt this simple cancer cure immediately? Why not have Medicare pay for the treatment? Why not direct research funds to improving treatment by eliminating fungi and parasites by electromagnetic impulses?

Donate to class-action lawsuits, not cancer research

If all Canadians directed the money they now donate to research of cancer and other diseases towards legal action instead, we could do without government funding for court action. Those who oppose implementing alternative health care treatments should be made to defend their action in public. If opponents to alternative health care had to justify their actions to an independent court body, they would back down and laws would be changed.

The trial and persecution of Gaston Naessens and Dr. Joseph Krop demonstrate medical suppression of two doctors, neither of whom had anyone register complaints against them. At the same time, many doctors with a track record of public complaints are protected by the medical association. The medical association uses the courts against dedicated medical doctors and alternative specialists. Why don't the people, with the government, use the courts against the medical association in return?

Effective cancer cures are available now. All we need is the freedom to use them and acceptance by Medicare to cover the costs.

The Supreme Court of Canada, if faced with a court action, would have to review the evidence, and public awareness would help reduce the awesome power of medical propaganda.

Form political action groups by electoral districts

Being elected and reelected means everything to a politician.

The Canadian government makes it easy to organize people according to electoral districts and smaller groups according to polling divisions. Just telephone 1-800-267-7360 at Elections Canada and ask for a *Polling Division Map* of your electoral district. For four dollars, you will receive a nine-square-foot blueprint map of your electoral district with all polling districts indicated.

With this map you can organize your electoral district according to polling stations, and organize voters so that voters in your district take a common course of action and vote strategically to ensure freedom of choice in health care. Start by making a directory of existing alternative health services in your riding and working with them. Build a community within your electoral district that focuses on health reform and the quality of life

When the government appoints a person to run in a riding, and supports his election, that person will be more obligated to the party than to the people. That's not democracy. That form of government is called an oligarchy, and was common in ancient Greece. It is more or less a modified form of a dictatorship. In a true democracy, the people must select who runs for office. Public apathy destroys the capacity of democracies to function.

By taking the initiative to work politically in your riding, your success is not dependent upon the success or failure of a central location. It is far more difficult to suppress a grass-roots movement than a centralized movement. You can obtain information and electoral maps concerning all electoral districts in Canada on the Internet at *www.elections.ca*. For a list and phone number of all elected members of parliament, contact the Public Information Office, Library of Parliament, Ottawa, On. Canada. See SOURCES index for details.

For another source of information on the Internet for federal ridings go to http://libertarian.ca/english/enride.htm. This 20-page list gives you electoral districts by province, current M.P., political affiliation, phone, fax and email address.

Phone your elected Member of Parliament or Congress, meet with him or her, and voice your opposition to suppressed cancer cures and waste of tax revenue. Ask your representative to do something and demand a reply. Make him or her become involved too. That's their job.

Help put an end to the monopoly and abuse of tax revenues by mainstream medicine. If you have experienced improved health through alternative methods, paid for from your personal income, demand that money you paid out for treating your condition be considered equivalent to taxes, and applied as a credit against your personal income tax. Take this information to your Member of Parliament and ask him to bring it up in the legislature. Try to establish how much money you saved medicare by avoiding medical costs.

When you fill in your annual tax return, send copies of your receipts. Request the examiner to accept your health care expenses as tax credits. Why not? You have saved the health care system money. Draw attention to this vital issue but do not do anything illegal.

I hope this research on the true cause of cancer and suppressed cures will cause you to take political action to help bring about change in the politics of medicine. The two go hand in hand. The information on effective cancer cures would be far more valuable to you if mainstream medical doctors were free to use these methods and Medicare covered the cost.

The problem of suppressed cancer cures and waste of tax revenues will not go away without a struggle. I would like to quote Barry L. Lynes one more time. This reference is taken from the Sarasota ECO report and the information is pertinent to all nations today.

In the 1950s and 1960s, a terrible example of tyranny of medical interests conspiring with high-ranking U.S. government health officials and bureaucrats was played out. Despite substantial public outrage, the "cancer establishment" stuffed their bad science and their insider agenda down the American people's throats. Over a period of time, the facts of the health officials' outrageous contempt for the public interests and a significant grass roots people's movement was lost or forgotten. However the pattern of ignoring the people's legitimate rights, abusing the public health responsibility, and suppressing viable alternative cancer therapies was to be used again and again in the decades which followed. The clear pattern of bureaucratic tyranny is still being used today.

Therefore the "history lesson" described here is one about which today's health activist fighting the same good-old-boy cancer establishment monster and its institutionalized evil should know. Why? Because being naïve to the well-developed and sophisticated tricks employed by the American Medical Association, the Food and Drug Administration, and the American Cancer Society can result, as it has for decades, in tortuous procedures usually followed by death for millions of innocent people who have developed cancer. This tragedy and on-going crime scream for mass public recognition, hard nosed media reporting, and then decisive political and legal action to end it once and for all.

If we were to replace the word American with Canadian in the above quotation, the statements would be equally as true. We are all victims of a worldwide crime syndicate.

U.S. Attorney-General Janet Reno recently indicted Hoffmann-LaRoche Ltd. and BASF AG, two pharmaceutical giants, for worldwide price fixing of vitamins. Assistant Attorney-General Joel Klein is reported to have said: *"The criminal conduct of these companies hurt the pocketbook of virtually every American consumer."*

The U.S. government action shows it is possible to take action through the courts. An international organization of people and governments is needed to attack the Head Office of Cancer Cure Suppression wherever it is located.

Organizing people to fight for reduced tax abuse

The following plan of action is proposed as a starting point for new visions towards healthcare.

The Internet can bring people with a common purpose together. I have therefore started a web site called *New Vision Inc.org.* This web site will provide you with an opportunity to work with others in your area as well as to connect easily with other groups. New Visions Inc. creates a common web-sight address with territories according to electoral districts. The web sight serves as a communication center.

New Visions stands for setting new goals for society and government to protect the interests of the public and environment before that of business.

Incorporated stands for business. Businesses make profit, and profits are needed to fight for a stronger presence in daily politics. Each electoral district will establish a business office with a team of directors to manage community owned businesses for profit. Businesses will include any product or service the district wishes to provide for the customers in their area or distribute on the Internet to other districts. Alternative health care products would be only one type of product.

Organization reflects that this is an organization of businesses and non-profit groups combining public efforts for social changes.

Our home page is designated as newvsionsinc.org/ho for New Vision Incorporated Head Office. An electoral district in Canada or the U.S. can be identified as nvixxxx. The last four digits being used to identify your electoral district. In this way, all regions are organized according to existing electoral districts within one organization.

The home page *(under construction)* contains a list of all 301 Canadian Federal Ridings and 504 Senate Districts in the U.S. You can also connect to home pages of other organizations seeking political, economic, or environmental reform. Businesses and organizations may place a web page within the designated nvixxxx code for their immediate area so that people can locate suppliers for products and services. You can promote your business locally or internationally. The organization will operate on business profits, not donations or fund-raising. As a member of New Visions Inc. you will have an opportunity to increase your business and fight for greater freedom of choice in health care.

Every electoral district will function as a business/political association, with activities focused on making profits by providing products and services to the people of that district. The four proposed business activities are as follows:

Business: refers to being legally incorporated as a business. The goal is to make profits to finance political action and provide products and services not readily available in your district. The overall focus will be to build a network of alternative health services and suppliers to import, manufacture or grow natural health products, and support existing businesses and professionals in the alternative health field. Funding for non-violent protests and organized boycotts are also a possibility.

Politics: To take an active part in local politics by nominating representatives for political parties, electing the most suitable candidate and maintaining influence with those elected. To help influence federal government decisions regarding health care and environmental pollution with lobby groups and court action where suitable. People elect a politician once about every four years to represent the district. Lobbyists influence him or her continually. The new business will register government lobbyists to compete with other businesses and association lobbyists.

Community: To supply the people in your area with alternative health clinics, to educate consumers regarding health matters, and create public confidence in alternative services. This would include collecting data to identify and screen out unethical practitioners and product providers. Establishing a strong communication links with E-mail and E-commerce, newsletters, newspaper, radio and T.V. would also be important work of this function.

Business Management: To successfully operate your NVIO district, maximize use of available human resources, and provide a means to communicate and organize voters for a strong common front leading to greater freedom of choice in health care and better health services, reduced taxes, and less waste of tax revenue.

Your goal is to organize a sufficient number of voters in your riding to convince your Member of Parliament (or Congress) that his or her political career rides on meeting the needs of people rather than meeting the goals of big business, lobby groups, and personal interest groups. If you can organize a sufficient number of voters to swing, or possibly swing and election, you will be heard.

Our goal is to give people more say in government as well as save taxes and improve health care. Our method is to counter the lobby process, break the medical monopoly in health care and stop exploitation of public funds through continuous abuse of health care.

It is time to take action NOW

Take a moment and think of the benefits or losses if you take action verses the benefits or losses if you do nothing.

Past generations did not have the Internet to organize the public for political reform. We do at this time. Past generations did not know the cause of cancer. We do. This is a unique opportunity that we cannot afford to miss.

We suffer now from the failure of past generations to impose freedom of choice in health care into the constitution. This failure is now leading to the destruction of the democratic society they fought and died for.

As a university student, I learned that democracies are a middle-class institution designed to protect the interests of the majority from the wealthy minority. Old wealth was based on land and taxation of those dependent on the landlords. New wealth from industry and trade created a large middle class. These groups created our first democracies. A wealthy middle class sustains a democracy. No middle class; no democracy.

The present business environment is creating a new class of super wealthy multinational business owners who evade taxes by off shore tax havens and by lobbying government officials for incentives. The existing middle class is being taxed into poverty levels. The existing route to new wealth is to exploit public taxes for health care services and provide massive international trade taking advantage of low-cost production in third world countries.

No democracy has lasted more than 500 years because public apathy and political corruption resulted in a return to a dictator type of government with power in control of the few. Once a dictator becomes established, it is very difficult to regain lost freedoms. The majority of those who supported the dictator suffer the same fate as those who resisted him. They all lose freedom, and suffer a reduced standard of living.

The medical monopoly, more than any other single institution, is wasting, exploiting, and destroying middle class profits. Allow me to repeat Dr. Hari Sharma, who said in 1993: "Management experts predict that within a decade, health care costs will cancel all corporate profits and bring the capitalistic economy to a halt." This decade ends in the year 2003.

The most recent calculation according to newspaper reports, place the U.S. cost for cancer therapy at 110 billion dollars annually. More than $2 billion per week in one country for treating one infectious disease. When the capitalistic economies fail, what type of society and social order will we have? Who will be in control of our health care? What freedoms will we have?

David Suzuki and Holly Dressel have published an inspiring book called *From Naked Ape to Superspecies.* In this book, the authors bring attention to the problems of modern day society and place the blame directly on the movement toward a global economy. The problem is not freedom of speech, the problem is freedom of access to the mass media. Perceptions are controlled by mass media, and perceptions are reality, even if they are not the truth.

I believe people must become involved in a class action suit to gain access to the mass media. Businesses, such as *Adbusters,* who specialize in spoofing false advertising, find they cannot buy time to advertise. In *From Naked Ape to Superspecies* (Page 2680, we read:

> The right to communicate is one step beyond freedom of speech. "Freedom of speech simply means that you're allowed to stand up in a park on a box and say what you want to people who are passing by." Lasn explains. "But freedom of speech doesn't give you access. The really important battle of our Information Age is the battle for access. And if we can win this battle and win the right to communicate legally, then I think we have a level playing field between citizens and corporations. We would be able to talk back to the corporate image factory. We would be in a position to create alternative futures and to pursue alternative visions, and eventually create the sort of world that we need rather than the sort of the world that the corporations are trying to railroad us into at the moment."

The capacity for a small group of people to control and distort the flow of information over a wide range of media is something to be feared. On the other hand, it could also be turned to an advantage to promote the truth if people were organized and became the major influence in the media.

30: A new vision for the 3rd millenium

Like most other people, I would rather spend time with my family, go to the lab and do research in my field of genetics, or pursue my hobbies. But I have children and grandchildren. I have a profound stake in the future. I'm only one person, and I have no illusions or conceits about saving the world. But I hope my grandchildren will never look at me and tell me, "Grandpa, you could have done more for us." If we adults fail to put the environment on the front burner, our children and their children will not have any hope of experiencing the abundance and diversity of life's creatures that existed when we were still young. I have read the statistics on contaminated water, asthma and cancer rates, allergies and immune problems, climate change and the loss of top soil. I realize that the very things that give our children health, and even life, are in jeopardy.

Author David Suzuki and Holly Dressel wrote the above statement in the introduction to their 1999 book, *From Naked Ape to Superspecies* (Page 3).

I find it applies equally well to my situation, except my hobbies and specialties are in the field of inventions. There is a close relationship between our polluted environment and rising health costs. Something must be done now for the sake of future generations.

Do you share these thoughts concerning future generations? If past generations had resisted the medical monopoly, and enshrined freedom of health care in the American Constitution or Canadian Charter of Rights, we would not have these medical problems today.

David Suzuki and Holly Dressel also wrote: "we would be in a position to create alternative futures and pursue alternative visions" if we had equal access to the media. I say lets pursue alternative visions to gain equal access to the media. It is the most critical step towards renewal.

I think it is safe to assume that most of humankind is now interested in a new vision for the sake of future generations.

We have a right to stop destruction of the earth's ecosystem.

We have a right to be interested in the future, because we must spend the rest of our lives there.

We have a right to freedom of choice in health care, because it is our health and our lives.

We have a right to criticize government mismanagement and waste of tax revenues because it is our money they are wasting.

We have the right to communicate and associate with others.

We have the right to take a diseased child out of the country for alternative health care. He or she is our child. The state does not own our children nor does the medical monopoly in health care own the sole right to administer health care.

We have the right to refuse toxic drug therapy such as AZT, if we do not believe in its safety. Doctors do not have the right to force toxic drugs into our children.

One by one, our fundamental rights are being taken from us.

As an association of free people in a free society, we have the right to access public communication channels that form public opinion and perceptions. We have the right to a level playing field to counter the corporate image factory. We have the right to counter false information and commercial propaganda that destroys our rights and our future.

In closing this section of the book, I would like to reflect with you upon the current situation and look into the future. What's in store if the present economic, political and medical systems continue to destroy our planet and limit our freedoms?

The concept that cancer is now predicted to kill one in three people, if they do not die of other diseases, is horrendous. Global warming with changes in weather patterns are destroying crop production and creating global eco-crises. Massive storms and droughts are common occurrences. How can we be optimistic in the future, as we watch the quality of life diminishing all around us?

If nothing is done to change our political-economic-medical complex (the system), the quality of life for the majority of the population will continue to spiral downward. The simplistic statement that says, "If we keep going the way we are going, we are going to get to where we're going", sums it up rather well. Where exactly are we going? Whose vision are we following?

The system is failing us. There are both good and bad people in every occupation, and this includes people in politics, business and medicine. How can new ethical leaders be encouraged to act to improve the system? How did we get into this situation? Commercial control of the mass media is one of the steps because it creates false perceptions. What are the others?

The most powerful force operates at the personal level. The system destroys the non-conforming individual.

There are formidable obstacles in the path of those in power who would strive to stop existing practices that benefit only those in power. These include loss of one's position and financial income, possible loss of camaraderie and respectability, loss of funding for business functions, and loss of credibility with associates and the public. Loss of life is another possibility not to be taken lightly.

Fighting for change is a difficult path only for the most courageous individuals who are driven by an inner quest to improve the human condition for others. These potential leaders will emerge only if there is an opportunity to succeed and survive. They have watched others destroyed by the system, with nothing to show for it. Right now, they are doing the best they can with what they have available. They are waiting for an opportunity to emerge.

They need the backing of a strong grass-roots organization to protect them and support them against an established bureaucracy. In my opinion, the only way for a meaningful change in the political-economic-medical system is for ordinary people to become involved in a competitive political-economic-medical system. Once the competitive grass-roots organization is established, ethical leaders in the field of politics, business and medicine will emerge and contribute towards a new vision. Those who are destroying the environment, suppressing cancer cures, exploiting tax revenues, creating false perceptions, and so on, can be booted out.

Why not create a competitive communications network on the Internet and other media to polarize public opinion? Why not create a competitive publicly owned and operated political-economic-medical system to fight for freedom. The people we elect are no longer in control of our economy and health care system. If they were, we wouldn't have these problems.

Motivating oneself to try accomplishing something new and potentially embarrassing requires belief in a cause, and belief that one will succeed or at least have a chance of succeeding. Four major factors come to mind.

1. Is it a worthwhile goal? Is it something I will enjoy doing? Enjoying the process is vital for staying with the job.

2. What are the rewards? A) in the process; B) in the outcome.

3. What is the cost in time, effort, and loss of other opportunities?

4. What may be lost if I don't bother to try?

If you show apathy for this vital need, others will also be apathetic as well. There is no middle ground. You cannot leave it to others.

Opening the door to your comfort zone will let people into your life. The process will enrich your life in many ways.

By overcoming your fears and liberating yourself, your actions and presence will liberate others. You will send a message to others that says it is okay to become involved and it is the right thing to do.

Instead of spending your days doing things that are important and urgent, you must also make time to do things that are significant for the future. You must help maintain an infrastructure for your freedoms. Doing significant things gives meaning and purpose to your life, because it applies to all people and all times. Getting involved in your community is urgent and important. Developing and building a new vision is significant.

What I am proposing is not another non-profit service club. It is a for-profit service club. It is a network of publicly run businesses that provide essential services, earn profits, and reduce the cost of living. For people with business skills, these are sideline businesses or retirement activities. Businesses are run by paid employees, but managed by volunteers from the for-profit service club. Profits are slated for public action rather than absorbed by individual owners and managers.

This is not a new idea that has never been tested. Rather, it is an old and proven idea. The Chinese army runs over 10,000 businesses making profits for defense expenditures. Labor organizations own apartment towers, commercial blocks, and restaurants. We need public businesses earning profits to build a new vision because businesses are the only source for these funds due to regulations confining activities of non-profit organizations.

In North America, any organization that is organized and run as a business to make a profit has tremendous advantages over non-profit organizations. Non-profit organizations are controlled by regulations and limited by volunteers and fund raising. Business organizations, on the other hand can earn huge profits, expense business meetings and travel costs, and expense seminars and trade shows. Profits can be used for any purpose, including political donations or lobbying of government officials. Doing business is always respectable, if the goals and methods are worthwhile. That's why I believe people should organize businesses to raise funds for financing community action.

Starting and building a successful business is made possible if the directors subscribe to the 4 Way Test developed by Herbert J. Taylor. This is not really a test. It's a way of life and a way of doing business. All decisions and actions must demonstrate four attributes. These are:

1. Is it the truth?

2. Is it fair for all concerned?

3. Will it build goodwill and better friendships?

4. Will it be beneficial to all concerned?

When management of a business follows these principles, businesses attract talented people to provide human resources, attract funding when necessary, and establish customer loyalty. With these three essentials, running a business successfully becomes a matter of applying normal business practices. Rotary International and Rotarians follow these principles, and Rotary International is the most successful associations of people in the world. Rotarians are a non-profit organization limited to fund raising activities, but they still raise billions of dollars for public use.

Businesses earn money, and money is required to accomplish goals. New Visions Incorporated is a concept that puts it all together. It is a meeting place for ideas and human resources with a common goal of survival and enhanced quality of life. It is an opportunity to create and follow a new vision for society. Whether we like it or not, business is the engine that drives society, and business profit is the fuel. In order to have a new vision, the middle class must retain control of the fuel. Taxes and tax abuse destroy the function of the middle class in society.

Group motivation is a very powerful force. Successful businesses are organizations based on great promise, self-realization and group motivation. The rewards are shared by all, and the process is made enjoyable by teamwork. Working with others to achieve worthwhile goals is the key to enjoyment and success. By forming business orientated associations, profits can be used to reward those who devote time and energy to achievement of worthwhile goals. Additional profits can be used to achieve public goals so that everyone benefits.

New discoveries are occurring at a rapid pace and more and more opportunities exist to develop and market new products, reach new markets, and increase profits. Increased world trade has placed too much opportunity for the concentration of wealth in the hands of fewer and fewer people. Most of these businesses operate from off-shore tax haven countries and do not pay taxes. That's why our economies and democracies are failing.

One way to stop the further concentration of wealth is for public grass-roots corporations to go into competition with the private corporations. A second way is for an organized electorate to stop the exploitation of tax revenues through government policies that reward foreign controlled international traders and monopolies. A third way would be to produce and market new products, at the community level, local regions, and internationally, through E-commerce.

The field of electronics and energy production, for example, present great potential for business profits.

Richard Gerber, M.D., author of *Vibrational Medicine, New Choices for Healing Ourselves,* writes (Page 364):

> Crystals hold the key to unlocking a vast new technology based upon the manipulation of etheric (ether or energy in space) energies for healing as well as other applications. Because the special geometric patterning, crystals are able to tap into universal energy patterns and frequencies that science is only beginning to discover. What scientists have not yet realized is that the ordered pattern of crystals, and their relationship to etheric fields, is similar to the ordered molecular structure of permanent magnets and their associated magnetic fields. Crystals, because of their inherent etheric fields, are a source of what Dr. Tiller would refer to as magnetoelectricity.

According to the *Encyclopedia of Space,* by the Hamlen Publishing Group, we learn that the satellite Explorer 12 was put into a very eccentric orbit to measure the earth's radiation zones. It discovered fields composed essentially of electrons evaluated at hundreds of thousands of electron-volts. The cause of these high energies is based on movement of the earth. We read (Page 544):

> .... Artificial satellites have shown that in the environs of our planet, up to a distance of seven terrestrial radii, there is not only a magnetic but also an electric field. The latter is produced by the

movement of the ionosphere in the earth's magnetic field. The process is similar to an electric generator.

The earth is a giant electric generator. Magnetic and ionic fields are a result. The northern lights illustrate the existence of an ionic field. The planet earth includes an electromagnetic field with an atmosphere filled with energy due to the spinning of the earth through the ether or plasma energy of space. The energy starts below the surface and extends into space. At the surface it is evident in the Brownian movement of colloids in water. In the atmosphere, lighting illustrates the electrical potential available from water molecules in motion. Richard Gerber suggests that liquid crystals can be used to harness etheric energy as a source of free energy and produce new inventions in the medical field. I believe he is right.

Scientists should be able to invent motors by spinning crystals through an ionic field and producing electricity, in much the same way spinning a coil of wires through a magnetic field produces electricity.

Medicine in the new millenium can be the study and use of minerals, crystalloids, and etheric or ionic energy to bring about a new age in health. This will not come from a drug-orientated medical monopoly nor from governments already strapped for operating funds.

The door is open for publicly organized businesses to research and produce these products, and distribute them without being limited by the existing political-economic system. The profits can be used to integrate with the system, compete with the system, and to reinvent the system so that new visions can be established to serve people rather than industry.

All elementary particles are created by motion and all elementary particles can be harnessed for energy because they are produced in limitless amounts through motion. Just as the clouds never run out of energy for lightning, humankind need never run out of energy for human needs.

Paramagnetism and crystal forms provide scope for harnessing free energy similar to the energy of lightning. New discoveries could open the door to a vast new world with non-polluting free energy and unlimited power to serve humankind. There are probably several methods to harness this free energy. The first issue is to believe it is possible and invest time and money to do so. People discuss these ideas at free-energy conventions and describe various ways how free energy devices may be built. Numerous books about 'zero-point' energy are available. Zero point refers to the energy level of space. At these conventions, I have observed demonstrations and seen artifacts that prove vast amounts of energy are available. See SOURCES for information on the *"Planetary Association for Clean Energy"* .

One of the more interesting concepts discussed at free energy conventions is that all energy particles have only one thing in common. They spin. They may spin clockwise (positive energy) or counterclockwise, (negative energy), but they spin. As soon as this spin energy is absorbed, the particle disappears. Energy or gas molecules that spin are called a vortex.

Someone blowing smoke rings in the air demonstrates the power of a vortex, as does a tornado. A vortex concentrates energy or molecules of gas beyond the level of adjacent energy or molecules. Rapid motion increases density. Energy is released when the vortex is disturbed.

If we imagine energy particles to be a vortex of the ionic or magnetic field in space, we can explain the nature of energy. A vortex exists as a concentration of ionic or magnetic energy, due to a disturbance from matter as the ionic or magnetic field flows around the particle of matter.

Let's use water as an example. Slowly push a spoon through a bowl of water and watch the two vortexes form roll away from each edge of the spoon. Notice that one spins clockwise, the other spins counterclockwise. As the vortexes collides with the container wall, energy is absorbed into the container wall. The same type of thing happens with a vortex of gas, or a vortex of energy.

The whole concept of energy and energy particles can be simplified if we imagine electrons to be a vortex of magnetic energy in a magnetic field or a vortex of ionic energy in an ionic field. The mysterious northern lights are vortexes of ionic energy vibrating at the frequency of light. The galaxy and sun provide the ionic and magnetic fields, and the spin of the earth provides the disturbance. One ionic field is disturbing the other.

Electrons are vortexes of magnetic energy. The nucleus of the hydrogen atom—the smallest nucleus known, creates one vortex. This is the minimum amount of disturbance to create a permanent vortex. The larger nucleus of helium creates two vortexes, and so on. The larger the nucleus, the more electrons it produces and appears to hold in its outer shells. The quantum theory falls into place as the minimum energy required to disrupt the existing energy fields or change an established electromagnetic bond.

There is no limit to free energy as long as the earth spins and rotates about the sun. Living things illustrate that this energy is free for the taking. Antennas on insects appear to function as energy collectors.

The great American inventor Nickola Tesla built a motor that appears to have converted ionic energy into functional electron energy. The motor consisted of a series of plate-sized disks, separated by the thickness of a washer. Steam was blown between the disks and energy was drawn off from the steam by these rapidly spinning the disks. The steam did not drive the disks like a turbine. The disks harvested energy from the steam.

Tesla built his car at the Great Arrow plant in Buffalo N.Y., and test-drove it during the late 1930's. Reports say that the box-like motor that generated electrical energy had two antennas. When these were extended, the motor produced more horsepower. The motor, or one like it, was described in Scientific American with great enthusiasm. The pollution-free motor could power a car across the continent on a single tank of fuel. Fuel was only used to start the rotor spinning and make steam. Once it was running, electrical energy was used to reheat the steam and spin the rotor. This invention could have revolutionized the world, but appears to have been suppressed for political and economic interests. It could still save our ecosystem and reduce pollution levels from combustion of fossil fuels.

Someone out there must still have the capacity to produce it now. The fact that it has not been introduced back into the marketplace can only mean that other devices such as this will be suppressed.

How did it work? The invention was suppressed so we really don't know. I theorize that it could be based on the paramagnetic quality of water. Remember, a paramagnetic substance takes on a magnetic charge in the presence of a magnet, but loses the charge as soon as the magnet is removed. By flowing steam through a magnetic field and the disks, the magnetic or ionic energy could be collected. Water is an inexpensive paramagnetic substance but other oxides could also serve this function.

If steam were passed through a powerful stationery magnetic field, the water molecules would take on a corresponding paramagnetic charge. By injecting paramagnetic steam between spinning disks, the paramagnetic charge would be transferred to the disks and drawn off as electrons. By forming the disks from one of the electron-accepting elements, such as sulfur, carbon, or phosphorus, and collecting them at one point in the disk's revolution, electrons could be drawn off in unlimited quantities. Just think of disk brakes on a car, or front wheel brakes on a bicycle. The brake-pad like device would draw off free energy to be delivered by wire for functional purposes. The energy would be very similar to that of lightning bolts that flow from clouds on a hot summer day, but seldom if ever from clouds in cold weather. Heating water molecules greatly increases their capacity to generate electric energy, probably because the ionic hydrogen bond is more easily broken.

This concept is no different than generating electricity from magnetic fields, except that it would be far more efficient because the magnetic drag would be absent. The ions are generated by the spin of the earth through the sun's gravitational field, and the ions are harvested without the need for thermal or nuclear energy to drive the generators. Pollution free energy would be the result. I know it sound far out and unattainable, but so have many other inventions that are now commonplace.

If one wishes to invent and prosper from a mechanical means to convert ionic energy to electrons, one must do so without trying to maintain patent ownership and exclusivity. Exclusive information and knowledge is easy to suppress. Information given to the public without controls in place cannot be suppressed. Society will not be ready for free energy devices until a new political-economic structure is in place. Alternately, inventions such as these, freely given to the public, could create a new vision for society and a new political-economic structure.

Society needs grass-roots public organizations that place the ecology and public good ahead of huge private wealth and power. The public must first organize and become a force in the economic-political system so that such devices can be produced and marketed. The public must lobby the government more effectively than business lobbyists are doing now. Inventors cannot produce these devices now because they cannot be marketed.

Why not help reinvent the Tesla motor or such a device and publish production details so that it cannot be suppressed? Every electoral district could have a free-energy machine factory, producing parts or machines and selling these pollution-free motors to the public as a business. Competition would generate rapid advancements and private businesses could also build them. These publicly owned businesses could compete with private interests because the majority of the consumers would recognize it is to their advantage to support the public sources.

The energy is all around us. All we have to do is harness it and do so in such a way that it cannot be metered, taxed, controlled or limited. By freely giving production methods to the public, and allowing energy-producing devices to be made in every major community, humankind's dependence on fossil fuels for energy could be eliminated. The continual concentration of wealth in the hands of the few fossil-fuel energy dealers would be reduced, and the world would become a better place for all. Even if these ideas seem too far-fetched to be practical today, there are hundreds of more practical ideas waiting to be developed. Why not develop new products through community owned businesses using the human and economic resources available in your community?

454 Section Three: Misinformation, suppression, and cover-up

If we start with a new vision, and start going in a new direction, and keep going in that new direction, we will end up in a new place. In order to reinvent society, it will take an organized public with goals, determination, wealth, and political influence. By becoming active in this endeavor, you can protect what you have, reduce taxes, improve health care, and so on.

If you are hesitant to become involved in a new endeavor, because you feel somehow inadequate for the job, you might consider reading the book, *How to Re-invent Yourself,* authored by Marcellus B. Andersen. Andersen, who lives in Toronto, conducts seminars and book publicity meetings throughout North America, instructing people on four main topics. These are:

1. how to renew your personal belief support system;

2. how to establish new relationships and better interactions;

3. how to start a new career and attain your goals; and

4. how to develop a clear purpose to life that inspires you every day.

Please see SOURCES for details.

There is a window of opportunity that is open now due to the Internet and scientific discoveries. There is an opportunity for the average person to secure a more abundant life through political-economic activities. The abundance can come from new developments in science and electromedicine, not simply by taking away from someone else, polluting the ecosystem, or mining the earth's resources. Imagine pollution-free motors running on limitless free energy. Imagine greenhouses growing healthy mineralized organic food with free-energy to help reduce costs. Imagine growing your own food in a private backyard greenhouse or in community owned businesses. Imagine free-energy heating and air-conditioning. Imagine free-energy transportation. Imagine desalinating the ocean for fresh water. The window of opportunity to reinvent society is in technology, the Internet, and existing public awareness that there is an urgency to do so.

By re-inventing ourselves as communities, we can reinvent the system. Instead of seeing ourselves as individuals, we should see ourselves as members of a team or network. As individuals, we can accomplish more by building an organization than by attacking the system. Organized into business communities, creating and using business profits for public, political, and economic goals, we can develop and follow a new vision. Having specific goals help. It all starts with a desire or a dream.

In 1995, I made the following statements as my introductory remark in a speech before several hundred people who had come to hear Dr. Hulda Regehr Clark speak in Toronto.

"Do you remember Dr. Martin Luther King saying: 'I have a dream. I have a dream. I dream of the day when the Black man in America will be free from racial prejudice and segregation'"?

Well, I have a dream too. I dream of the day when all men, women, and children in America, will be free from medical prejudices and medical suppression of alternative health care".

To my surprise, I received an immediate standing ovation. People want change. We will no longer be the subjects of prejudice and suppression. As you know, King organized and rallied his people and through non-violent protests, they realized their dream. America became a better place for everyone. We can do that.

I hope that you will make freedom from medical prejudice your dream too. If you have an opportunity to speak publicly about freedom of choice in health care, consider saying that you have this dream. Dreams of a new vision for society can come true, if we (the people) believe in them, and commit to do whatever it takes to realize the dream.

In order to maintain a dialogue with you, and for you to connect with others, I have started a web sight called www.newvisionsinc.org. This is an organizational web sight so that any person or group can connect with other people or groups and network to raise funds for political action. If you are a member of a service club or other non-profit organization, consider organizing some of your members into a business for the purpose of earning profits to support your goals.

I wish you the *best of health.*

GLOSSARY

Definitions have been adapted from various sources with comments added to explain relationship to the cancer process based on the microbial infection and current of injury theory as the cause of cancer.

Acetylcholine: chemical that serves as a neurotransmitter, communicating nerve impulses between the cells of the nervous system. Not involved in replication of DNA.

Ammonia: is a common gas with the chemical formula NH3 or one nitrogen atom with a valance of three chemically bonded to three hydrogen atoms. Ammonia dissolves readily in water to form ammonium (NH4). Ammonia destroys enzymes required for metabolism and destroys function of nerves leading to degenerative nerve diseases.

Anabolic process: Complex substances such as amino acids, digestive enzymes and immune system defenses are assembled from simpler components, with the consumption of energy. Both enzymes and energy are required in this process. Adequate cellular energy is the key to a strong immune system, digestive system, and good health. Cells that function on fermentation, instead of oxidation, lack energy to assembly normal cell-wall material.

Autonomic nervous system: part of the nervous system that controls involuntary functions, including the heart rate and activity of the intestines. This system controls repair of injury and initiates replication of DNA.

Bacteria: The overall chemical composition of the bacterial cell is very similar to that of all other types of cells of animal, plant, and microbial origin, which are capable of growth and replication. Bacteria thus possess the protein ribonucleic acid (RNA) and deoxyribonucleic acid (DNA), which are the major classes of chemical constituents for replication. Bacterial enzymes can control human cell function and modify replication cycles.

Blood clotting: production of semisolid mass of protein fibers and blood cells that prevents excessive bleeding after injury. Internal blood clots in ducts and storage vessels initiate cancer.

Bone marrow: soft tissue in the center of some large bones that manufactures red and white blood cells. Infection of bone marrow leads to production of mutated defensive cells and leukemia.

Cancer (1): is a disease (*according to defective gene theory*) that attacks the basic life process of the cell, in almost all instances altering the cell's genome (the total genetic complement of the cell) and leading to wild and spreading growth of the cancerous cells. The cause of the altered genome is a mutation (alteration) of one or more genes; or mutation of a large segment of a DNA strand containing many genes; or, in some instances, addition or loss of large segments of chromosomes. The probability of mutations can be increased many fold when a person is exposed to certain chemical, physical, or biological factors known as carcinogens. (*Note: The theory has never been proven.*)

Cancer (2): is a disease that occurs (*according to the current of injury theory*) when the normal process of repair to injury or natural growth causes DNA to replicate and new cells to form by division. During the process of division and assembly of the new cell-wall membranes, human cells that are infected with fungi or bacteria form a new cell-wall membrane that is mutated and subsequently rejected by adjacent normal cells. The repair process is not satisfied and the replication of cells continues, causing cancer.

Cancer Cells: Cancer cells survive due to the capacity of the cell to maintain fermentation of glucose for energy. Human cells can produce enzymes to switch naturally between oxidation and fermentation. Defective DNA is not involved in any of the cancer processes. Curing cancer includes destroying existing cancer cells as well as microbial infections.

Catabolism: a complex substance is broken down into simpler ones, usually with a release of energy. Enzymes are required to break down the molecules and eliminate the wastes. All chemical actions inside living things are catalyzed by enzymes. Viruses in cells are destroyed by catabolism if energy is abundant. Immune system deficiency is a catabolism deficiency.

Chitin: carbohydrate polymer of the simple sugar glucose. It is found in the cell walls of plants, and green algae as well as insects and fungi. The compound makes cockroaches 'crunchy'. Excess glucose in diets contributes to cell-wall chitin production of cancer cells. Processed grains are mainly glucose and should be avoided by cancer patients.

Connective tissue: tissue made up of noncellular substances, the extracellular matrix, in which some cells are embedded. Skin, bones, tendons, cartilage, and adipose tissue (fat) are the main connective tissues in organs such as the brain and liver, where they maintain shape and structure. Blood clots in connective tissue, due to injury, lead to cancers called sarcomas.

Cytochromes: several iron-containing compounds, the function of which is to carry electrons to molecular oxygen. Products produced by fermentation destroy these enzymes, stop the respiratory-oxidative process, and thereby cause death of some cancer patients through asphyxiation.

Dedifferentiation: cancer cells tend to lose differentiated traits and become more embryonic and primitive. (*See differentiation.*) Dedifferentiation indicates that cancer occurred after cells were developed and that cancer cannot be due to genetic defects during replication or differentiation.

Differentiation: cells with specialized traits are said to be differentiated. Cancer often occurs in cells after replication is complete, allowing cancer cells to be identified by the type of tissue that is affected.

Disease: is fundamentally a condition resulting from lack of essential minerals, vitamins and cellular energy to build functional enzymes and immune system defenses and enzymes to remove toxic waste from the cells. Lack of mineral balance is the one common denominator of all diseases, followed by fungal and parasitic enzymes and waste affecting cell function and cell-wall membrane components. Metabolic therapy is a cure for all diseases.

Enzymes: are protein catalysts for chemical reactions in biological systems. Catalysts control a chemical action in which exchange of electrons is involved, but not for the ionic hydrogen bond that is controlled by ionic energy. Enzymes are not consumed or destroyed by the chemical action. Heat, acids, or other enzymes and ionic fields degrade enzymes so they must be continually replaced. Enzymes are mainly translated from mRNA in the cytoplasm of the cells. Fresh and raw vegetables and fruit provide additional enzymes through nutrition.

Epithelial growth factor: (EGF) regulates the growth of cancer cells of epithelial origin. EGF is the primary enzyme initiating cancer in 96% of human cancers. Microbes have cell walls and produce EGF. Fermentation of trapped blood sugars in vessels and ducts allows microbial EGF to contaminate epithelial cell walls thereby causing mutations in the cell wall.

Epithelium tissue: tissue of closely packed layers of cells that form a surface or lines a cavity or tube. Epithelium may be protective (as in the skin) or secretory (as in cells lining the walls of the gut). Most cancers initiate in these tissues.

Estrogen: any of a group of hormones, principally estradiol, produced by the ovaries. Estrogens control female sexual development, promote the growth of female secondary sexual characteristics, stimulate egg production, and prepare the lining of the uterus for pregnancy. The menstrual cycle is the result of estrogen, and excessive amounts of estrogen can lead to a current of injury in sex-organ tissue.

Fungi: their bodies consist of slender, cottony filaments called hyphae; a mass of hyphae is called a mycelium. The mycelium carries on all the processes necessary for the life of the organism, including, in most species, that of sexual reproduction. 'Mycelium' can invade mucus membranes of human cells to contaminate the cell with 'mycotoxins' and injure cell-wall membranes to initiate a current of injury and replication of infected cells.

Gene: is a sequence of nucleotides that CODES in DNA (*forms codons*), with about 3% capable of receiving stimulants from enzymes and hormonal stimulants to produce functional products. The other 97% probably respond to ionic signals of the autonomic nervous system, as well as the vibrational frequencies of the intellectual, emotional, and cellular environment. Health through a positive mental attitude and a rewarding life style tend to maintain better health through mental and emotional stimulants received by repressed genes.

Genome: the full complement of genes, carried by a single set of chromosomes. The term may be applied to the genetic information carried by an individual or to the range of genes found in a given species. The human genome is made up of about 80,000 genes according to recent estimates.

Glucose: simple sugar, and the primary product of photosynthesis. It is polymerized to make cellulose and chitin. Formed from starch and carbohydrates.

Glycolysis: meaning metabolism or the breakdown of glycogen molecules (sugar) to release energy for cells. Two types are: *aerobic glycolysis* meaning with oxygen; and *anaerobic glycolysis*, meaning without oxygen.

Hydrogenation: a process introduced on a large scale in the 1930's for making margarine and shortenings as cheaper substitute for butter and lard. Epithelial cells require unsaturated lipid molecules, but hydrogenated oils do not provide the required characteristics for cell-wall respiratory and metabolic function, thereby leading to disease. Processed fats and oils, with demineralized foods is creating an undernourished, overfed, and overweight society.

Lymphatic fluids: the plasma, or fluid within the blood vessels; the interstitial fluid, or fluid which surrounds the cells; and the intracellular fluid, or fluid within the cells. Lymph fluid found in the lymphatic system is being drained from the tissues by lymph capillaries, which enter lymph vessels (lymphatics). These lead to lymph nodes (small round bodies chiefly situated in the neck, armpit, groin, thorax, and abdomen), which processes the lymphocytes produced by bone marrow, and filter out harmful cells known as macrophages. Swollen lymph nodes indicate your body needs detoxification, not an operation to remove the nodes.

Lymphocyte: type of white blood cell with a large nucleus, produced in the bone marrow. B lymphocytes, or B cells are responsible for producing antibodies; T lymphocytes or T cells, have several roles in the mechanism of immunity.

Meiosis: the process of cell division in which the number of chromosomes in the cell is halved. It only occurs in cells with a nucleus, and is part of the life cycle that involves sexual reproduction because it allows the genes of two parents to be combined without increasing the number of chromosomes. Meiosis demonstrates that replication of DNA does not occur until the two strands of DNA are joined and the ionic hydrogen bond is formed.

Mitosis: the process of cell division by which identical daughter cells are reproduced. During mitosis, the DNA is duplicated and the chromosome number doubled so new cells contain the same amount of DNA as the original cell. The ionic hydrogen bond is broken to allow replication.

Nucleotides: in DNA are sequences of molecules with nitrogen containing bases joined by a sugar-phosphate backbone. (*See pyrimidines and purines*)

Oncogene: A *theoretical* dominant gene that promotes cell division. An oncogene normally controls the cell cycle but leads to cancer when overexpressed. *Plays a key role in medical propaganda concerning the defective gene cause-of-cancer theory.*

Parasympathetic nervous system: division of the autonomic nervous system responsible for slowing the heart rate, decreasing blood pressure, and stimulating the digestive system. Nutritional deficiencies in electrolytes, toxins, and pollutants in the body can cause health problems to the autonomic nervous system. Also causes replication of DNA.

Phospholipids: any lipid consisting of a glycerol backbone, a phosphate group, and two long chains. Phospholipids are found everywhere in living systems as the basis for biological membranes.

Plasma: the liquid component of the blood. It is a straw-colored fluid, largely composed of water (around 90%), in which a number of substances are dissolved. These include a variety of proteins (around 7%) such as fibrinogen (important in blood clotting), inorganic mineral salts such as sodium and calcium, waste products such as urea, traces of hormones, and antibodies to defend against infection.

Polymerase: is the scientific word used to identify enzymes that assemble chains of nucleotides called *polymers*. Polymerase functions in replication of DNA but does not initiate replication. Enzymes function at the atomic level.

Purine: refers to the uric acid group of organic compounds in the body. The group gets its name from urine from which it was first isolated. Purines have a stable double ring structure. The DNA components Adenine and Guanine are purines because they have a double ring structure. See also pyrimidines.

Pyrimidines: are organic compounds that have a single ring structure. The DNA components Cytosine and Thymine have a single ring structure and are thus referred to as pyrimidines. In normal DNA, pyrimidines join only with purines. The concept that virus enter the genetic code to cause cancer can be disproved by the significant differences in structure of DNA nucleotides and all known viruses. Viruses have an outer shell consisting of protein.

Substrate: in digestion and assimilation of nutrients, chemical bonds in amino acids, and carbohydrates can be broken apart by removing hydrogen ions but a method is needed to keep the active hydrogen ions from recombining. Special enzymes produced by the cell are required for this function and a substrate is needed to combine safely with hydrogen. Ammonia destroys substrates required to maintain the citric acid cycle.

Yeasts: whether round or oval shaped, are unicellular fungi with a distinct cell wall, which form a psydomycel in contrast to the thread fungi. (psydomycel look like narrow balloons twisted into shapes). Yeasts multiply vegetatively by sprouting and/or splitting. Yeasts are part of the fungal kingdom, and taken as a group are the major cause of all degenerative diseases. Fungi are obligatory anaerobes that function as parasites in the body, and serve to reduce corpses to basic elements for renewal of life.

BIBLIOGRAPHY

Ali, Majid: The Journal of Integrative Medicine," Vol. 1, Number 1, Winter 1997. West End Avenue Suite 1H, N.Y. 10023; 212-873-2444

Anthony & Kolthoff: TEXTBOOK OF ANATOMY AND PHYSIOLOGY, The Mosby Company. 8th Edition, 1971

Appleton, Nancy: LICK THE SUGAR HABIT ISBN 0-89529-386-2

Asimov, Isaac: ASIMOV'S NEW GUIDE TO SCIENCE ISBN 0-465-00473-3

Atkins, P. W: MOLECULES, Scientific American Library, 1987, ISBN 0-7617-5019-8

Becker, Robert; Gary Selden: THE BODY ELECTRIC, ISBN 0-688-06971-1

Bird, Christopher: THE LIFE AND TRIALS OF GASTON NAESSENS, 1990, ISBN 2-921138-02-6

Cantwell, Alan Jr.: THE CANCER MICROBE, 1990, Aries Rising Press ISBN 0-917211-01-4

Carter, James: RACKETEERING IN MEDICINE, 1992 ISBN 1-878901-32-X

Carpenter, Jean: STOP AGING NOW, ISBN 0-06018355-1

Callahan, Philip: PARAMAGNETISM; REDISCOVERING NATURE'S SECRET FORCE OF GROWTH, ISBN0-911311-49-1

Clark Dr. Hulda Regehr: New Century Press,

THE CURE FOR ALL CANCERS, 1993, ISBN 1-890035-00-9

THE CURE FOR ALL DISEASES, 1995, ISBN 1-890035-16-5

THE CURE FOR ALL *ADVANCED* CANCERS, 1999, ISBN 1-890035-16-5

Chinery, Scott: HUMAN GROWTH HORMONE, L & S Research, P.O. Box 1577, Toms River, N.J. 08753-0550

Chopra, Deepak: QUANTUM HEALING Exploring the Frontiers of Mind/Body Medicine. ISBN 0-553-05368-X

Costantini, M.D, Heinrich Wieland, M.D. and Lars I. Qvick, M.D: FUNGALBIONICS, The Fungal/Mycotoxin Etiology of Human Disease,
Vol. I, ARTERIOSCLEROSIS ISBN 3-930939-00-2
Vol. II, CANCER ISBN 3-930939-01-0

Coult, D. A: MOLECULES AND CELLS, 1966, Longmans Green & Co.

CRM Books: BIOLOGY, APPRECIATION FOR LIFE, ISBN 87665-163-5

Dale, T: TRANSFORM YOUR EMOTIONAL DNA, ISBN 9-9652947-6-5

Day, Charlene: THE IMMUNE SYSTEM HANDBOOK, ISBN 0-9695781-0-5

Diamond, Harvey: YOU CAN PREVENT BREAST CANCER, 1995, Promotion Publishing, ISBN 0-9636328-1-7

Dubois, Charlotte & John Lubecki: THE END OF CANCER, 1995, ISBN 884030-00-9

Erasmus, Udo: FATS AND OILS, ISBN 0-920470-10-5

Erdman, Robert: THE AMINO REVOLUTION, 1987, Simon & Schuster, ISBN 0-671-67359-9

EXPLORE Magazine: Explore Publishing, P. O. Box 1508, Mt. Vernon, WA 98273. (206) 424-6025

Grace, Eric: BIOTECHNOLOGY UNZIPPED, Promises and Realities. ISBN 1-895579-45-7

Gerber, Robert: VIBRATIONAL MEDICINE, ISBN 0-939680 7

Gerson, Max: A CANCER THERAPY, The Cure of Advanced Cancer by Diet Therapy. ISBN 0-88268-105-2

Guyton Authur: M.D. TEXTBOOK OF MEDICAL PHYSIOLOGY, W.B. Saunders Co. ISBN 0-7216-4394-9

Hamlyn, Paul: THE ENCYCLOPEDIA OF SPACE, 1968, SBN: 600012050

Heinrich, Elmer G: THE POWER OF MINERALS, The Rockland Corporation, 1-800-421-7310

Hoffer, Abram: "Journal of Orthomolecular Medicine," 1992, Volume 7

Hoffer, Abram: HOFFER'S LAWS OF NATURAL NUTRITION, ISBN 1-55082-095-8

Igram, Cass: EAT RIGHT TO LIVE LONG, ISBN 0-911119-22-1

Kamen, Betty: THE CHROMIUM DIET, SUPPLEMENT AND EXERCISE STRATEGY, 1990. ISBN 0-944501-03-6

Kaufmann, Klaus: SILICA: THE FORGOTTEN NUTRIENT, ISBN 0-920470-24-6

Lakhovsky, George: THE SECRET OF LIFE, Cosmic Rays and Radiations of Living Things. ISBN 0-932298-86-9

Langer, Stephen: and James F. Scheer: SOLVED THE RIDDLE OF ILLNESS, ISBN 0-87983-357-2

LaPage, Geoffrey: ANIMALS PARASITIC IN MAN, 1963, Dover Publications, Inc. Library of congress # 63-17908

Levine, Joseph and David Suzuki: THE SECRET OF LIFE, ISBN 0-7737-2744-2

Lewis R: HUMAN GENETICS CONCEPTS AND APPLICATIONS, 1997, W.C. Brown Pub.

Locke, David M: VIRUSES; THE SMALLEST ENEMY, Library of Congress 71-185103 (1974)

Luria, Salvador: LIFE, THE UNFINISHED EXPERIMENT, LOC 72-1179

Lynes, Barry: THE CANCER CURE THAT WORKED! Fifty Years of Suppression Sixth Printing, 1997, Marcus books, ISBN 0-919951-30-9

Lynes, Barry: THE HEALING OF CANCER The Cures, the Cover-ups, and the Solution NOW! ISBN 0-919951-44-9

Master Formula Booklet: FEEL BETTER BOOKS, 1-800-656-7606

Marchand, Charles: THE THERAPEUTICAL APPLICATIONS OF HYDROZONE AND GLYCOZONE, 1904. Reprinted, 1989, by ECHO2O2, INC.

McGraw-Hill: MULTIMEDIA ENCYCLOPEDIA OF SCIENCE AND TECHNOLOGY: "Bacterial Physiology and Metabolism"

Mason, E.B: HUMAN PHYSIOLOGY, 1983, Benjamin Cummings Publishing ISBN 0-8053-6885-X

Martin, D.W. Jr: HARPERS REVIEW OF BIOCHEMISTRY, 19th edition, 1983, ISBN 0-87041-037-7

Martlew, Gillian: ELECTROLYTES THE SPARK OF LIFE, 1994 ISBN 0-9640539-0-X

McCabe, Ed: OXYGEN THERAPIES, A new way of approaching disease. 1988, ISBN 0-9620527-0-1

McGrayne, Sharon: 365 SURPRISING SCIENTIFIC FACTS, BREAK-THROUGHS, AND DISCOVERIES. 1998, ISBN 0-471-57712-X

Morgan, Peter: HOME MEDICAL ENCYCLOPEDIA, 1992

Moss, Ralph: CANCER THERAPY The Independent Consumer's Guide to Non-Toxic Treatment and Prevention. ISBN 1-881025-06-3

Motz, Lloyd: THE UNIVERSE, Its beginning & End. ISBN 0-684-14239-2

Mudd, Chris: CHOLESTEROL AND YOUR HEALTH, The Great American Ripoff! ISBN 0-9624515-1-7

Murray, Richard: BASIC GUIDE TO UNDERSTANDING CLINICAL LABORATORY TESTS, ISBN 1-882657-01-2

Passwater, Richard: A. GTF CHROMIUM, ISBN 0-87983-272-X

Philpott William: CANCER, The Magnetic/Oxygen Answer, Choctaw, Oklahoma 73020 Phone 405 390-3009

Picken, Laurence: THE ORGANIZATION OF CELLS AND OTHER ORGANISMS, 1962 Oxford Press in Great Britain

Pearson, Durk: LIFE EXTENSION, A PRACTICAL APPROACH, ISBN 0-446-51229-X

Perot, Ross: INTENSIVE CARE, 1995 ISBN 0-06-095172-9

Sahley, Billie; Birkner, K. M: HEALING WITH AMINO ACIDS, Pain & Stress Publications, San Antonio 1997 ISBN 1-889391-07-7

Schroeder, H: THE TRACE ELEMENTS AND MAN, ISBN 0-8159-6907-4

Scientific American: SCIENCE DESK REFERENCE, 1999, ISBN 0-471-35675-1

Sears, Barry: MASTERING THE ZONE, 1995 ISBN 0-06-039150-2

Sharma Hari: FREEDOM FROM DISEASE, 1993, ISBN 1-895958-00-8

Smith, R. E; P.K. Smith; H. Bigelson: YOUR CURE FOR CANCER, ISBN 1-57901-030-X

Soyka, Fred: THE ION EFFECT Electrically charged particles in the air may control your moods, health and sense of well being. ISBN 0-7704-1512-5

Stern, Jess: EDGAR CAYCE THE SLEEPING PROFIT, 1967, ISBN O-553-26085-5

Stites D.P: BASIC AND CLINICAL IMMUNOLOGY, 4th edition, ISBN number 0-87041-223-X

Suzuki David & Holly Dressel: FROM NAKED APE TO SUPERSPECIES, 1999 ISBN 0-7737-3194-6

Tayler, Herbert: THE HERBERT J. TAYLOR STORY. ISBN 0-87784-836-X

Thomas, John: YOUNG AGAIN How to Reverse the Aging Process, Plexis Press ISBN 1-884757-77-4

Trull, Louise B: THE CANCELL CONTROVERSY, Why is a possible Cure for CANCER being suppressed. 1993, ISBN 1-878901-1

Vance, Judi: BEAUTY TO DIE FOR, The Cosmetic Consequence, 1998, ISBN 1-57901-035-0

Varmus Harold, and R. Weinberg: GENES AND THE BIOLOGY OF CANCER, ISBN 0-7167-5037-6

Wallace, Bruce: THE SEARCH FOR THE GENE, 1992 ISBN 0-8014-2680-4

Washnis, George: DISCOVERY OF MAGNETIC HEALTH, 1998 New Edition; ISBN 0-9639560-9

Weinberg, Robert A: ONE RENEGADE CELL, ISBN 0-465-07275-5

West, C. S: THE GOLDEN SEVEN PLUS ONE, 1981 ISBN Library of Congress No. 81-86099

Whang Sang: REVERSE AGING, 1984 Siloam Enterprises 560 Sylvan Ave., Englewood Cliffs, N.J. 07632

Willner, Robert: DEADLY DECEPTION; Proof that Sex and HIV absolutely do not cause AIDS, 1994, Peltec Publishing Co. Inc. 1-800-214-3645

Yarrow, David: FIRE IN THE WATER, How minerals become biology. ISBN 1-928820-02-6. USA (941) 426-1929.

INDEX

If you would like to have us send information on this book to someone, please fill in the name and address and fax or mail the information to us. Or, if you would like to purchase books for resale, please see order form for details and send in your purchase order.

Dealer inquiries invited from:

book retailers, wholesalers and distributors

cancer associations

health action groups

health care professionals and product dealers

political action groups

Please fax request for information on business letterhead.

800-656-7606
(905)-945-2180

www.newvisionsinc.org

BOOK ORDER AND REFERRAL

Quantity pricing in effect. Inform your customers, friends and relatives.

CANCER The Cause, Cure and Cover-up by Ronald Gdanski

LIST PRICE (per book)

1 to 4 books: $24.95 U.S. $34.95 Cdn.

WHOLESALE PRICES: (per counter display of 5 books)

   1, 2 or 3 displays: (less 35%) *($16.22 U.S. or $22.71 Cdn./book.)*

                    $81.08 U.S. / display

                    $113.58 Cdn. /display

Case Price: (4 or more counter displays—20 books (4 displays) per case)

   1 to 35 cases: less 50% *($12.47 U.S. or $17.47 Cdn./book.)*

                    $249.50 U.S. /case

                    $349.50 Cdn./case

DISTRIBUTOR PRICE 36 cases (144 displays-720 books) per pallet.

           Minimum one pallet. Inquire for details.

TERMS: Prices and packaging subject to change without notice.

        Shipping and taxes additional. FOB Grimsby, Ont. Canada

        Shipping weight approx. 1 1/2 pounds or .6 kilo per book.

        Indicate choice of delivery: Parcel Post, CanPar, UPS, Transport

        Payment with order or COD. Net 30 with established accounts.

VISA and Master Card accepted by phone or E-mail.

Card number: _____

Name: _____

Street: _____

City: _____

Prov/state   _____PC/ZIP_____

Phone/Fax   _____

Email: _____w.w.w. _____

Feel Better Books and Tapes

P.O. Box 124B Beamsville, Ontario. Canada, L0R 1B0

Phone FAX   1-800-656-7606   (905) 945-2180

Email at www newvisionsinc.org

Please send FREE information to the following people.

(Photocopy this page and fax or mail it in to have information sent out.)

Referred by: _____

Name: (print) _____
Street: _____
City: _____
Prov/state_____PC/ZIP_____
Phone & Fax _____
Email: _____

Name: (print) _____
Street: _____
City: _____
Prov/state_____PC/ZIP_____
Phone & Fax _____
Email: _____

Name: (print) _____
Street: _____
City: _____
Prov/state_____PC/ZIP_____
Phone & Fax _____
Email: _____

Feel Better Books and Tapes

P.O. Box 124, Beamsville, Ontario, Canada L0R 1B0

FAX 1-800-656-7606 or (905) 945-2180

Email   @www.newvisionsinc.org

SOURCES

(Work in progress. Suppliers are invited to submit listing information. Additional pages will be added as needed in future printings.)

714X Video Cerbe Distribution Inc., Rock Forest, Quebec. Phone (819) 564-7883, fax 564-4668 or Internet at http://www.cerbe.com.

Center for Cell Specific Cancer Therapy (CSCT) in the Dominican Republic by calling 1-877-741-2728. See also www.csct.com .

Elections Canada for electoral district maps. Phone (613) 992-4793, fax (613) 992-1273.

The Multi-versa Health Strategy, Coville, Penelope & Briglio, Kathleen: A self-instructional course (16 Chapters) in natural health care and managed recovery. 1999, Feel Better Books: 1-800-656-7606. Internet at www.trafford.com.

Dr. Hulda Clark Video of Toronto Seminar 1995, or books by Dr. Clark: Feel Better Books, 1-800-656-7606

How to Re-invent Yourself, Inspiring Strategies of Personal Renewal, by Marcellus B. Andersen, ISBN 0-968468-0-9 Contact Bowdens, 1-877-269-3367

NAP New Action Products, 33 Baker Road North, Grimsby, Ont. L3M 2W9. 1-800-541-3799 (Trace minerals, herbal combinations, zappers, etc.)

Ludde Protocol Video 604-925-6486 or fax 604 925-0135.

OZONE and the Politics of Medicine Threshhold Film Inc. (30 minute VIDEO) (604) 873-4626

Planetary Association for Clean Energy, (books and newsletter) 100 Bronson Ave., Suite 1001, Ottawa, Ont. K1R 6G8. (613) 236-6265, (613) 235-5876

TRACE-LYTES and CAL-LYTE mineral supplements

USA (941) 426-3375. Canada NAP 1-800-541-3799)

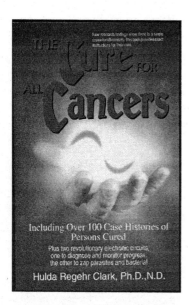

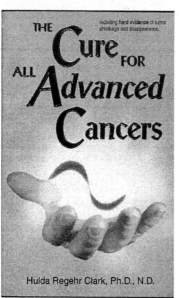

We believe cancer is caused by a combination of four conditions:

1. Nutritional deficiencies and pollutants leading to the loss of oxidation metabolism in normal cells;

2. Invasion of membrane cells by virus, fungus or bacteria resulting in benign growths and the switch to fermentative metabolism;

3. A break in the membrane resulting in the normal repair mechanism causing these cells to replicate in order to repair the membrane.

4. Continuous mutation of cells during meiosis resulting in cell-wall trait mutations. Membrane cells are rejected to form tumors, leukocytes do not function, causing leukemia, and fractured bones do not heal.

It follows that the cure for all cancers is to eliminate the conditions that cause cancer and to return the cells to their original oxidative metabolism:

1. Cleanse the cells, organs and lymphatic system of pollutants and parasites. Avoid new toxins and reinfection.

2. Replace the essential minerals, vitamins, oils, carbohydrates and amino acids through nutrition.

3. Avoid all fungal food and mycotoxins that support fungal parasites.

4. Have faith that your God-given life force has enough intelligence to heal itself if given all that it needs to do so.

Books available from Feel Better Books and Tapes 1-800-656-7606

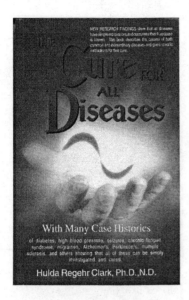

If someone says there is no cure for your disease, can you be sure he knows all there is no know about it?

Some medical researches now believe that all degenerative and so called autoimmune diseases are the result of fungal infections, mycotoxins or other contaminants disturbing cell and organ function.

The immune system does not develop fully until months after birth. Early childhood infections agents become accepted as self by the immune system and remain dormant until conditions allow for them to thrive.

Antibiotics taken to cure illness results in the reliance of the immune system for more antibiotics when needed. The immune system becomes dysfunctional for that problem. Supporting the immune system by eliminating resident parasites and cleansing the cells will result in normal health.

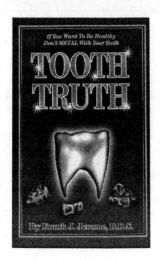

Consider mercury fillings to be time bombs in your body. Amalgam fillings need replacement from time to time because the toxic metals have leached out into your food and saliva. They become toxins in your cells and lead to chronic fatigue and other diseases.

Root canals may lead to chronic infections that leach mycotoxins into the blood stream. Take the time to know and understand this vital issue. Don't destroy your future health by filling a cavity with 50% mercury or gold plating an infection.

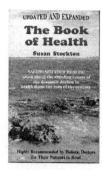

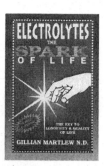

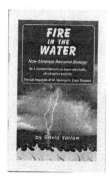

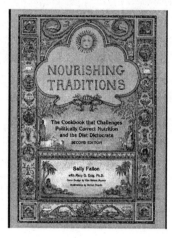

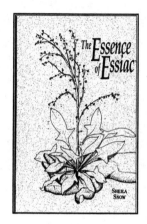